Freedom

SLIM FOR LIFE!

from the

Diet Trap

JUICE MASTER
JASON VALE
★★★★★

HARPER
thorsons

Also by the author:

The Juice Master's Ultimate Fast Food

Chocolate Busters: The Easy Way to Kick Your Addiction

Turbo-charge Your Life in 14 Days

7lbs in 7 Days: The Juice Master Diet

Juice Master: Keeping it Simple

Juice Yourself Slim: Lose Weight Without Dieting

5lbs in 5 Days: The Juice Detox Diet

The Funky Fresh Juice Book

HarperThorsons
An Imprint of HarperCollins*Publishers*
77–85 Fulham Palace Road,
Hammersmith, London W6 8JB

www.harpercollins.co.uk

and *HarperThorsons* are trademarks
of HarperCollins*Publishers* Ltd

First published by HarperThorsons as *Slim for Life* in 2002
This updated edition published 2014

10

© Jason Vale 2009, 2014

Jason Vale asserts the moral right to be
identified as the author of this work

A catalogue record of this book is
available from the British Library

ISBN-13 978-0-00-728492-4

Printed and bound in Great Britain by
Clays Ltd, St Ives plc

Contents

Appendices

'The Best Book I Have Read on the Subject for Twenty-five Years'

I sent the manuscript for this book off at 12 noon on a Wednesday, and at 2 p.m. the following day I got a call from the first and only publishers I had sent it to. The first thing the editor from HarperCollins said was, 'This is the best book I have read on this subject for twenty-five years', followed by, 'It's like a cold glass of water on a hot summer's day.' I was flattered, to say the least, but I knew at the same time that the information was pretty groundbreaking. Luckily, the editor at HarperCollins wasn't the only person to think the book was extremely different to everything else out there and I have received thousands of emails from all corners of globe, saying how the book has completely changed their lives. The problem is there are so many 'diet' and 'health' books on the market that it's all too easy to group them together. Luckily, through no press or advertising, *Slim For Life* has grown through word of mouth alone and is now not only a best-seller, but is even quoted in some medical papers.

Don't Listen To Me

My words cannot possibly encapsulate the ways in which this book has helped so many people, so before we begin, here is an extremely short selection of the very genuine unsolicited emails and reviews we receive on a daily basis. Please make a point of taking the time to read them as every aspect of this book is here for a reason. I sincerely hope this small selection helps to inspire you, now that you have bought the book, to actually go on to read it. After you have read this short section I will finish the introduction explaining what you have in store so that you fully understand the nature of my writing and you get the most from the book.

A whole new way to look at food

'Since reading this book twelve months ago i have lost 5 stone [31 kg], my skin and hair looks amazing and i am full of energy! This book is truly life changing. it's not the sort of "Same old ..." diet book which tells you to weigh out 3 oz [368 g] of cottage cheese every day, it actually changes the way you think about food and explains why you're hooked on certain foods (and un-brainwashes you too!). i started by reading another of Jason's books — *The Simple Way To Stop Eating Chocolate* — as i used to eat way too much chocolate. Now it's been fifteen month since i've had any and i've not missed it for a second! i'd recommend these books for absolutely everyone, fat or thin (my slim boyfriend has read *Slim For Life* and it's changed his views on food too!)'

J. Bramwell

4 stone in 4 months

'From reading this book in May and adopting most of the principles
within it i have gone on to lose 4 stone [25 kg] in as many months
and feel better than i have in years. The book is very informative yet
easy to read and something about the way it is written makes you
want to take heed and actually cut out many foods from your diet
(something i never thought i could do!!). i have never written a
review before but for this i had to make an exception, this many
people can't be wrong!'

J. Ainley

Another one of the converted

'This book is a life changer. i am a 52-year-old male who has been
on a diet for the majority of those years. i have lost 5 stone [31 kg]
three times and other large amounts along the way. And every time
i've put it back on and more besides. i've reached goals at Weight
Watchers, Slimming World (i was Suffolk's only male consultant
there) and other slimming clubs. i read Jason Vale's book on the
27th of December (yes in a day) and i'm cured of ever being on a diet
again. i will never weigh again. i will never drink diet drinks tea or
coffee again. i will not eat cakes, chocolate, or the foods i now
know to be damaging. in what amounts to a month (in which i have
juiced every day and eaten well) i feel a whole lot better and am
sleeping at night (i used to get up to eat), i have so much more
energy and my trousers are falling down. if you are thinking about
buying this book you would be a fool not to. This book is a
godsend. Thank you Jason Vale. if anybody buys this book on my
recommendation and reads it from start to finish i will be a happy
man because i too will have made a difference. it works!'

M. Howe

'the best book i have read on the subject for twenty-five years'   vii

Buy this book and transform the way you think about health

'This book isn't just about what to eat, it's about the psychology of health, and it's something everyone should read.

'i'm not fat and i never have been — but this book has given me more power to improve my health than anything else i've read in the last decade. i used to be addicted to certain types of foods — usually those loaded with sugar. Even though i looked healthy to most people i struggled with low blood sugar on a daily basis and i experienced massive mood swings because of the food in my diet. So i was delighted when i read *Slim For Life* because it helped me understand why i was hooked on all sorts of junk, and it gave me the simple solutions i needed to take my health to a whole new level.

'if weight loss is your goal, i'm sure *Slim For Life* will help you get what you want. And if you're already slim, you should still read this book because it will help you stay in shape for the rest of your life without feeling stressed or under pressure.

'i'm now free from the food trap, and i owe massive thanks to Jason Vale for writing this terrific book.'

17-year-old life change

'Before i read this book i had spots — a lot on my forehead and some on my cheeks and back. But within a few weeks of adopting Jason's easy ideas ALL my spots disappeared. i'm a 17-year-old who read this book when i was 15 so i'm sure if i can do it anyone can do it. i was never fat but i binged all the time (and i mean all the time!) on crisps, chocolate, McDonald's, chips, Coke, white bread etc. i don't eat any of that rubbish any more and i never will again. At first i was scared of giving up these foods but by the time i finished the book i never wanted to touch them again. Thanks a million Jason — you're so accurate when you say that this book is for people who want to be slim for life and not just for a week. Great book, great advice, great life changer.'

I could print an entire book from the thousands of testimonials I have had from this book alone. These were just a few and I hope they have provided even more reason to read the book. One thing you should know before you get stuck in is that my basic writing style isn't to everyone's liking. I fully understand and appreciate this, but my aim is not to win literary awards but to genuinely make a difference in the area of health and addiction. My aim is also to reach as many people as possible. Not only will my sometimes basic style annoy some, at times, but I also repeat myself constantly throughout the book. I do this as a form of hypnosis and re-conditioning and it is all meant for a reason. We have been bombarded for years with emotional messages from what I call **BiG FOOD** and **BiG DRiNK** in a bid to lure us in and trap us. We have the space of one book to reverse all of that brainwashing and the repetition of key points is one of the best ways to achieve our goal.

THIS IS NOT A BOOK ON JUICING!

I would also like to make it clear that unlike many of my other books, this is not a book on juicing and smoothie making. In fact, if you don't want to go near a juicer after you finish this book you don't have to. Yes I will talk about juicing and yes I think it's a truly wonderful *tool* to the land of the slim and super healthy, but it's not 100 per cent essential. I want people to fully understand that although I am also known as, 'The Juice Master', this new version of *Slim For Life*, *Freedom From The Diet Trap*, doesn't rely on juicing as a prerequisite to lifelong slimming and health success. I am hoping that after you read this book you will want to get fresh juicing into your life and use it as a tool to lifelong good health, but if you don't you will still have success.

This version of the book is slightly different to when I first wrote it and there are a couple of new chapters too, but the message and impact is still the same. If you have read the book before the new format and few bits of new information may well make re-reading it easy and worthwhile. It's like an old film you've seen before, many aspects you would have forgotten and it's good to revisit some aspects again to *remain* free from the food and diet trap.

Read the book with an open mind and read at least a chapter a day until you finish. I realize that it's hard to imagine how a simple book can make such a massive difference; especially if you have tried God knows how many different methods before. However, after reading thousands of letters from people all over the world, I can guarantee you cannot read this book with an open mind and not make a fundamental change to your diet. You will also never see food or the industry in the same light ever again.

I wish you every success and if you get time I would love to hear from you.

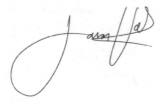

1

OH NO! NOT ANOTHER DIET BOOK!

That's right – what you are holding is not another diet book. In fact, if you're looking for something that is the complete opposite to the misery, deprivation and ultimate failure of dieting – then you have finally found it.

This book is not just for people who are overweight either; it's for anyone who has ever had the slightest issue with food, which – in today's processed food and image conscious world – pretty much covers everyone I think. And it's also not what I call a 'state the obvious' book either. What I mean is, I'm not going to spend the time we have together stating the mind-blowingly obvious to you about certain foods or treating you like some kind of moron. That was one of the things I hated about eating the wrong foods, being overweight, feeling tired, lethargic and unhealthy myself – people assuming that just because I was thick physically, it automatically made me thick mentally. My doctor at the time was one of the worst for this and was head of what I call 'The State The Bloody Obvious Brigade'. He would say things like, 'You're eating too much of the wrong types of foods, you don't exercise enough and you should lose weight. If you changed your eating habits and exercised more you would feel better and be slimmer.'

Well no shit Sherlock! It was the same when I used to smoke 40–60 cigarettes a day; my doctor would say, 'It's killing you and costing you a fortune, you'd be richer and healthier if you quit.' Once again – no really, what a revelation doc, hadn't figured that one out, now you've pointed that out I'll just extinguish this last one and I'll call it a day.

Some doctors are not the only members of the 'State The Bloody Obvious Brigade' either; it appears most health books, diet clubs and people in general are also lifelong members of it. We've even got people like Gillian McKeith who, when confronted with a 5 ft (1.5 m) woman weighing in at 20 stone (127 kg), feels the remarkable need to see a sample of their poo before suggesting the appropriate measures. The appropriate measures not surprisingly being to eat less crap, increase fruit and veg intake and exercise more. Information which would hardly come as a surprise to anyone who hasn't been on another planet all of their lives and information which would hardly be a surprise to the 20 stone (127 kg) woman either.

Then you have some members of the 'diet guru' world saying you can actually eat anything you like and be 'thin' as long as you 'eat when you are hungry', and 'stop eating when you are full' – as if anyone who is overweight doesn't try to do this all the time. Is it possible that our compulsion to overeat just may be caused by the type of foods we are eating? Isn't it also possible that it takes a shed load of food for some people to ever feel full?

What all members of the 'bloody obvious' fail to realize is **we're not stupid**. We all know that things like chocolate, cola, coffee, cakes, crisps, ice cream, alcohol, milkshakes, and things like fast-food burgers and fries are not good for us and make us tired, ill and fat. We are also aware that fruit, vegetables, nuts, seeds, grains, fish etc. are all good and would keep us slim and healthy. We also know that a good dose of daily exercise makes us feel good and helps to keep us trim. I'm not being funny but who on earth doesn't know this? However, my point is: does just knowing this help you to actually stop the unhealthy foods and change your eating habits in favour of the good stuff? Does the knowledge that daily exercise is wonderful for you help you actually to get up and do some? No. If it did you wouldn't be reading this book, you would have already done it. And that's the problem. The instinctive knowledge that these foods are bad might make you think more about how much of them you are eating and thus make you try to control your intake of them on a consistent basis, but it doesn't stop you *wanting* them or, most of the time, having them. It certainly didn't stop me.

That is why I was 30 lb (13 kg) overweight, badly asthmatic (took both the blue and brown inhalers, taking up to sixteen puffs a day), covered from head to toe in a skin disorder called psoriasis (at one stage I didn't have an area of skin which wasn't affected in some way) and had all the genuine energy of a comatose dormouse. The only reason I didn't get even bigger and sicker was because I was always on a diet. The yo-yo king, that was me – always fighting a constant battle not to eat too much of the wrong kinds of foods; always using a degree of willpower, discipline, and control to keep my health under some kind of control; always doing spats of 'healthy eating' and exercise to 'keep the weight off'. I hated it every time and always rewarded myself at the end of the nightmare with the very same stuff that caused the problem in the first place. I was more than fully aware that the foods I was eating were causing my physical problems – fat, lethargy and asthma – but the truth was I was psychologically hooked at the time and simply didn't know what to do in order to escape. On the surface it appears obvious and logical, but addiction and logic have nothing in common. As already stated, logically we know what to do, but addiction totally transcends any degree of logic.

So, if you thought you'd picked up a health/slimming book that was simply going to tell you that you should eat more fresh fruit and veggies, drink their fine juices, do more exercise and cut out the crap from your diet, you are very much mistaken. The reason? You already know you should do this and so does every one else.

THE FOOD AND DIET TRAP

What you need, therefore, is not a lecture on the bloody obvious, which will get you nowhere, but a full understanding of what I describe as 'The Food and Diet Trap'. You need a full explanation of why you *do* eat the foods you eat – even though at times it goes against your rational judgement – not why you shouldn't. You need to know exactly how the physical effects caused by certain 'foods' and drinks affect your thoughts – how they cause cravings and *additional* hungers and how to rid yourself of them. You need to know exactly what is happening, both physically and mentally, when you eat things like refined sugar, refined fat, cakes, muffins, chocolate, coffee, cola, diet drinks, dairy products, etc. You also need to know precisely how the **BiG FOOD** companies manipulate and condition you into buying what I describe as 'drug foods', yes *drug* foods. You need to know how these drug-like food and drinks companies will do whatever it takes to get you – and keep you – hooked on their 'brand' of junk*ie* foods and drinks. You also need to fully understand that many of the foods which we have been told by those we trust to do the right thing – governments in particular and their 'food groups' – are excellent for our health, are in reality causing us harm. You need to realize that **BiG FOOD** have **BiG POCKETS** and what is going on in the **BiG FOOD** and **BiG DRiNK** world will astonish you. Much of what I know I am not even allowed to print and it's more than a bugbear I can assure you. If I put down half of what I knew I would get hammered (perhaps even literally). But what I can print will give you at least enough incite to make an informed decision as to whether you continue to give **BiG FOOD** your hard earned money.

DIGGING OUR GRAVES WITH OUR FORKS

It's worth knowing that what we put into our mouths in the name of food and refreshment is now the biggest cause of disease and premature death in the Western world. And **BiG FOOD, BiG DRiNK** and **BiG PHARMACEUTiCALS** aren't really that troubled, as long before you are spent, you have spent ... a lot! **BiG FOOD** makes you sick and **BiG PHARMACEU-TiCALS** have plenty of people to sell to, in the name of making you better of course.

And that is what this book is about – *everything* you ever needed to know about The Food and Diet Trap. The manipulation, the con tricks, the addiction, the control, the false advertising and everything you genuinely need to know to break free from it.

And when I say free I mean *really* free: free to move; free to eat what *you* genuinely choose to (instead of that choice being subconsciously made for you) free from restrictions; free to think for yourself; free to look at people eating junk*ie* foods without any desire to do what they are doing; free from eating a load of crap and then wishing you hadn't; free never to go on a diet again; free from having to exercise control over certain foods on a constant basis; free from having to use willpower; free to wear what you want; and totally free to live the rest of your life in a slim, sexy, vibrant, and energy-driven body. It's the kind of freedom no amount of money can buy; it's the kind of freedom many dream of but never reach. It's the kind of freedom which can be easy to achieve, but only once the brainwashing and conditioning has been removed and you have a clear route out.

The Past Doesn't Equal The Future

It also doesn't matter what you have tried in the past or what you have been through, anyone – and having dealt with thousands of people of all ages from all over the world – I do mean *anyone* can find it easy and enjoyable to change what they eat and be slim *and* healthy for life. All you need is an open mind and the conviction to finish the entire book. Most people who buy books of this nature don't even finish them and then complain that it was 'something else that didn't work for them'. This book really is different from any other food/diet/health book you've read on this subject and I am very, very excited to share this information with you and I know it will make a difference. However, the only way it can make a difference is if you do three things:

A) Read the book with an open mind
B) Finish the book
C) Follow the simple set of instructions at the end

Many of the points in the book are repeated at various times. This is deliberate. I ran an addiction centre for many years and addiction psychology is what this book is all about. The only reason why I repeat certain points is to help remove the years of brainwashing and conditioning by **BiG FOOD** and **BiG DRiNK**. It may jar at times, but please have faith in the fact I know what I am doing. The book is a form of hypnosis. I make sure that the key messages are placed at precise intervals in order for you to make the change effortlessly. Many people can't even pin-point what it was about the book that made the difference, they just know that after reading it they felt completely differently about certain foods and drinks (as the short selection of reviews and testimonials in the introduction to this book shows). So please don't get caught up with what some in the U.S of A would annoyingly describe as 'Analysis Paralysis' – where you get so caught up trying to analyse something that it prevents you from getting the message and thus the result you are looking for. The book has many chapters, most short and punchy and all designed to keep you reading. I am not here to win any awards with the written word and yes plenty will be repeated throughout and my style will bug some for sure; just have faith and all will fall into place.

So first things first, before we get into the real juicy aspects of the book it is important to understand fully …

2

THE FLY SYNDROME

**'if you always do what you've always done,
you'll always get what you've always got'**

I don't know who originally said this now overused saying but they were bang on. I call it The Fly Syndrome.

Have you noticed how flies keep banging themselves against the same pane of glass in a desperate attempt to get out? And they continue to do it even when there is an opening just above them. Why don't they just fly slightly higher and set themselves free? The answer is very simple – they cannot see that there is a simple way out and believe that what they are doing will eventually set them free. And this is exactly the same for the overweight/unhealthy person who keeps going on diets or special exercise programmes that they hate in order to be slim and healthy. They simply cannot see that there is an extremely easy alternative. They honestly think that if they just keep doing the same thing for long enough that this approach will eventually set them free. But, just like the fly, simply doing the same thing over and over again will not produce a different result and will not set them free. I know because I did more or less the same thing over and over again expecting to get a different result.

However, what if the fly decided to go to a 'positive thinking fly seminar'? What if they went on a motivational fire walk to get all ...

motivated and stuff? What would happen then? Well nothing. All that would happen is you would now have a very excited, determined and positive fly who still couldn't break the glass. It doesn't matter how many times the fly repeats a positive mantra to itself along the lines of, '**i CAN DO ANYTHiNG i SET MY MiND TO**', unless it sees the gap at the top, physics mean the fly will **NEVER** break the glass, regardless of what the bloody hell it says to itself and no matter how determined and positive it is. What the fly needs is clear to anyone observing the poor bugger banging its head on the glass over and over again. It simply needs to understand the position it's in and simply change its approach. It's not difficult for the fly to get out, it's only difficult while it tries to escape by thinking it can break through the glass.

Exactly the same goes for anyone in the food trap. Whether you know it or not at this stage, the likelihood is you are in the trap yourself (to whatever degree) and you can do all the affirmations, positive thinking and be as determined as you like, but it won't set you truly free – as you've no doubt experienced in the past. You may get slimmer and healthier at times using this approach but it won't stop you wanting junk*ie* foods and therefore having to exercise constant control not to have them. In other words, you will still be mentally locked in the food trap.

I used to think that if I was managing to exercise control over my intake of certain foods it meant I was in control. I now see that if you are *having* to exercise control on a consistent basis it means you are in reality being controlled, and if you are being controlled you are not free. It's the constant need to exercise control on a daily, weekly or monthly basis that is one of the nightmares of the food trap (more on this later).

What you require is an incredibly easy escape route, and the exciting news is you're reading it. I know it's hard to believe a book can make such a difference, particularly if in your mind you have tried so many things in the past, but I promise you it can. The truth is it's actually frighteningly simple to change what you eat and get slim, in the same way it's simple for the fly to escape. The main problem is not only have we been conditioned and brainwashed to eat certain foods and drinks, it is almost taken as read that the whole business of losing weight is difficult. It isn't – **IT'S EASY!**

I totally agree that it may be hard to believe at this stage, but again, it's time to stop being a fly and open your mind to the fact that it's more than possible when you approach it in a very different way. The reality is it's feeling sluggish, living with excess fat and ill health and constantly either trying to control your food intake or bingeing that is hard work.

BACK TO FRONT

This is where most people have got it wrong, as I did for many years. We believe that health is hard work – that we will have to go through some degree of torture to achieve the body of our dreams. Many of us think that it's just easier to eat junk foods and stay unfit rather than go through the tremendous amounts of willpower, discipline, and dedication – not to mention pain and hard work – we believe are necessary to achieve good health. That's why we don't get excited and look forward to getting slim and healthy – we assume that we will have to suffer in some way. We have been conditioned to believe that, and every time we try and fail we simply confirm this false belief. That is exactly what I used to believe too. I now realize that a life of junk food, being unfit, hating the way you look and feel on an ongoing basis, and lacking in confidence is not easier – and it's certainly nowhere near as enjoyable as feeling alive, clearheaded, healthy, physically and mentally vibrant, and loving the way you look and feel.

We have a lot to get through and a lot of subjects need to be covered in order for you to break free. I want you to feel fantastic and live a quality of life, health-wise, that many people simply dream of. This book really is a catalyst to you getting there. There will be points in the book where you will want to stop, where you think you've read enough and that you 'get it', but please, please …

DO NOT ATTEMPT TO CHANGE YOUR EATING HABITS

Do not go off 'half cocked' – you need to be armed with all the correct information and instructions, otherwise in no time at all you could very easily switch to what I call 'diet' mentality. You need a full understanding of all junk*ie* foods and drinks first and how they affect your body and mind. Only then will the mental instructions that will guide you out of the food trap make sense and prevent you from having to use your willpower, or as I call it 'the diet recipe'. That way you will not just be free, but you will feel free from the start and love the journey. So – in case I haven't yet mentioned it enough – please finish the entire book if you want true freedom from the food trap without having to diet ever again. And while I'm on that subject let me explain why diets (in the long run) do not work, can never work, never will work, so that you can finally feel totally free to …

3

NEVER GO ON A DIET AGAIN

Let me ask you a question. If I told you I had discovered a way to lose weight and gain health, would you be interested? Well, perhaps. However, if I explained that the method involves months of physical and mental torture, that you would have to opt out of life on a regular basis and feel miserable and deprived for months, that it would make you irritable, and involves incredible amounts of willpower, discipline, and control – and, oh yes, I nearly forgot the best bit:

The method has a 95 per cent failure rate

Would you still be interested in trying it? In fact, would you invest incredible amounts of time, energy, and money in anything that guaranteed a 95 per cent failure rate? I would have thought nobody in their right mind would do such a thing, and that is exactly the problem – many people are not in their right (frame of) mind. That is why millions of highly intelligent people 'diet' despite knowing that at the end of their 'hard work' and misery there is a 95 per cent chance it will all have been for nothing – and most are fully aware of this fact before they begin.

I'm not knocking them either, for I am certainly in no position to do so. After all, I tried many, many diets myself. When I look back, I wonder why? Did it not dawn on me after my second diet that this mental approach to getting slim and healthy for life was not going to work? A definition of madness is to do the same thing over and over again and expect a different result. 'But I've tried several different diets' you say. But have you? I thought I had tried many different diets but are they ever really that different? They all involve feelings of sacrifice, misery, and deprivation. They all involve varying degrees of control and willpower. They all make you feel guilty when you're eating and down when you're not. They nearly always fail. They usually make you gain more weight than you had to begin with (if you're on a weight-loss diet). This is not one specific diet that I'm talking about – it's all of them. All diets are shining examples of the fly syndrome.

Despite knowing this, we still think that the next diet will be 'it' and seem willing to try anything, no matter how ludicrous or life threatening it may seem in our often desperate need to get to the land of the thin. Since the original F Plan diet (and we all know that the F doesn't stand for fibre) we have tried eating grapefruits before every meal on the 'grapefruit diet' and even reached (or perhaps retched would be a better word) for that delightful smelling and tasting cabbage soup first thing in the morning on 'the cabbage soup' diet. Then we had the 'wedding dress diet' (but what happens after the big day?), the 'Champagne and caviar diet' (you don't lose any weight, but you're so plastered you don't actually care) and the 'egg diet' (which involved eating eighteen eggs a day – no I am not kidding). Then, of course, there was the Hay diet (where you should never mix protein and carbohydrates together or you will internally combust) and the numerous 'eat nothing but protein diets'. This is where we were expected to believe that eggs and bacon swimming around in fat was in some way better for us than a piece of fruit. As mad as it sounds, even some rational thinking people went for this one. Do you lose weight eating *nothing* but protein? Yes. Is it healthy? **NO IT IS NOT**. You can often spot a high protein diet follower, they often have a giant head on a twig like body. After the nothing but protein came The South Beach Diet, and once again we were allowed to eat fruit and some carbs, hooray!

Then came the hugely popular GI (Glycaemic Index) diets, but keep up because GI is already 'so last year darling', and it's now been replaced by the many GL (Glycaemic Load) diets. It appears GI didn't work after all and it's the Glycaemic Load that's important now. (Hope you're keeping up with all of this). At least South Beach, GI and GL have some good basis in nutrition, but all sorts of mad 'quick fixes' have entered the fray. Have you heard of The Baby Food Diet? Yes we have intelligent grown adults eating baby food to get slim. It appears that whatever a 'celebrity' does, we all blindly follow, even if logically it's completely bonkers. Take the Thumbnail Diet. Of all the ones I have spoken about so far, this perhaps takes the biscuit. This is where you get to eat anything you want (sounds good so far but wait) … providing it is no bigger than your thumbnail and you must eat every fourteen minutes. Who worked out the precise science behind eating a thumbnail of food every fourteen minutes (not fifteen, heaven forbid don't round it up!), I will never know – but the word crackers springs to mind.

And let's not leave out things like the Cambridge diet, Slim Fast and all the other 'nutritious' shakes that promise weight loss in supersonic time. Then we have the many calorie-counting diets; the Kensington diet, the 'see' food diet, the Eat Fat Grow Slim diet (where you had to drink oil before each meal – again not joking), the 'sex diet' (yes there is one – best of a bad bunch I'd say, and more fun than eating cabbage soup). I could go on and on and on, but all of the above, even the Thumbnail seems incredibly sane compared to, wait for it – the 'Fresh Air' diet. Yes, let me repeat that –

THE FRESH AIR DIET

I wish I was joking, but it is perfectly true. This really is 'Extreme Dieting' and I believe the most dangerous 'food movement' (or non food movement) on earth. It isn't actually called 'The Fresh Air Diet', but 'Breatharianism'. It is a lifestyle popularized by an Australian woman called Ellen

Greve, or Jasmuheen, as she is better known. Greve claims she hasn't eaten since 1993; yet, she admits 'she drinks herbal teas and confesses to the occasional "taste orgasm" involving chocolate or ice cream'.

She claims not to eat the food but simply every now and then get the 'taste'. The fact that three of Greve's followers have starved to death while adhering to the Breatharian way of life, doesn't appear to dissuade her. In 1999 the Australian television programme *60 Minutes* tested her ability to live on 'prana', the 'Light Of God'. After just four days, Dr Berris Wink – president of the Queensland branch of the Australian Medical Association, urged her to stop the test. He wanted to stop the test because, according to Dr Wink, Greve's pupils were dilated, her speech was slow, she was dehydrated and her pulse had doubled. Funny how when tested she couldn't live without food or water for four days yet claims not to have eaten anything since 1993! Believe it or not she's not the only one at it either. One Wiley Brooks, who heads up 'The Breatharian Institute Of America', is equally as bats in my opinion and there are many, many more. This is obviously the ultimate *diet* and I am amazed they haven't been shut down. How on earth can you encourage people to 'live on light' and not be accountable if anything happens to them? In a world where the holy grail appears to be a Size Zero, surely these people need bringing to book.

Clearly 'Breatharianism' is beyond extreme and obviously mental, but I think we have all been guilty of trying some pretty ludicrous diets over the years. But why do we do it? Why do we jump on one diet after the next, regardless of how irrational they are? In truth, don't we already know exactly what we need to do in order to drop the weight and get healthy? Wouldn't it be fair to say that you could write down at least ten different ways to lose weight that – *if you followed them* – would all work? Could you not also design yourself an exercise programme that – *if you followed it* – would make you lean and fit? I think that we are intelligent enough to realize that if we ate nothing but cabbage for three weeks we would lose weight (and most of our friends probably) and that if we ate loads of fruit and veg and drank the fine juices they contain, we would all be extremely healthy.

I knew exactly what to do to get into shape and get healthy, I don't know anyone who doesn't. What I didn't know was how to stop eating crap and be happy about it. I knew how to stop eating rubbish and be miserable about it – I had a Gold medal in that one – but how the hell do you change what you eat and be happy about it? The problem is, we have all simply been going about it the wrong way.

TELL ME WHY I DON'T LIKE MONDAYS

When I started any of my diets I would almost immediately suffer, not physically but *mentally*. I would always start my diet on Monday (when else?). I think if people just *stopped going on a diet they would instantly eat less crap anyway*. Think about it. When I made the declaration that I was going on a diet on Monday, I would go into 'food freefall'. I would eat as much rubbish as I could possibly cram in from the Friday onwards declaring to the world, 'It's okay, I'm going on a diet on Monday'. So I would always eat a lot more than I would have normally eaten if I hadn't made the conscious decision to 'diet' in the first place. I would then go shopping on the Sunday and buy a trolley full of fruit and veg. Have you noticed how immediately judgemental we become when we have a load of good food in our trolley? We start eyeing up other people's trolleys and if they have a load of sugar and fat laced 'foods' and drinks and they don't look the picture of health and have a little hyper child with them, we start thinking, 'well no wonder, what do you expect'. All this and we haven't even bought the food yet, let alone actually eaten the stuff!

I would then wake on the Monday and immediately start to think of all the things I couldn't have. I would 'hang on in there' using all my might and willpower. To be fair I had usually stuffed myself so much over the weekend in preparation for the dreaded day, that I was usually okay most of the first day. But then out of the blue, usually late after-noon, a little voice would start chipping away and my desire for some-thing naughty would kick in. This is when I would use as much resolve as I could to resist temptation, which normally meant going to bed early in an attempt to sleep the craving away. Halfway through Tuesday and the inevitable 'I've picked the wrong time' would rear its ugly head. This would be rapidly followed by 'The bomb could go off tomorrow' and 'What's the point of living?' and I'd be back where I started. Well not quite – usually I'd then eat more than normal to subconsciously make up for lost eating time.

On other occasions I would not call it a 'diet' but simply say 'As from Monday, I will start to eat healthily'. Now I am sure that whoever invented the fridge hated fruit and veg. There is that drawer at the bottom to put your veg in so that you can conveniently forget that it's there – only to rediscover it days later when it's beginning to make its own way out! You then throw the mouldy veg in the bin with the declaration, 'I forgot all about that, if I'd have remembered I would have eaten it. Oh well, let's go get a take-out – it doesn't matter because I've decided to make a fresh start ... on Monday.' Recognize the pattern?

I never once got excited about getting a slim physique and gaining health because of the hell I thought I had to go through in order to achieve that goal. I never once looked forward to a change of diet; it was always a feeling of dread. I was defeated before I started. We should all, if we think about it logically, be very excited when we are about to change what we eat in order to get the body of our dreams. But if you are psychologically hooked on certain 'foods' and you believe that you gain something from them – pleasure, comfort or whatever – then those foods, even if you know they are also making you fat and ill, do not become less precious if you are forced to do without them. As you have no doubt experienced, they become the most precious thing in the world. Your entire focus is on either eating them or not eating them – as a result you experience the same mental tug-of-war that so many people think they have to go through.

The problem with this is there is only so long that anyone can 'hang on in there' and experience this often nightmarish mental tug-of-war. No wonder I never succeeded on a diet. No wonder it has such a high failure rate. And that is the real problem with diets – you effectively force yourself to do something which you do not want to do in the hope that you will reach what you do want – i.e. your ideal weight or optimum health. But all the time you are doing something you don't want to do you are having an internal, and often external, tantrum. One side of your brain wants the fat producing 'foods' and the other half doesn't because you want to look and feel better: 'Yes I will, no I won't' – it's a constant mental battle. There is only so long any sane person can do this before they say 'Sod this for a game of soldiers, life's too flipping short!'

WHEN ARE WE EVER FREE?

And at what point do we ever feel free from this mental battle? I use the term 'free' to describe not having to worry about the food we eat or having to exercise discipline and control over our intake; I mean truly free to eat what we want, whenever we want, free from guilt and restriction. So, when are we free? The minute the diet is over? I would say no. Because, when the diet is over we then start to eat the same crap which made us miserable in the first place and in no time at all the battle starts all over again. And every time we diet we end up with a bigger battle on our hands. When you have been knocked down just once it's easy to pick yourself up. If you keep getting knocked down you end up thinking 'what's the point in getting back up?'

The answer is to remove the very thing that is knocking you down – this is not simply the type of food itself, but more the conditioning, brainwashing, and misinformation that is the cause of why we put this crap in our mouths. All these factors, as well as the diets themselves, combine to create the belief that life would not be as enjoyable without junk and drug-like foods. That life would be 'dull' and 'boring' if we ate healthily and did exercise; that people who do this are boring, no-hope health freaks who have forgotten how to really live; that it is a 'constant battle' to be healthy and maintain your ideal weight. I used to believe this rubbish too.

Two of the main weight loss clubs in the world also perpetuate the belief that it's a lifetime battle – so much so that you have to attend their meetings every week just to make sure you are still on track, that you haven't 'fallen off the food wagon'. Yes I am talking about Weight Watchers and Slimming World. Now, before I go on, I must say that I am fully aware that both of these organizations have helped many, many people throughout the world and if you get a good 'leader' at your meeting place, they can be extremely effective. However, I also know that however admirable their motives might be, they are often instilling in the person with a 'food problem' the notion that they will have to try and 'control' their weight forever. They usually imply that almost no matter what they do, for them, it will be a constant lifelong battle.

TOTALLY POINTLESS

Weight Watchers used to have a 'points system'. You were awarded certain points per food and at the time they probably thought it was a revolutionary system. However, did you know that as far back as the late Thirties and early Forties there was a very similar points system used for restricting people's intake of food? It was called the 'Rationing' club! Yes, when food was scarce in the war people were given ration books and were allocated what were literally called 'Personal Points' for each day. You were allocated a certain amount of points and each food had a 'value' – sound familiar? The big difference was, no one was in the rationing club voluntarily and no one was pleased to be losing weight either. The whole business of counting the 'points' value of certain foods and rationing yourself accordingly is nothing short of madness. I bet there was not one single person in the war who ever thought they would see the day when people would actually pay for the privilege of deliberately restricting the amount of food they were allowed by counting 'points' – especially in times when food is in abundance.

Most diet clubs give the impression that if you don't do things like count points and attend weekly meetings you will binge and go back to your old 'habits'. Overeaters Anonymous (yes there is such an organization) take the idea of the 'constant battle' even further by suggesting that the 'problem' is due to some kind of weakness inherent in *you*, rather than with the drug-like foods and drinks themselves. They suggest you are born with an 'overeating gene' and they have a twelve-step programme to help you 'cope with' your disease. Yes, that's what they call your problem – a disease. The twelve-step programme is to help you *cope with*, not cure, your disease. For as far as they are concerned the disease is caused by something in your genes and there is no known cure. You were born with it and there is nothing you can do about it. How's that for setting yourself up for failure? That to me is the same as seeing someone sinking in quicksand and saying that the reason they're sinking is nothing to do with the quicksand but it's because they were born with a quicksand sinking gene. Yes people will sink at different rates depending on many factors, but surely if you can get someone out of the quicksand, they are cured? (more on this later).

DO AS I SAY ... NOT AS I DO

Due to our often desperate desire to lose weight, it appears we are willing to take advice from virtually anyone – regardless of whether or not they are ill and fat themselves. Many of the 'leaders' running the now over 12,000 slimming clubs in the UK are often 'yo-yoing' themselves. They are often *still* constantly having a battle with food, their health and their weight. One person who actually owns one of the biggest slimming clubs in the UK is reported to be overweight themselves – that's the founder!

It is true that you don't have to be a great football player to be an excellent football manager, but when it comes to this subject it is extremely important. For example, if you went to a 'stop-smoking' therapist to quit smoking and they had a cigarette hanging out of their mouth, would you listen to a word they have to say to you, even if the advice was correct? Clearly not. Don't get me wrong, I'm not picking on these people (after all, I know what it's like to be in the food and diet trap and it's really not that funny to be constantly struggling with your health, weight, and food intake), I just think it's very hard for anyone to get truly free from this whole diet and food struggle nightmare, when the people teaching haven't done it themselves. Remember, it's not about simply losing the weight, it's about getting slim and free. That way the change is easy and is one for life.

The overall position of the 'diet' industry seems pretty clear then. When it comes to weight loss and changing eating habits we have only two choices:

A) Use willpower, discipline, and exercise control *forever*, or
B) Run out of the will to control, say 'sod it', binge — then after the binge go back to trying to control again for a while.

What a life!

It seems to be a no-win situation – miserable when you are allowed to eat the crap and miserable and deprived when you're not. However, despite what we have all been conditioned to believe, there actually is an alternative and, as I have said, you are reading it. The best part of all is that when you see it clearly, when you see just how ridiculously easy it can be and indeed how obvious once pointed out, it will be one of the biggest 'light-bulb' moments you will ever experience

The diet mentality doesn't just apply to people who are overweight either. There are many slim people who want to change their diet because they want to feel fitter and healthier and have more energy. But they too have the same problem. They want to be healthy, but they also want to eat crap. So they have to force themselves to do something which they do not want to do in order to reach their goal. Many overweight people think all slim people are happy campers, but often they are having the same mental battle with food as they are. They too believe life would be nowhere near as enjoyable if they ate healthily.

One of the main reasons for this false belief is often the diet itself. Diets often encourage us to believe that life is a nightmare and boring without our 'usual' foods and drinks and wonderful with them. But I feel a touch of amnesia sets in. Obviously when we are not on a diet we are happier than when we are on one; but we are still not happy. That is why we want to change isn't it? It doesn't seem to occur to us that even when we are not on a diet we are still more miserable than someone who doesn't have to worry about their intake of food, their health or their weight. It wasn't only when I was consciously on a diet that I had this 'I want to eat, but I wish I didn't' mental tug-of-war. The truth is I always had it to some degree. I was constantly trying to control my intake of certain foods. On a diet I just had to try and control it even more than usual – which simply made me much more aware of it.

it is having to exercise control over your intake of food on a daily basis that is the problem.

You shouldn't have to control what you eat, you should be free to eat whatever you want, whenever you want, without having to worry about your health or weight. We have all been doing it for so long we have come to accept it as the norm – but it's not normal to have to exercise enormous amounts of control on a regular basis. For example, non-smokers can smoke whenever they want – they just don't want to so clearly there is no problem. It is only smokers that have the problem of trying to control their intake that have a smoking problem, non-smokers have their freedom – the freedom of not *having* to smoke. Even those smokers who have stopped but still crave them all the time aren't truly free either; they are still exercising control not to smoke. It is only those people who have smoked, stopped and don't miss them who are truly free.

I can overeat whenever I want to, but I just don't want to anymore. I finally have true freedom around all food. Wild animals have this freedom too. In fact we are the only creatures on the planet that do this control and dieting stuff. Why? Because we have television, radio, and so-called 'experts' telling us what we should eat and often when we should eat. Unlike us, wild animals rely purely on their natural instincts. We also instinctively know exactly what to eat and when to eat. Our problem is that we have an intellectual brain that can easily be 'washed' by people with all kinds of vested interests, either status or financial. However, if we were left to our own intuitive devices we would all be eating healthily and no one would have a 'food problem'.

DIETS TREAT THE SYMPTOM – NOT THE CAUSE

Diets *never* solve a food problem – they ultimately make it worse for most people. The second you go on a diet you feel deprived. You are usually no longer 'allowed' to eat the foods you love or you have to restrict yourself from eating a certain amount of them. The situation is that even if you do manage to 'hang on in there' and reach your weight 'target' or 'goal', what happens? You 'reward' yourself … with what? Yes, the very 'foods' you have been longing for in the quantity you have been dreaming of. You have been incredibly 'good' and you feel you deserve a 'treat' for all the effort you have put in for all this time. The problem is the 'feel good' time is pretty short lived. In no time at all you soon realize that you are once again packing on the pounds. Once this dawns on you, the no-win situation rears its head again. You either let the food floodgates open, or you try to exercise immense control over your intake once again. The point I am making is simple – you are never truly free. All you have in fact 'treated' yourself to are feelings of guilt, self-loathing, lethargy, a body you hate, and a lifetime desperately trying to control your intake of certain foods. And how do we try and solve that problem – another diet!

We need to start understanding that excess fat is a physical 'symptom' of a psychological problem. The real issue is mental – *not* physical. Diets aren't designed to change the way you think, they are simply designed to change either what you eat or how much you eat, not how you see certain foods. Diets are designed to treat the excess fat (the physical symptom) but they do nothing to address the real issue, which can solve the problem for life. Because diets only treat the symptom, inevitably the situation ultimately gets worse.

Hit The Roof

For example, if I had a leaky roof and rain was falling onto my ceiling tiles, pretty soon it would show. If I simply replaced the ceiling tile, I can feel good for a while, but soon the tile would need replacing again. However, because the cause of the problem hadn't been addressed (the hole in the roof), the situation would naturally get worse. The hole in the roof would get bigger and more tiles would be affected. I could keep replacing more and more tiles and on the surface all would look good, but in reality far from solving the problem I am always making it worse. All I clearly need to do is fix the roof and I would never have to replace a tile again. Exactly the same principle applies here. Remove the brainwashing, conditioning, and false beliefs about certain foods and drinks while exposing **BiG FOOD** and **BiG DRiNK** for what it is, and you get to the root cause of the problem. Once you remove the *mental* cravings, you have removed the need for any willpower, thus removing the cause. Once the cause has gone, the symptoms (excess fat) soon start to disappear and so to does the need ever to go on a diet again.

DIETS CAN MAKE YOU FAT!

Another major problem with restrictive diets is that they often aren't nutritionally thought through and many times you literally starve your body. If you deliberately stop yourself eating when your body is genuinely screaming for food, you are fighting against the most powerful instinct in the world: survival. No wonder people find it hard. When you do this, your body's metabolism slows down; yes *down*. If it keeps going at the rate it is with such a small amount of food coming in, you will die very quickly. This is why the minute the body senses that there is a severe lack of food coming in, it assumes you have no choice in this decision (after all no other creature on earth would restrict in times of abundance). And rather than let you die, your metabolism slows *down* considerably to conserve energy. At the same time, the body stores even more of what you do eat as fat as it senses lean times ahead. Because the fat is needed, the body even begins to burn muscle tissue, which is a bit of a bugger as muscle helps to burn excess fat – so a double whammy. In fact, virtually every time you go on a restrictive diet you lose muscle tissue and gain more fat cells. Once you gain fat cells they never die, they simply shrink. This is why it is so much easier for people who have been overweight in the past to gain weight again ... *rapidly*.

MORE BIG FAT PROBLEMS

When the 'diet' is over (which normally happens either when you say 'sod the diet' or you somehow manage to reach your physical goal) your metabolism is still working much slower than before you started the diet. It will increase again, but gradually – which is why it is important to build food up again slowly and not overeat. However, as most people are chomping at the bit for the diet to end so they can 'live normally' again, any chances of a *gradual* increase in food is pretty slim. In fact, any 'end of diet' period is usually followed by a massive meal – either to celebrate the achievement, or to illustrate the fact that 'life is too short so sod you all ...' etc.

Having acquired a slower metabolism, you now go back to eating exactly the same amount of food you ate before you started the diet. What happens? You put on *more* weight than before you started the diet – and, it seems, a lot faster than it took to shift it. This is not simply your perception either. A study carried out on a group of rats in 1986 showed that by the time they did their second diet, the weight loss was half of what it was the first time and, wait for it, the weight was put back on **THREE TIMES AS FAST**. This is happening to millions of people around the world as we speak. The problem is it's a cause and effect chain reaction, for when you see the weight rapidly piling on again you once again think that it's time to do something about it – what? Yep the latest **DIET**.

Now I understand why dieting, as well as the addiction to certain foods and drinks, makes people fat. They often contribute to the problem people are trying to solve. It is only in fairly recent times that people have reached over 500 lb (227 kg) in weight. One family in the US –

The Woods family – weighed in at 1 tonne – yes **ONE TONNE**. And if you think we are talking about a large family (so to speak), we are talking a combined weight of just *four* women. One girl, Terriny Woods, was 41 stone 12lb(over 260 kg) and she was just 15 years old at the time. Yes 15 years old.

If you keep going on a diet and then binge directly afterwards, your body will produce more fat cells, your metabolism will not know what the hell it's doing and your system will store more fat in case you starve it again. This is the cycle people repeat again and again. Physically and mentally diets can be a nightmare. You never break free from the constant mental battle of trying to control your intake of certain foods or certain amounts of food. Nor do you break free from the many physical problems they create – all that happens is you become totally obsessed with food. You're not happy when you feel you can't eat and you feel like crap after you do it. It's time to stop this madness. It's time to fix the leaking roof once and for all and stop replacing the tiles.

The Medical 'Solution'

There are of course many people who have been through the dieting mill and have realized this is not a long-term solution. At the same time their excess weight, as well as ailments related to their obesity, often cause people to take much more drastic measures than simply trying the latest diet. The increase in weight loss surgery and weight loss pills has exploded over recent years. Big people are big business and there are many people making billions of pounds by preying on their insecurities and desperation – all in the name of 'medical help' and 'genuine care' you understand. While I am all for some short-term medical intervention in many areas of 'disease', I see no place whatsoever for weight loss pills. And when I say no place, I mean no place at all. Even weight loss surgery, in some *very* desperate cases, can at times be the only solution to save a life and I can see at least a debate for it. However, these all new all-dancing and singing 'weight loss solution' pills are never the answer. Weight loss drugs are no longer aimed simply at the morbidly obese and given by GPs *only* as a last resort to those who really do feel they have tried everything else and would possibly die otherwise. Unfortunately things have got so far out of hand with the weight loss drug industry (as indeed I believe it has with the whole drug industry no matter what the disease) that I think it's now safe to say we are without any question on the verge of ...

4

PHARMAGEDDON

Never in history have we seen so many drugs being handed out so willy-nilly to so many people for so many different things. Every pill sold, means more money for **BiG PHARMACEUTiCALS**. And one particular 'disease' is now more of the holy grail for **BiG DRUGS** than almost any other – obesity. With millions of people getting bigger by the day while craving the land of the thin more and more, the desperate need for a 'quick fix' is now at an all time high. And what better quick fix than a simple pill?

In 1998, the NHS (National Health Service) gave out 20,000 anti-obesity pills. Just seven years later in 2005 that figure rose to 880,000 pills, the figure will almost certainly be over 1 million pills today. This annual cost to the NHS was £690,000 in the late 1990s and is now nearly £40 million. Yes **FORTY MiLLiON POUNDS** of your tax money going directly into the hands of the pharmaceutical companies, and the figure is growing daily. The government justify the ever increasing costs by claiming, '… the benefits to the economy outweigh the cost to the NHS', they go on to explain, '… a lot of illness can be avoided by using these pills to aid weight loss'. Exactly what illnesses have ever been 'cured' as a direct result of the introduction of so many weight loss drugs I don't exactly know, but no doubt there will be some 'scientific data' to back up such claims and if there aren't it wouldn't be too difficult to get some. I also haven't seen a reduction of people gaining weight either, which given all you have to do is take a pill, is surprising. If these weight loss drugs are, as they often purport to be, 'the easy solution to fat and obesity', and given we are in an obesity epidemic, why don't they simply give them to everyone so we can all live a 'fat free' and disease free life?

Well the simple answer is they aren't exactly the 'magic bullet' some purport them to be. What is extraordinary is that each anti-fat drug comes with a little side note explaining something along the lines of 'can help to lose weight in conjunction with a diet and exercise programme'. Now, stop me if I appear nuts here, but doesn't that defeat the whole argument of these fat drugs? Aren't they apparently there as a last resort for those people who have tried everything else and now have no choice but to seek medical help? Aren't they surely designed for people who have failed on the diet and exercise front? People who, for whatever reason, cannot tap into the right mind set to change their diet and exercise more? If that is the case and they are only meant to be given to such desperate people (after all, drugs should always be the last resort) and if these drugs are only effective *with* a change in diet and an increase in exercise, how can they possibly work for the group for which they are intended? Do these pills somehow miraculously inspire people to change their diet and get on the treadmill? If so, they really are miracle drugs. I get images of perhaps a three-dimensional tablet acting like a motivational cheerleader/speaker inspiring people to eat well and exercise. Seriously, think about it. If these drugs *don't* help people lose excess weight by simply taking them, regardless of any change in diet or physical movement, then what's the point of them? Even if they did enable an *odd few* to lose a *little weight* without changing anything else, are the potential risks of taking any drug and changing the fine chemical balance of the body worth it and what on earth do these pills do to get to the cause of the problem?

WONDER DRUGS

Coincidentally, as I write this small chapter, yet another 'weight loss pill' has come onto the market and only yesterday I was on the radio talking about it. I say coincidentally, but as they are coming out faster than the rate of stealth taxes, it's not really that much of a coincidence. What's fascinating about this particular one is the fact that for some reason it has been approved in England, but rejected by the FDA (Food and Drug Administration) in the US because the safety of the drug was not demonstrated. The first question I have is an obvious one. How can a drug be okay for humans in the UK but not for those in the US? How can it be cleared on a scientific level here and yet not on a scientific level over there? I was always taught that science is 'fact', when of course I now know it's 'opinion'. In the *opinion* of the FDA it is, at time of this writing, not demonstrated as being safe and in the *opinion* of those in England it is fine. When I say fine, it doesn't seem to matter that this drug – Rimonabant – has noted possible side effects which may include suicidal thoughts. However, as always, the counter drug argument of 'it does more good than harm' soon starts after any negative drug press.

Dr Ian Campbell, medical director of the charity Weight Concern said, 'You have to balance the risks with the advantages of quality of life improvement. Rimonabant has a role, it should be used with care but directed towards the right patient it can be effective and safe.' However, he also goes on to say that the drug should not be used in people being treated for depression or with a recent history of depression. However, unless once again I have lost leave of my senses, the people for whom the pill is directed are more than likely going to be depressed aren't they? If you are obese and so desperate that you are willing to take a drug which has the potential for suicidal thoughts (even if the chance is extremely small), wouldn't it be fair to assume there's a huge chance that person is already depressed? The medical profession will no doubt look to see before prescribing that the individual has no history of depression. But again that would be based purely on their medical records. If so, we need to ask, how many people go to their GP with depression for being overweight? And surely the ones who do are the very people who the drugs are designed for, aren't they? Yet, it is recommended that this drug should not be taken if you are depressed, which begs the question, who exactly are these pills meant for? Deliriously happy obese people perhaps? But if they were over the moon with their weight, why would they seek medical assistance to lose weight? Can you see how mental the whole thing is when you start to look at it? It's even more insane when you think the US committee of experts who reviewed studies of Rimonabant from all over the world, told an FDA hearing that the drug is associated with an increased risk of suicidal thoughts – *even in those with no history of depression.* Studies also highlighted significant increases in anxiety, insomnia, and panic attacks in patients given 20 mg of the drug compared with placebo.

This is far from the first time weight loss drugs have been put under the adverse drug reaction (ADR) spotlight. Over the years many of these 'medically approved' weight loss drugs have had reports of all sorts of side effects ranging from random anal leakage to even death. But at least up until now you had to see your GP first before you could get hold of them. At least it was down to a professional to make a qualified judgement as to whether you should be given such pills and whether the chance of any adverse drug reaction, in their opinion, would be outweighed by what they hope will be a reduction in the patient's weight. However, as from the spring of 2009, the way with which people get hold of some weight loss drugs will all change. For the first time in history in the UK you will be able to buy the first ever 'over the counter' weight loss drug – Alli. No prescription – no doctor's appointment – no assessment, just walk into your local chemist and get your drug. Given that we are in a world where thin is the new black, I feel the decision to license this drug as an OTC (Over The Counter), will prove to be one of the most reckless in the history of medicine. The potential for 'drug' abuse here is on a scale as yet unknown. After Alli was launched in the US in 2007 it sold 75 million in the first six months alone, which gives us some kind of idea of what's in store here. I would also bet this will not be the only OTC weight loss drug either; once this comes along the floodgates will open and getting hold of your weight loss drug will become as normal as buying an aspirin (by the time you read this book it may already have happened). The dangers to anyone with a shred of common sense are painfully obvious, especially as you can also buy these pills on the Net too. Teenagers for one will no doubt get hold of these and chances are, with no one checking to see how many people are buying and taking, will take much more than the recommended dose in the delusion they will lose more by taking more (no doubt many adults will also do the same!). Losing weight is one of the biggest obsessions teenagers and many adults have and to produce a drug that anyone can easily buy without any checks with a promise of weight loss is unwise to say the least.

What's crazy is both the FDA in the US *and* now the FSA (Food Standards Agency) in the UK, gave the drug the all clear to be sold over the counter, expressing the benefits far outweigh any possible risk to health. But in order for this drug to be cleared the FDA and FSA would have had to come to the conclusion that the drug is both safe and effective – the criteria all approved drugs have to pass. But, ignoring the moral issue of having a weight loss drug as an OTC and God knows how many people who may well abuse it, I question it on both the other fronts. Firstly it stops the absorption of some fat soluble vitamins like A, D, E, and K. The body is such a finely tuned machine that you simply cannot brush aside the effects this will have on the overall health of the body; effects which may not become apparent for many years. On top of this, the drug works by stopping the body from absorbing some of the fat you eat in food. This sounds like good news, but a) it's not necessarily fat that makes you fat (as I will illustrate a little later) and b) it is essential the body *does* absorb fat. (They aren't called '*essential* fatty acids' for nothing after all). Also the actual weight loss effectiveness of the drug has been brought into question too. There was even one report that showed an average of just one pound of weight loss in an entire month. A loss hardly worth risking a bit of random anal leakage for, which, just so you know, is one of the potential side effects of this particular weight loss drug. In fact, GlaxoSmithKline recommends that Alli users wear dark pants and keep spare clothes available at work until they 'have a sense of any treatment effects'. Yes, such are the chances of 'steatorrhea' – oily, loose stools – and fecal incontinence, frequent or urgent bowel movements and flatulence, that the makers suggest you wear some dark pants just in case something happens unexpectedly. Seriously, is it me or has the world gone completely bonkers? Clearly there have also been many studies with Alli that have shown significantly more weight loss than the 1 lb (0.45 kg) in a month I quoted a second ago, but is having to wear dark pants just in case something foul unexpectedly comes out of your bum really worth it?

I could write an entire book on just weight loss drugs alone, but the point I want to illustrate is once again what on earth do any of these pills do to get to the *cause* of the excess weight problem? What can they possibly do to stop someone's *desire* for certain foods? It may stop someone eating certain amounts of fat through fear of a sudden 'soiling of their pants', but what on earth does it do to stop the excess consumption of refined sugar – the *biggest* cause of excess bodily fat there is? What does it do to stop them even *wanting* fatty foods but just not having them through fear? Even if someone does lose weight taking any weight loss drug, if nothing has been done to change the way that person perceives what they eat or the way they eat, then what on earth stops them piling the weight back on when they stop taking the pill? Doesn't this work in exactly the same way as the 'fad diets' many in the dietetic and medical profession slag off so readily? Aren't these over the counter diet pills a 'quick fix' solution? Once the 'quick fix' is over, it's back to the same pattern of behaviour which caused the problem in the first place. Once again, excess bodily fat is a *physical* symptom of *addictive psychological* problem. With that in mind, please rest assured that in my opinion there will never be a weight loss pill that can possibly send you to the utopia of a Food Freedom mentality and so the land of the thin.

Shortly before going to press the European Medicines Agency (EMEA) recommended the suspension of the marketing authorization of Accomplia, as Rimonabant is known as in Europe, because its 'benefits no longer outweigh its risks'. This despite the fact that the drug was cleared by NICE (National Institute for Health and Clinical Excellence) for use as a last resort on the NHS only four months earlier.

Under The Knife

People's desperation to get to grips with their weight and health doesn't simply stop at radical, nutritionally unsound, diets or suspect diet pills. Going under the surgeon's knife is getting more and more popular. In the United States alone, 177,600 operations were performed in 2007, according to the American Society for Metabolic & Bariatric Surgery. One of the most common operations and now probably the most widely talked about is gastric bypass surgery. This works by making your stomach smaller and removing part of your bowel to make your digestive system shorter. This was also the operation Fern Britton famously had and it's not for the faint hearted. Personally I feel Fern Britton was given a hard time when it came out her dramatic weight loss was not simply down to diet and exercise, as she had apparently claimed, but rather surgery. I don't think some realize how low and desperate someone has to get to even contemplate surgery for weight loss. Gastric bypass surgery can be potentially life threatening and is usually used in extreme cases only. However, due to what they deem as the 'success' of such operations, the plan is to extend this 'opportunity' to those who aren't necessarily morbidly obese (large chance of dying as a result of their weight), but just obese. Please understand that the way obesity and morbid obesity is measured at the moment is using an antiquated system known as BMI (Body Mass Index). This ridiculous system doesn't take into account muscle mass and is completely inaccurate in many cases. This system even shows the extremely muscular and well-toned rugby player Jonny Wilkinson as obese! Pretty soon you will have slightly overweight people (who according to the BMI scale are obese) getting this surgery. It's also worth knowing that we are already in a position where many children are now going under the knife for obesity, yes kids.

Once again though I have the same question – does this treat the cause or the symptom? Unlike drug pills I can actually see an argument for some types of weight loss surgery. There would, I believe without question, be some people who would be dead now without it. However, this type of treatment is getting more and more popular and for some, far from being the last resort, it can be seen as the 'easy' solution and one of the first things they try. Easy is not the word I would use for this operation, stomach bypass or any similar procedures. Remember, these operations don't stop you *wanting* certain foods; you just can't eat as much of them. So you still want to, but you can't. This, for many, is a form of living mental torture. Many get around the problem by simply blending a load of junk food with some liquid and drinking it instead. So they are still often having their sugar and refined fat fix, just in a different form or chewing the same crap very slowly. This is why there are some people who despite operations like this, still have problems losing weight. One lady lost just 1 lb (0.45 kg) in the seven weeks following her stomach bypass op. She spent £6,000, went through the nightmare of being under the surgeon's knife to have her stomach strangled, yet still has exactly the same problem as before. She still battles every day with the mental cravings she has for the chocolates, cola, cakes, and all the other artificial sweet things that are causing the problem – and she still consumes them. She is still on a permanent mental diet – still constantly trying to fight a desire to eat and drink certain foods. And exactly the same can happen with jaw wiring, the stomach 'pacemaker' (yes there is one) or any of the other drastic surgical methods used to try and shift the fat.

When In Doubt – Suck It Out!

Then we have those who don't fancy the idea of their stomach being stapled and having to restrict what they eat, and opt for a bit of liposuction. No willpower, discipline, and control needed here, simply let them knock you out and suck the fat out. You then leave hospital so battered and bruised you feel like you have just gone ten rounds with

Mike Tyson – but at least you're thinner! Your skin is the biggest organ of the body and when you start cutting it open and sucking fat out, it simply cannot be a good thing to do. And, like all the other weight loss methods I have mentioned here, liposuction again does absolutely nothing to remove the *psychological addiction* to certain foods and drinks and desire for them. All it does is treat the physical symptoms of being mentally locked in what I describe as 'the food trap'.

Set Yourself Free

What's required is a very different approach. The irony is, as I will keep mentioning throughout this book, that the whole process of changing what you eat in order to get slim and healthy and to stay slim and healthy is ridiculously simple. The problem is we have all been going about it the wrong way for so long we are all totally convinced that there isn't an easy way. We all strongly believe losing weight will require tremendous amounts of willpower, discipline, and self-control for life. We think if we don't possess such strengths, we will need to seek out pills, patches (yes there is a weight loss patch!), or the fat hoover to help us get thin. However, just because we believe something is difficult to virtually impossible – and even if that belief is backed up by 99 per cent of the population – it doesn't make it so. If I can simply a) change this false belief and b) show you an extremely easy way of thinking that will set you free around food in a way you possibly haven't felt in years, freedom is yours.

This process cannot only be easy, but also enjoyable. The answer is not to starve yourself, cut yourself open, pop a pill or staple your stomach, but to change the way you think about the 'foods' in order to successfully, not go *on* a diet, but …

5

CHANGE YOUR DIET

When I was unhealthy, tired, lethargic, and fat, I knew, as we all do, that if I ate plenty of fruit, vegetables, and salads I would be slim and healthy. The problem was I actually hated vegetables and salads. I had fruit every now and again – summer mainly – and even then only the odd orange. As for salads, somehow I don't think the token side salad, which I hardly touched, really counted. The main difficulty I had was that I simply didn't like the taste of vegetables and salads and they just never seemed to satisfy. Even the fruits I did eat didn't seem to satisfy me the same way as steak and chips. Besides which, I had always been conditioned to believe that if you ate that 'rabbit food' you were being boring. No, my regular diet was comprised of steak and chips; McDonald's; Burger King; chocolate; crisps; a big 'hearty' breakfast; tons of tea and coffee; loads of white bread and butter; big helpings of white pasta; egg or beans on toast; hot dogs; Sunday roast. In fact, you name it I ate it – *as long as it wasn't green!* I often looked at well-prepared, beautiful-looking salads and thought, 'I really wish I liked that, but I just don't'. If I could get as much pleasure and satisfaction from eating fruit, salad, vegetables, and drinking carrot juice as I do eating steak and chips and drinking Coke, then I would do it – who wouldn't?

Well it transpires you can and the change really is simple. I know at this stage that may sound like rubbish, especially for those who have tried 'everything' in the past, but I did say at the start that an open mind is vital for success here. Not only will you get just as much pleasure and satisfaction from your new way of eating, but infinitely more so. These days I wouldn't even let you pay me to eat a McDonald's or Burger King, yet for years these were my 'brand' of food and I ate them daily.

When I wake up in the morning now and head straight for my juicer and blender, I do so not because I 'have to' or because I need to lose weight due to some restrictive diet. I do so because I wouldn't dream of doing anything else now, it has bizarrely become my choice; I actually want to do it. When I choose a meal at a restaurant now I actually look for tasty salad!

I am writing this with some surprise because a few years ago, the first thing I 'had' to do in the morning was stick the kettle on to give myself a caffeine 'boost'. I now know this was to try and get me over my junkie food hangover (more about that later). I would then eat a big bowl of cereal, several rounds of toast and maybe a couple of boiled eggs. At the weekends my breakfast consisted of everything that was on offer at JJ's café. The great British breakfast – the bedrock of a good heart attack as they say.

I used to have images of people who owned a juicer, drank carrot juice and ate leaves. One which perhaps you have at the moment. I would think 'What sad, boring people – what on earth do they do for fun?' But how deluded was I? As if I was having enormous amounts of fun being a fat, tired, and lethargic person, hating the way I felt and looked on an almost daily basis. As if I was enjoying a life where I was constantly battling with my intake of food or the latest 'diet'. I believe this is where we all have got it wrong. I always thought that if I *stopped* eating the junk I would be making a sacrifice and if I did eat overeat and/or eat junk it was somehow a wonderful life. I thought if I drank fresh juice, ate good food, created the body I wanted, felt light, and had the energy I required to live my dreams that I would somehow be missing out, I would be making massive sacrifices to get what I wanted. But the question is, what sacrifices? I don't think we ever stop to actually ask that very important question. Whenever I overate it would always be followed by thoughts of, 'I wish I hadn't done that' or 'why did I do that'. I never really enjoyed the food either as it would be gone in seconds. I was eyeing up the next mouthful before I had eaten the one on my fork! I was setting myself up for a lifetime of misery, lethargy, and being overweight all for literally *seconds* of what I thought was genuine pleasure – even though I hated myself soon afterwards. I would hardly call that a fair trade off.

I often felt bloated after eating a pile of what I deemed as 'the most pleasurable food on earth'. My physical problems were clearly caused by the amount of the foods I was eating and the quantities I consumed. These foods would always seem nice in my mind before I ate them, but as soon as I did, I wished I hadn't. That's not true satisfaction; it's the complete opposite.

Since changing my diet I now see the truth – there was nothing special about these foods at all, it was one incredibly clever illusion, one which I believe has deluded millions around the world. Like any illusion, it appears extremely real until it gets shattered. That is precisely what this book is about; page by page it will gradually chip away at the illusion until it is completely shattered and that 'light-bulb' moment will be yours for the taking.

Contrary to what we have been conditioned to believe it is *extremely* easy to switch your diet as opposed to going *on* one, we have all simply been looking at the wrong way for so many years we find it hard to believe it can be ridiculously easy.

A Sweet Change For The Better

For example, I know many people who used to love sugar in their tea and at the time would never drink it without, but now wouldn't pay you for a cup with even a grain in it. Why not? What has changed? The tea and the sugar have always remained exactly the same. The difference is they have simply trained themselves to like tea and coffee without sugar. The process is not hard; in fact it usually takes all of a week to get used to any new taste. The week is not painful, just a bit strange at first like any change. The coffee without sugar does not taste wonderful at first but after a while it soon starts to taste better to the person than it did with sugar in. The point that I am making is that the vast majority of people who make this change, would now never drink tea or coffee with sugar in it again. Not because they can't, or because they are being forced not to, but because they have no *desire* to any more. This is an extremely important point to understand in order to reach 'Food Freedom' mentality. They aren't on a 'no sugar in tea *diet*'. In other words they don't stare longingly at people adding sugar to their tea and feel envious because they can't have it. The reason for this is simple. They *can* have sugar in their tea, but are now choosing not to. Diet mentality is one of, 'I want, but I can't have' (which is enough to drive anyone of strong will, crazy. Yes *strong* will, I will expand on this later) but when you change your diet you have a, 'I *can*, but I don't actually want to' mentality. When you have this mentality and have *changed your diet* as opposed to gone *on a diet*, there is no need to use any form of willpower, discipline, or self-control. In fact, those who do stop sugar in their tea and have done so for a little while, act as if you have poisoned them if you put some in (which in a way you have). The point is clear and simple: by changing their brand they will *never* have to use willpower, discipline, or self-control not to have sugar in their tea again. In other words – they are genuinely free to choose.

YOU CANNOT HAVE FREEDOM OF CHOICE WITHOUT THE FREEDOM TO REFUSE

This is a theme I will be repeating throughout the book – 'you cannot have freedom of genuine choice, without the freedom also to be able to refuse'. It is interesting to observe that people who are mentally *on a diet* detest it so much because they feel their genuine freedom of choice has been removed. What they don't seem to realize is that in many cases they aren't actually genuinely choosing to eat the foods causing the health and excess fat problems anyway. They often want to stop the diet in order to get back to the freedom of choice they believed they enjoyed. This is an illusion for, as I will repeat, you simply cannot have genuine freedom of choice without genuine freedom to refuse. If people could simply choose to refuse, then diets would be obsolete and no one on earth would have a weight problem. People would simply exercise their genuine freedom of choice to refuse. If you could genuinely choose to have or not to have, then you wouldn't be reading this book. The reality is our choices are being made for us. BiG FOOD and BiG DRiNK – just like the tobacco companies over forty years ago – are adding chemicals to our 'food' and 'drinks' in order to make us feel hungrier faster. Haven't you ever wondered why logically you just couldn't simply stop eating certain things, even when it has gone completely against your intelligent rational judgement?

Addiction and logic don't go together, if they did no intelligent person would have ever smoked after it became clear it causes cancer and nobody would continue overeating and/or eating rubbish knowing it makes them fat, ill, miserable and can cause premature death. Logically, if this type of eating made people happy, everyone who is overweight would all be leading blissfully happy lives.

BRITAIN'S FATTEST TEEN

Coincidentally as I write this book a teenager has made front page headlines in the *Sun* newspaper in the UK. Georgia Davis has the unenviable title of being 'Britain's Fattest Teen' weighing it at 33 stone (209 kg) at only 15 years of age. Consuming between eight to twelve thousand calories a day it's easy to see how she got to be that big. The big mistake people make, including Georgia herself, is that it is not her choice to eat like this. There is no way on earth this poor and desperate girl genuinely chooses to eat the amount she does and be the size she is. If she had genuine freedom of choice she would simply stop eating so much rubbish and switch to fruit, veggies, and salads. Doctors have told her 'she could drop dead at any moment', no doubt believing a touch of 'stating the bloody obvious' would somehow help her. If anything, trying to scare any kind of addict off their drug rarely if ever works, in fact it usually has the opposite effect. For example one of the times a smoker will reach for a cigarette is when they are stressed and uptight. I remember my doctor telling me that if I continued smoking my lungs would collapse. I was so scared and stressed when I came out what do you think was the first thing I did? Yes – light a fag to help calm me down! The same principle applies to drug food. You tell someone like Georgia that she will die unless she changes, it won't help her. She will simply find somewhere to cut off from the world and eat. Why? Because, as I will repeat, addiction and logic have no place together. Georgia said, 'I can't walk any more than a few steps without getting out of breath and a few months ago I developed type 2 diabetes. When I look in the mirror I feel sad and go to my bedroom and cry. I know it's partly my fault. But it's so hard to stop eating.'

But it's not hard to stop eating apples, bananas, grapes, cucumber, sardines, or spinach – even when people love these foods. Why? Because they are not drug-like foods and they don't create a hole, they *genuinely* feed the body. Georgia went on to say, 'Food is like a drug. Some people choose heroin but I've chosen food and it's killing me.'

But that's the point; no one actually chooses to be a heroin addict any more than they choose to get hooked on certain foods. The more you try to fill the hole with the substances creating the hole the bigger the hole gets. All that has happened to 33 stone (209 kg) Georgia is the hole has got out of all proportion and the only thing which appears to give any degree of satisfaction is an enormous amount of the same. This poor girl knows it's killing her, knows it has caused her to have diabetes and even knows she could drop down dead at any moment, yet she still continues to struggle. This is because telling her what she is doing is killing her is the same as telling someone in quicksand they are in fact in quicksand and should get out. **SHE KNOWS!** This girl knows all the reasons why she shouldn't eat all this rubbish daily, what she doesn't know is what compels her to do so against her rational judgement. And that is precisely what makes this book so very different to any 'diet' book you have ever read and is precisely what will enable you to break totally free.

It is interesting to see that Georgia Davis said that eating is 'like a drug' to her. What I am saying is that it's not simply 'like a drug to her', it is a drug and it is a drug to millions of people all over the world. This is due not to some inherent weakness in those millions of individuals, but the addictive nature of the drug-food itself. It is true that not everyone who smokes cigarettes becomes heavily addicted, but nearly all are addicted to some degree. The same applies to drug-like foods and drinks. Not everyone is this heavily addicted, but millions are certainly addicted to some degree. This is not the nature of the people but the nature of the substances themselves. And it's not 'food' *per se* that they are overeating and 'using' as an emotional crutch, it's *drug*-like food that people become addicted to and use to try and feed an emotion. After all I don't see too many people attending Apple Anonymous or going to weekly meetings to try to stop eating broccoli do you?

This is why I disagree so vehemently with people like Paul McKenna. While I admire much of his work in other areas, I cannot agree with his 'I Can Make You Thin' principles due to the addictive nature of the foods themselves. Paul suggests you can eat whatever you like as long as you eat only when you are hungry and stop eating when you are genuinely full. But that's like saying to a smoker on twenty cigarettes a day that all they have to do to avoid cancer is to cut down to one cigarette a day. While the advice itself is correct – after all I don't believe anyone would actually get cancer smoking one a day – if you have ever smoked you will know that actually trying to smoke just one a day when you have been on twenty is virtually impossible. And if you did manage it, you wouldn't be happy, you would just be wishing your life away waiting for that one cigarette. It's the same with drug-like food. Anyone who is already hooked on a certain amount can't just 'cut down' or 'eat slowly' and 'stop when they feel full'. In fact these drug-like foods often trigger an almost uncontrollable urge to binge and overeat. How many times have you thought 'just the one' chocolate or biscuit and before you know where you are you have polished off a great deal more?

Georgia Davis cannot stop eating when she is full because she never feels full. In the same way your body builds up an immunity and tolerance to a drug, it does the same with drug-like food and drink. You end up needing more and more in order to try and fill the hole and void the drug itself has created. Georgia's problem is she *does* eat when she feels hungry, the problem is she feels hungry most of the time due to the addictive nature of these foods and drinks. What Georgia ultimately needs is to starve the false hungers and create a genuine one. Once that happens *then* and only then can the advice of 'eat when hungry' and 'stop when full' be effective.

MILLIONS TRAPPED

I need you to realize that the trap you find yourself in, the one I found myself in and the one millions are in all over the world is simply a result of clever marketing and chemicals designed to make you feel ultimately dissatisfied. They create a hole, which appears to be filled with more of the same, yet in reality the hole gets bigger till in the end you don't ever truly appear to be able to fill it. The irony is we believe this empty feeling can only be filled with more of the same rubbish, which is perhaps the biggest aspect of the illusion – as you will discover.

The 'food' business is the same as any other and **BiG FOOD** simply wants to sell more. They will only do this by removing genuine nutrients (to create a malnourished body which always demands more in a desperate need for the right nutritional requirements) and adding chemicals, which compel an otherwise intelligent person to eat certain things and eat more than they would ever do in their rational mind. Despite 15-year-old Georgia's immense size, the main reason for her insatiable hunger is malnutrition. She, like millions, is overfed but undernourished.

If you *change* your diet and don't go *on a diet* – in the same way as when a person gets used not to having sugar in their tea and coffee – you never have to think about your diet again. You will be free to genuinely choose what you put into your body and you won't be a slave to, or victim of, the **BiG FOOD** system.

I want to make this point clear: I am not being 'good' drinking freshly extracted vegetable juice daily and skipping the junkie food in favour of good wholesome foods, I choose to do it – it's my regular diet now. The people who no longer take sugar in their tea have no desire to go back and I have no desire to go back either. This whole 'being good' is a nonsense way of thinking anyway and is part of the 'diet trap'. For example, are you being good for not taking heroin? Do you feel proud of yourself because you haven't sniffed glue today? If you did feel proud then it would mean that you indeed have a glue problem. I am not proud of myself for not stuffing myself with crap today, I just don't want to eat this stuff as my main diet any more. Unlike a conventional diet (in the restrictive sense), I can eat and drink whatever I want, whenever I want, I no longer have to put restrictions on myself. The difference is that I just do not want them any more. I am not being 'good' for eating what I do, it is now my genuine choice to. I am not continuing to do what I do to lose weight, because I'm already slim, and I'm not doing it to stay slim – I'm doing it because it is now my brand and I love it!

YOU WILL LEARN TO ENJOY ANY FOOD OR DRINK YOU HAVE ON A REGULAR BASIS

A few years ago I would never have believed that I could literally train myself to love fruits, salads, vegetables, and their juices. I even love avocados now, a fruit I absolutely detested before. However, as macrobiotics has been teaching for years, you will adapt and learn to love any food or drink you have on a regular basis (I am unsure if Brussel sprouts are included in that mind you). That is something I would have dismissed in an instant a few years ago, but there is a great deal of truth in it. Years back I tried some Chinese herbal medicine in an attempt to clear my skin of psoriasis. The best way I can describe the medicine is tree bark. I had to boil what looked like bits of tree and forest detritus in water twice every day. To say this stuff stank would be putting it mildly and it tasted as bitter as a winter's night in Halifax. I hated it to say the least, but I drank it as I was willing to try anything. As I drank this warm muddy-looking water, I would hold my nose and try not to be sick – it really was that bad. Here's my point: within one month, not only did I get used to the smell and taste – I actually began to like it. This is why changing your diet of food is going to be a breeze, once we remove the brainwashing, conditioning, and trickery of **BiG FOOD** that is. Nothing you switch to will taste and smell anything like tree bark so the adjustment won't take anything like a month and you certainly won't be holding your nose and trying not to be sick during it. In fact, most of the things many of you will already love. But it really doesn't matter if at this stage a main course salad and some vegetable juice sounds about as appealing as a fortnight's holiday in Afghanistan. Once all the brainwashing, conditioning, and misinformation regarding your diet of foods and drinks has been removed, and you have the correct mental tools on exactly how to change your diet easily, you will be amazed at what will happen and how easy and enjoyable it can be.

You Health Freak!

This doesn't mean for one second that once you change your diet all you will be able to eat is salad and fruit – so don't panic. Halfway through the book you could well start to think it's all about eating grass, which is why it's so important to finish the entire book. Trust me, at the end you will be about to eat **ANYTHiNG** you want, whenever you want to eat it. The key here is to remove the brainwashing and conditioning and expose **BiG FOOD** for what it is, so that your *genuine* choice will be not to have the rubbish nor give your hard earned money to **BiG FOOD** and **BiG DRiNK**.

I never dreamt that one day I would go out for a meal and actually want a main course of fish or avocado salad – that I would choose it over everything else. I never thought that I would be in a position where I would have vegetable juice daily, seriously, *vegetable juice* – you would never have thought it. I never imagined that I would go out of my way and actually pass by McDonald's or Pizza Hut to get to a juice bar or find something healthy. I certainly never thought that I would look at people eating crap with genuine pity as opposed to total envy, as I used to when *on a diet*. I just feel very lucky that I changed my diet when I did. I often seriously wonder where I would be now if I hadn't.

CHANGING YOUR EATING HABITS

Just as important as your diet is the *way* you eat. In order to get and stay 'Slim for Life' and to increase your chance of a longer life, it is vital to learn the process of eating just to the point of being almost full. It has been shown many times over that the lighter the burden put on the digestive system, the longer – on average – a person lives. This principle is key to lifelong slimness.

It takes about twenty to thirty minutes for the body to acknowledge it has all of its nutritional requirements, so if you eat until you are full you have overeaten. This is also why it is so important to chew your food thoroughly, as it gives the body a chance to acknowledge it is going to be fed. The enzymes in your mouth are more powerful than those in your stomach, and it is essential to use your 'natural blender' (your mouth) before swallowing to signal the right digestive juices in your stomach. It seems odd that people say they love their food so much, and that is why they find it hard to change, yet it's the very thing they miss out on every time. Think about it. Most people are on the next forkful as they gulp down the previous unchewed mouthful. They are completely missing their food already!

A study carried out by the University of Osaka, Japan, and published on the website of the *British Medical Journal*, illustrated that people who eat quickly and eat until they are full are three times as likely to be overweight than those who eat slowly and leave the table without feeling completely full. The study, led by Professor Hiroyasu Iso, suggests that the manner of eating too quickly – and until absolutely full – is a significant factor in the obesity epidemic, as it overrides signals in the brain which would normally tell the person to stop eating. Dr David Haslam, GP and clinical director for the National Obesity Forum, said, 'The great dietary gurus of a century ago stressed the importance of chewing food for a long time and eating slowly, and these messages are even more important today.'

CHANGING YOUR DIET GIVES YOU CERTAINTY

I know for certain that I will never be overweight again. I know for certain I will never go on a diet. I know that I will not have to worry about whether I am getting the correct nutrients. I have energy, I feel light, I wake up and actually feel awake, I feel mentally sharp, I have regained confidence I had no idea I'd even lost, and I now wear whatever clothes I want. In short, I am what some people would describe as a 'health freak' and it is just simply the best feeling in the world and I wouldn't trade it for any amount of money on earth.

The reason I have written this book is because I also know for certain that once you fully understand every aspect of the 'diet trap' and follow a few simple instructions, you too will change what you eat and you will love it. Everyone has it within their power to change their diet for good – because it's easy. Forget everything you have tried in the past and everything you have heard or read about food – let's start with a clean slate. No past to drag with us or dwell on, just a compelling future to look forward to.

I have designed this book so that at the end you will not only want to change your diet, but you will literally love the process. And that tends to be one of the main problems people have when they think about changing what they eat. They feel all doom and gloomy before they even start; as if they will be missing out and making a huge sacrifice by making the change. If you change your diet for life and totally change how you look at your old diet then you will never feel as though you are missing out for one simple reason – it will suddenly dawn on you that you aren't.

In order for you to see this clearly, and before we even attempt to make any changes, we need to debunk the clap-trap that you've been bombarded with for years about food and health. 'Stuff' that is now stored in your head and your conscious and subconscious doesn't even question it as fact, it just takes it as read that it is. The biggest problem is we believe a lot of what we have heard over the years about nutrition, diets, and health because it is put across by 'experts'. The question I want you to ask is: is it possible that some of the experts were taught incorrectly themselves? Is it possible that we just have too much information about food and nutrition? Is it possible that we have literally been blinded by science? Is it possible we have over complicated the issue so much that we can't see the wood for the trees?

I ask you to set aside what you believe to be 'fact' and read what I am about to write with an extremely open mind. It is time to simplify the whole business about what we should eat, what quantity we should eat, what time we should eat and what is best for us by unloading our minds of pieces of so-called vital health information, which, plain and simply ...

6

WE DON'T NEED TO KNOW!

What is your body fat ratio? What is your resting heart rate? Do you know? What is a bioflavonoid? What is riboflavin? Do you know? How many calories are there in a banana? How much protein do you need daily? How many vitamins are there? What is the best source of calcium? What does vitamin K do for you? Which has more vitamin C – an orange or a green pepper? What is a ketone? How does ketosis work? Do you know which foods contain vitamin P? What is your body mass index? What is your metabolic rate? If you do not know the answer to these questions – good! We don't need to know.

A little over one hundred years ago we didn't even know what a vitamin was, but we still got here didn't we? A gorilla doesn't know how many vitamins or minerals there are in a banana or whether it contains any calcium or protein: why don't they know? Because they don't need to know!

There are no nutritionists or dieticians in the wild, how do they cope? How do animals manage to keep so fit and excess fat free without knowing things like 'their resting heart rate' or without ever wearing a heart rate monitor to show what 'zone' they are in? With no dieticians on hand or fitness instructors, it almost makes you wonder how on earth they know what to eat to be healthy or how to stay trim and fit. Well I say it makes us wonder, but that's not true. We fully expect all wild animals on earth to *instinctively* know what to eat, when to eat and what to do to be fighting fit. We don't expect them to have to read books on the subject of food or to seek 'qualified' advice. We are under no illusion at all that their intuition, provided by whoever or whatever created us, is the best guide to health and healing foods.

So this begs the question, why do men and women, who are apparently the most intelligent beings on earth, not expect to know these simple things for ourselves? Why is there so much confusion over what we should eat and how to get fit? The answer is simple really; too much knowledge; too much advertising; too much peer pressure; too many conflicting books; too many people with letters before and after their name; and too much brainwashing and conditioning from people with vested interests as their number one focus.

There is no advertising, brainwashing or 'intellectual' knowledge in the wild. Animals eat foods that were specifically designed for them. They also eat when they are genuinely hungry and they stop when they are full. They are perfectly happy eating the diet laid down by nature for it fully furnishes their body with everything it needs and they love the taste and smell. Wild animals are also not concerned about how much they weigh on a daily basis, nor what size fur they are. Why? Because all of their own kind are the same size and shape. If a giraffe became extremely abnormally fat would we need to test its blood pressure, put it on a scale or take a sample of its poo (Gillian McKeith!) to see if something was wrong with it? Or do you think that *intuitively* we would just know?

When I look back it seems strange that despite being what I consider to be a reasonably intelligent person, I would do things like jump on a set of scales to see if I was packing a bit too much on the weight front. Did I not already know? The only reason I jumped on them in the first place was because I already knew I had, I just wanted to know by how much. Again, could I not see by how much? Did my bulges not tell me? Did the fact my shirt buttons were popping not tell me enough or the fact I couldn't squeeze into my jeans? All weighing scales do is confirm the obvious to us and to everyone else around us. As mental as this sounds I would even get on the scales slowly sometimes in a desperate, nonsensical attempt to weigh less. Did I honestly think that by getting on the scales slowly I would not be as fat as I was? What the flipping hell was wrong with me? After working with hundreds of thousands of people from all over the world over the years it was somewhat of a relief to see I wasn't the only one who did such incredibly bizarre, irrational things. I believe all the 'intellectual' knowledge we are bombarded with makes us do things that are flipping bonkers. When I see your average bloke running around the park or on a treadmill with a heart rate monitor around their chest and looking at their special watch to see if they are keeping in the 'fat burning zone' I do wonder if we have all taken leave of our senses.

Talking of which, here's a perfectly true story which illustrates what I mean. A friend of mine was on one of her many 'diets' some years back. On visiting her about a week or so into her 'new' diet, I noticed that there was a large chocolate cake, half eaten, on a plate next to her. To be honest I was quite glad because I know what a complete waste of mental torture time diets are. I asked her if she was still on her diet (assuming she wasn't) and to my surprise she said 'yes'. I said what about the half-eaten cake? What I heard next has gone down in history: 'It's okay', she explained 'because I weighed myself before I ate it and I weighed myself afterwards and guess what? – there was not an ounce of difference'. I wish I was joking, but that really is a true story.

I realize that most people haven't done something as bats as that in order to justify their intake of food, but there are hundreds, if not thousands, of perfectly intelligent people going places on a weekly basis and actually paying for someone to weigh them – paying for someone to tell them what is already painfully obvious to them and everyone else. Although it may not seem like it at first glance, weighing yourself all the time is certainly on a par with the half a cake thing.

I went to Weight Watchers many years ago for a couple of meetings. The 'leader' was actually very good. But seriously, what the hell were we all doing there? We were standing in line waiting to be weighed. At the time I attended if someone had lost weight from the week before, they would ring a bell and the group would do what I call a 'Ricky Lake'; they would literally clap and yell. Now I am all for encouraging and giving praise, but what about those who hadn't lost any weight. You feel bad enough as it is going in to one of those places – the last thing you need is to be made an object of pity. I am aware that Weight Watchers no longer do the bell thing, but they do still weigh you, along with nearly every other diet group.

Scales chain you to a diet mentality and they can be deceptive. Sometimes people look slimmer and feel healthier, but when they jump on the scales they see little or no change and so start to feel depressed. But we should sod the scales, it's how you look and feel that is the real measure of success. What many people fail to take into account, and the reason I am so against the antiquated BMI scale, is that:

Fat takes up five times more room on the body than muscle but muscle is a lot heavier than fat

If you drop fat but *increase* your muscle, your scales could well stay the same, but your shape is so much thinner. Weight is not the issue, it's all about the physical *shape* you are in. To free yourself of diet mentality you will also need to free yourself from the scales. Go for the 'look and feel' measure of success, it's a lot more accurate. Throwing away your scales can be one of the most liberating processes in gaining freedom from the diet trap.

We not only use scales to weigh ourselves, but also to weigh the food we eat in order to try to control our calories – and again we have been doing this for so long we don't question the sanity of it. But seriously, what are we doing? You don't ever see a gorilla weigh bananas before it eats them to check it's not overeating and you certainly never see a squirrel weighing its nuts (OK perhaps a bad analogy).

'A CALORIE IS A CALORIE' IS A LOAD OF OLD TOSH

The problem is that we have seen people doing these things for years so we just tend to follow suit without questioning what we are doing. Calories are a great example. Calories are one of if not the most meaningless gauges for health we have ever obsessed over. Unfortunately, the 'how many calories does that contain' mantra is so ingrained in us, that many people find it difficult to nigh on impossible to let it go. What is a calorie anyway? Do you know? Does anyone who hasn't studied this subject in depth know? It's actually the amount of energy (heat) needed to raise one gram of water by one degree centigrade. In other words – we really don't need to know. Again there is not one wild animal alive that knows how many calories are in the food they are eating for the same simple reason – they do not need to know. They don't know the recommended daily calorie intake for a female or male version of their species either, they just seem to know what to do – how very odd. I wouldn't mind if the amount of calories we consume is a guaranteed way of controlling obesity, but it isn't. Between 1976 and 2000, Americans lowered their fat consumption by 11 per cent and also lowered their calorie intake by 4 per cent. Yet what has happened to the weight of that particular nation? Obesity has risen by 31 per cent in the same period, proving two major misconceptions:

A) The fat you eat doesn't add up to fat on you, and
B) The more calories one eats doesn't always mean more fat on you

I do realize that because we have been in the 'calories are king' mentality for so long there will no doubt be many people (particularly those in the nutritional field) who will be barking at the book at this moment. I did say an open mind was required for this book and that I would be challenging some strong beliefs. The point, however, is not so much to disprove the calorie theory, but to illustrate the nonsense of it all: intelligent humans staring at packets of snacks at lunch time declaring to whoever will listen its calorie content. In truth, knowing about calories, even if it were true, hasn't got us anywhere. Other than obsession and obesity.

If you are thinking that we are better off knowing about all aspects of nutrition and calories, ask yourself why? We apparently know more about 'nutrition' now than ever in history, yet heart disease is still the number one killer disease in Western society and we suffer from more self inflicted diseases than any wild animal on earth.

We not only worry about this nutrition 'stuff' but industries have been built on our fears. We spend millions of pounds on vitamin and mineral tablets every year in the UK alone. And why are we popping pills and rattling down the street? Simply to try and counter the effects of the processed and de-natured food we are consuming. But what about the pills themselves, haven't they also been processed in some way? Aren't they also de-natured? I had a journalist from a famous magazine recently ask me as I was making a wonderful smoothie, 'Is this a good replacement for vitamin pills?' I thought she was joking, but no. It appears we are so far removed from nature that some people now think fresh fruit and veg are the 'alternative' to vitamin pills. I did point out that vitamin pills are indeed meant as an alternative to real nutrition, but it went completely over her head. I am not against all supplements or indeed all vitamin and mineral pills – with over farming unfortunately in twenty-first century Britain it's often the only way to make up for the shortfall of vital minerals in our food. What I find crazy is the fact we have bastardised our food so much that we now have vitamin pills – when you think about it is kind of crazy. The danger here more than anything is that people believe as long as they get some vitamin pills down them they are free to eat crap. This is the real potential danger of such pills.

Blinded by Science

Did you know there are 40,000 phytochemicals in one tomato? What is a phytochemical? It's a name for a vitamin that they haven't formally named yet. Are there really 40,000 vitamins in one tomato?

I don't actually know and I don't care because as long as I get it into my body, I don't need to know. Who counted them anyway? Your body doesn't care whether you call them vitamins, minerals, bioflavonoids, or zookinoids – it simply wants them and desperately needs them.

Fruits and vegetables, as a whole, contain *every single vitamin and mineral* that we have found a name for and God knows how many more we haven't. They apparently keep finding new and amazing disease-fighting agents in all fruit and veg. Recently they've discovered some real beauties. Ever heard of beta-carotene? Well now they've found alpha-carotene. They have also discovered phenols, indoles, aromatic isothiocyanates, terpenes, and organo-sulphur: all of which are part of the new category of 'anutrients'. **NEW?** These scientists can shove together whatever letters they like but what they have found is far from new. They seem to want to get the credit for something nature produces. Fruits, vegetables, nuts, and seeds have been the same since the dawn of time and everything we need to furnish our bodies is to be found within them. When they do discover a 'new' phytochemical in a partic-ular fruit or vegetable they tend to try to isolate it, extract it, recreate it, process it, and put it in a pill. That is the equivalent of taking just one spark plug and the oil from a car in the belief you have found the most important components of the vehicle because it can't run without them.

BLAH! BLAH! BLAH!

Most of the time they also try and blind us with science by using what I call blah, blah, blah language. I am talking about people who will use the longest, most obscure words available to describe something which is actually very simple. However, they have studied it for many years, have spent flipping great wedges of cash on their education and are going to let you know they have by completely losing you in whatever text they write. I call it blah, blah, blah language.

It is about time we all took our brainwashed heads out of the sand. We just do not need to know what our ideal weight is (according to some man-made scale). We should not be weighing our food to see how much we should eat. Nor do we need to concern ourselves with vitamins, minerals, bioflavonoids, our body fat ratio, our resting heart rate, nor how many calories are in the bag of crisps. It is time to simplify the whole business of eating and health, remove the fear of changing your diet, and find physical and mental freedom for life. We will not achieve this by worrying about vitamin K, B6, C, D, K, Z, protein, calcium, or what foods are low fat. We will achieve our goal for life by *not* concerning ourselves with all this nonsense, but rather by removing the many years of brainwashing, conditioning, and manipulation by **BiG FOOD** and tapping into our genuine freedom of choice.

You already know why you shouldn't be eating the foods you are and why you should eat the foods you are not. However, that doesn't matter because everybody with a food problem knows this too, yet this knowledge does not help them. It certainly didn't help me. All it did was add pressure and make me feel stupid and weak-willed. And what would I do if I was under pressure, feeling down or a little stressed? Yep – **EAT!**

The problem is that although we know all the benefits of making the change, we also believe that we have to go through pain to get there and stay there. As I will repeat throughout this book, you will not have to endure any pain at all because it's easy to lose weight, gain health, have the body of your dreams and all the energy to enjoy it. You simply need to get into the right *frame of mind*, then you can easily get into the right *frame of body*. You will only have to suffer a lifetime of pain if you *don't* make the change – not if you do.

So now you know what you don't need to know, but in order to remove all the brainwashing and release you from certain 'junkie foods', there is a lot you really do need to know. The first and most important thing is the nature of the diet and food trap. What really compels us to eat things that we then regret almost instantaneously? What makes us eat foods that we know for certain are causing excess fat, ill health, depression, stress, and premature death? In other words …

7

WHY DO PEOPLE EAT JUNK FOOD?

The answer is very simple. It is a combination of just two reasons:

1) **The advertising, brainwashing, conditioning, and mind manipulation we have been subjected to since birth (the mental side).**
2) **An empty insecure physical feeling due to malnutrition, withdrawal, low blood sugar, or a combination of the three — caused by the 'food' and/or drinks themselves (the physical side).**

These two factors add up to addiction.

The good news is that virtually any kind of addiction, contrary to extremely popular belief, is easy to kick. However, it is only easy to kick once you have a full understanding how that particular addiction works and the nature of that particular trap.

The main problem is the first of the two factors: the many, many years of conditioning, brainwashing, mind manipulation, and total misinformation that we have been subjected to by the advertisers and so-called experts on the subject of health. This is really the cause of the problem and this is what needs to be *fully* removed in order to gain freedom. The lethargy, excess fat, health problems etc. are simply *symptoms* of the cause.

Fat Profits

It is time to wake up and realize that the livelihoods of many people depend on keeping us none the wiser when it comes to just how harmful and addictive certain foods and drinks can be. It is often their job to keep you hooked – without your knowledge of course – on what I will continue to refer to as drug foods or junkie foods. They are constantly trying to change the way you think in order to give you the very false impression that *you* are choosing to eat and drink their druggy-like foods. As I mentioned earlier, and as I will repeat, you cannot have freedom of choice without the freedom to also refuse. When do we know it's our genuine choice?

The tobacco companies played the same game for years. They kept very quite about the fact that their product is addictive, controls lives and kills people – and all the while it was advertised on television and radio (and of course the government got its share of the profits). Many doctors even suggested smoking to their patients as a good way to relieve stress from their lives. Doctors at the time were actually suggesting a known stimulant will relax a person. It is now known that many tobacco companies were deliberately adding chemicals to tobacco in order to make then even more addictive. My question is a simple one: is it possible the same thing is happening in some areas of the food and beverage industry? Is it possible that there could be some unscrupulous characters in the industry who would, like the tobacco companies, deliberately add chemicals to their food simply in order to make them less satiating and thus sell more to an unsuspecting public?

We have a situation where it is fairly widely accepted that the vast majority of 'food' sold in a McDonald's isn't exactly the healthiest on the planet. Yet some years back, planning permission was given to have a McDonald's in the grounds of the Tower of London. **BiG FOOD** often have good contacts and, like the tobacco companies of old, they seem to be able to get their food sold in the most unlikely of places. Having a McDonald's in a sacred place such as the Tower Of London is bad enough, but did you know there's even a McDonald's in Guy's hospital in London? Yes, a McDonald's in a blooming hospital!

You may think it's unfair to put junk food in the same category as cigarettes. After all cigarettes kill people, often control their lives, cost them a fortune and are highly addictive. But where exactly is the difference? As a nation the UK spends £7 million a day on fast food. Second only of course to the good ol' U.S of A. This money is spent on 'foods' that are known to be addictive and are known to cause all kinds of diseases, including cancer and heart disease – the two biggest killers in Western society. Just table salt alone is known to kill over 40,000 people a year in the UK, that's more than 100 people a day. This is virtually the same number as alcohol. White refined carbohydrates and refined sugar are known to be a major cause of diabetes and a whole host of other diseases (which I will explain later). Aspartame (the artificial sweetener found in diet drinks etc.) has been linked to ninety-two different adverse symptoms and all kinds of health problems. This stuff is known to tighten blood vessels, cause additional thirst and has even been linked to brain tumours. Yet not only is it being sold as a 'food' stuff, but is promoted as a product that will help people who have a weight problem. (I will cover aspartame and products like it in depth later so you'll never want to touch them again.)

The point is this, in my estimation the wrong kinds of food overall actually kill more people than all other drugs combined. And yes that includes heroin, crack, cocaine and even cigarettes. Yet there is not one single drug food product that has a warning on it.

We banned direct cigarette advertising, yet **BiG FOOD** spend literally billions advertising products that have been linked to major diseases and hardly any restrictions are put on them. These are 'foods' that can and do cause premature death, just like cigarettes; control people's lives, just like cigarettes; and products which, I estimate, slowly kill two-thirds of those who are hooked on them (which is *more* than cigarettes).

You cannot open a magazine, switch on your TV, or go to the cinema without being bombarded with images of drug-type foods. The government of course is not about to do anything about it as they earn billions in tax revenue from people's addictions to these heart-disease causing, stroke-inducing so-called foods. Their argument is always the same and runs along the lines of 'people are not stupid, they know the facts, we advise them to eat five portions of fruit and veg a day. If they choose to eat junk, then it's up to them'. Yet they make it law to wear a seat belt. Why isn't it our choice then? Because people are not addicted to putting on or leaving off their seat belts, but they are addicted to trashy foods. To say to someone like Barry Austin, (reportedly the fattest man in Britain) who I believe, at the age of 29, was 50 stone (317 kg) in weight and had a 82 in. (208 cm) waist, that it's his genuine choice to be like that is ludicrous. Given the genuine choice I imagine he would love to end his addiction to crap foods and he would love to be slim.

You Black Tar Nicotine Loaded Bastard

One of the major problems with 'food' addiction is that the problem is visible because the most common symptom for many (although not all) is excess fat on the body. Think about it: no matter how many cigarettes someone smokes, they're never called a black tar, nicotine-filled git or a cigarette-smoking bastard are they? Yet along with food addiction go the names and scathing attack on our characters: we get called gits and pigs – we're never just fat are we? This is why so many people don't reach obesity – because of how they will look. But they still have a food problem and are still constantly battling to control what they eat.

I used to feel very proud of myself if I managed to be good for a few days, or if I managed to control my intake of chocolate to the point where I only had it at weekends. I often used to cut down on the coffee and biscuits – put myself on the 'food wagon' if you will. There are people who do manage to exercise extreme control over their intake of trash food, but this is an awful way to go through life. If you have to exercise control over something, it must mean that that something is controlling you. It is the need to exercise control that means you are not in control as I alluded to previously. Confused? Let me put it this way. I do not have to exercise control over my banana intake, if I needed to discipline myself with my bananas then I would have a banana problem. For years smokers thought it was their genuine choice to smoke (in fact some people still retain this belief). However, when the ban came in and smokers were forced to stand outside their workplace in the freezing cold in order to get their fix, they started to realize they were not choosing to smoke, but *had* to (I know first-hand as I used to smoke 40–60 a day).

I do not know one single person who has to exercise control over their apple intake. Why? Because it is not a drug food. No chemicals have been added deliberately in order to compel you to overeat them. There is a natural cut off point. I also don't know anyone who would have the slightest problem getting rid of apples from their diet if a doctor told them they caused heart disease, lethargy, weight gain, and premature death. Yet there are hundreds of thousands of people who, if you told them the same thing about coffee, chocolate, alcohol, crisps, or fast-food burgers for example, would say, 'Up yours, life's too short' and continue eating them. Why? Because they are drug-like foods that compel people to want more and more, even if it goes against their rational judgement. Whether you actually have more and more is neither here nor there, it's the *wanting* more that causes the real problem – the need to exercise control.

TOTALLY WIRED

Some unfortunate people have lost the ability to exercise control over what they eat or drink. It was reported that Barry Austin was told he would die unless he slimmed, and he went through the drastic measure of having his stomach stapled. I also understand that when he was 19 he had his jaws wired together which lasted for four months and he lost 4 stone (25 kg) in that time because all he could consume was soup. I imagine his life was hell, especially at Christmas when he saw all the beautiful food laid out in front of him and knew he couldn't take part.

Can you imagine the torture he must have been going through? Apparently, his family liquidized his roast dinner and pudding for him to drink but on seeing the mush he was supposed to drink, his desperation was such that he ripped the wires out with wire cutters, leaving his mouth bleeding in agony. Do you think he goes through all this for a hamburger because he simply likes the taste? Is it possible that there is more to it? Is it possible he is simply mentally and physically addicted to drug foods in the same way a nicotine addict is addicted to cigarettes? It is not just possible but once we start to really look at it, it becomes obvious. It is not his genuine choice to do this – given the choice he would just eat healthily. Given the genuine freedom of choice we would be free to eat what he wants to eat. He doesn't want to eat that rubbish, he is just compelled to – for reasons unknown to him

The reason I have used Barry as an example is to illustrate the point that often it is not our genuine choice to eat certain 'foods'. We have simply been conditioned and brainwashed by **BiG FOOD** and **BiG DRiNK** on both a mental and physical level to the point where we get upset and even angry if we feel we can no longer eat certain things, even if those foods are making us ill. Unless you start to realize what is going on, you are in danger of remaining in the food and diet trap for life. The point of this book is to set you mentally free, so that you can eat whatever you want to and not what someone has conditioned you to in order to boost their bank balance. This can only happen if you fully understand how **BiG FOOD**, the very people who are peddling drug and junk foods, go about their business.

AD – FABRICATED

How do you sell a product that is of very dubious quality, is unhealthy and is contributing to (and in many cases causing) major health problems? Good old advertising of course. We have been programmed and conditioned to consume drug-like foods and drinks. That is why people think it's normal to eat these foods. But then didn't people think it was normal and sociable to inhale cigarette smoke a few years ago too?

Let us not underestimate the power of all the advertising and conditioning either: it works. Our brains are very clever computers, but they can also be programmed just like any other computer. Unless we learn to run it effectively ourselves, there are many, many people who are paid tremendous amounts of money to run it for us – and they do. That is why we have such a strong belief that fruit and veg are for boring people who don't want to 'live'. After all with Pepsi Max you can go snowboarding, skiing, bungee jumping, and 'Live life to the max – Pepsi Max'. Then of course we all know that 'A Mars A Day helps you work, rest, and play' and that 'Breakfast at McDonald's makes your day'. I can't ever remember hearing 'Live life to the max with a fresh mouth-watering Mango Max' or 'An apple a day helps you work, rest, play and helps prevent cancer' or 'Breakfast at a juice bar, stimulates the mind, feeds the cells, helps to lift the waste from your body and really does make your day that little more alive and vibrant'. Incidentally, if breakfast at McDonald's does make your day – **YOU REALLY DO NEED THIS BOOK!**

MIND CONDITIONING

The Russian physiologist, Ivan Pavlov's famous experiment illustrated just how easily we can be conditioned. It has been well documented, but for those of you who are not aware of the experiment from the 1890s I will explain it very briefly. He starved his pet dog for three days, then, when he gave it some food, he rang a bell at the same time. After that, every time his dog felt genuine hunger, Ivan would put some food down and at exactly the same time he would ring a bell. He didn't simply do this once or twice, but over and over again until it became a conditioned response: food/bell, food/bell, food/bell. In the end (and this is why I am using this analogy) even if the dog had already eaten and could have in no way felt genuine physical hunger, when the bell was rung the dog would look for food and literally begin to salivate.

Advertisers for drug and junk food know the power of this and they use it to sell you food when you are not even hungry. Have you ever been driving along, not even thinking about food, when all of a sudden you see the two golden arches of the McDonald's sign and felt hungry? Or do you remember when you were a kid playing in the street, not thinking of food at all, when all of a sudden you heard the sound of the ice cream man and decided you felt hungry? **WELL THAT'S THE BELL**. Going to the cinema means popcorn and a drink: **THAT'S THE BELL**. Easter – a chocolate egg: **THAT'S THE BELL**. Christmas – turkey or pudding: **THAT'S THE BELL**. It's 11.30 a.m. – time for a Diet Coke break : **THAT'S THE BELL**. Going to get petrol? – time for a pastie, or a bar of chocolate and soft drink: **THAT'S THE BELL**. Elevenses – time for a cup of tea (and a biscuit of course): **THAT'S THE BELL**. Watching football – must get the beers in: **THAT'S THE BELL**.

The fact is we react to a thousand different bells without even realizing it. The way they link in a bell is to advertise it over and over again. Sometimes they even include a specific time to take their product (as in the cases of Diet Coke break at 11.30 a.m. or After Eight mints). This is why they pay people like David Beckham and Britney Spears millions for a 30-second commercial to advertise products like Pepsi-cola. They link their 'feel good' music to a product that has nothing to do with feeling good.

Do you remember this?

'When your carpet smells fresh your room does too so every time you vacuum remember what to do. Do the shake and vac and put the freshness back, do the shake and vac and put the freshness back …'.

I would be surprised if you don't, because it was the most successful advertising campaign of all time for a household cleaner. The point I am making, and sorry if this freaks you out, but the last time that ad was on TV as an actual advertisement was well over twenty years ago. Twenty years ago and yet you probably remember it like it was yesterday – why? Because they beamed the song again and again and again until in the end you couldn't help but sing it and buy the product. This is why I make no apologies for repeating certain points throughout this book. I know it can jar and yes I know it can drive people nuts. However, it is the only way to remove the bells and create new empowering ones. It is the only way to *de*-brainwash you. So if you think, 'He's said that already' – I know, it was genuinely intentional and is based on the same principles **BiG FOOD** use to hook you. I am simply using the same technique to un-hook you.

The products we are dealing with here are not household cleaners, but ones that can literally destroy people's quality of life and reduce their life expectancy. They are products which – if consumed in large enough quantities – have been proven to undermine confidence, depress, and disable people. They can also enslave them. Oh, and of course, let's not forget that in the long run they can also potentially kill you.

We are constantly being bombarded with so many 'trendy' images for junk food. The junkie food outlets have all become fashion statements. We have McDonald's, Burger King, Pizza Hut, KFC, Ben and Jerry's, Häagen-Dazs and Starbucks, to name just a few. It has literally become a 'designer label' business. Is it any wonder that so many people are under the misapprehension that junk is where the pleasure is? That crap foods are a treat and fruit and veg are boring? Things have got so bad that we now believe that it is 'normal' to eat this rubbish and 'abnormal' to eat healthily. After all, if you do eat healthily on a consistent basis you are referred to as a freak, a health freak to be exact.

These images and beliefs have been drip-fed into our computer brains since we were born. Of all the bells, these are the most detrimental. Many television programmes and virtually all Hollywood films are also playing their part. Product placement is huge in the film and television industry, especially for drug-like foods and drinks. The coffee chain Starbucks, for instance, are now a major placement in many of the Hollywood Blockbusters. The movie *You Got Mail* should have been called You Got Starbucks. Hollywood has an entire department devoted to product placement, and specific agents to get your product in the latest blockbuster. And if they can get the actor to drink or eat the product it's a hit. It's one thing getting Superman thrown into a huge Coke sign, but if they can get him to drink it – **BiNGO!** In the film *Austin Powers*, the lead actor mentioned Heineken and sales of the beer went up by 15 per cent – hardly a coincidence. The last few movies in the James Bond franchise have plugged a variety of products, too.

BiG FOOD product placement and advertising's main objective is to sell the idea that you can feed emotion and make yourself happy with their particular food or drink. If someone's boyfriend leaves them on a TV show, the first thing to come out is the ice cream. If a child is depressed we can cheer them up with a chocolate bar or 'treat' them to a McDonald's. The problem is that we end up believing it. Not only that, but we all play our part in keeping the chain going: 'Tidy your room and you can have an ice cream', 'If you are good, you can have a chocolate bar', or perhaps worst of all 'If you eat your vegetables, you can have a treat'.

We have all been conditioned to believe that effectively poisoning ourselves with crap food, often devoid of nutrition, is a reward, a treat, a comforter and a genuine pleasure from a very early age. Sadly it's those who care for us most who are often the biggest culprits. To compound the message we have sounds and images beamed into our computer brains confirming what we have been taught. Every holiday seems to have a strong bell that revolves around food: Easter means chocolate eggs, birthdays mean cakes, Christmas equals pudding and so on.

The main reason why most people in Western society are caught in the food and diet trap is because it is an exceptionally easy one for people to fall into. Years ago it was very easy for people to fall into the smoking trap. This was largely down to everyone believing it was not only okay to smoke at the time, but that it was very sociable and had no harmful effects (well the masses believed that – the people in the know always knew). Everyone now knows that smoking causes cancer, and it is widely seen as anti-social. The tobacco companies therefore have to work harder and harder to get people hooked on their product. This is why with such a declining market in the West, the tobacco companies are expanding into developing countries – as if they don't have enough problems as it is.

However, unlike 'real' drugs, drug-like foods are seen as genuine food, and most of us have been on this junkie stuff from a very early age. In fact, if you were not breast fed there is a good chance you have been on junkie and drug foods ever since you were born. Even if you weren't on rubbish from the second you left the womb, it wouldn't have been long before you had your first fix.

Think about it – at what age would you give a child a cigarette? Never I guess, but 16 at the earliest. What about an alcoholic drink? Well it varies, but usually we wouldn't dream of anything less than double figures. What about junkie or drug food? Now we begin to see the problem. It seems perfectly normal to feed children junkie drug foods from a very early age. Not only is it seen as normal, but this drug-like food is seen as a treat; as a reward – so much so that you are seen as a baddie if you refuse to give them some. At the same time we are bombarded with billions of pounds' worth of advertising that is cleverly designed to keep people hooked on (or to change their brand of) drug-like food.

The biggest problem, and this is where you really need to open your mind, is that the so-called food itself seems to confirm everything we believe. Our minds are often easily deluded because of a physical chemical reaction in our body – a reaction which seems to confirm the advertiser's message and what we believe to be true. It is this element above all which we need to understand in order to break truly free. There have been some very clever and successful mind manipulation techniques used over the years with many aspects of people's lives, but none have affected more people or had more impact on our lives than …

8

THE FOOD TRICK

There's an old saying, 'you can fool some of the people some of the time but not all of the people all of the time'. But **BiG FOOD** and **BiG DRiNK** have almost managed to pull it off.

As you are no doubt aware, all businesses are out to increase their profits. How does any business sell more of the same product to the same person? Simple: by making them believe that they need it, that it will benefit them, and that their life would be incomplete in some way without it. The drug food industry is no different to any other. Their objective is simply to sell more food.

However, logically this shouldn't be as easy to do as it would be with something like clothes for example. You can, after all, keep buying clothes and very rarely, depending on the size of your house, will you run out of room for them. Even if you do run out of space, you can simply throw the old ones away and make room for the new ones. The fashion industry survives by making you believe the clothes you already own are no longer in vogue and you must buy more in order to fit into our fashion conscious world.

But how can they do this with food? Unlike clothes and storage your body does get full. You are after all either hungry or you're not. If you eat a certain amount your body gets what it needs and you no longer feel hungry. Well that's the theory anyway and that is exactly what happens when you consume genuine highly nutritious natural food, as I now know. However, what if **BiG FOOD** and **BiG DRiNK** found a way to remove many elements of genuine nutrition from what they sell and add chemicals which actually make you to feel hungrier than you would normally feel? What if they found a neat way to create 'false hungers' and thus a way to sell more of the same food to the same person? What if they found a way to make a person believe the only thing which can fill the hunger they feel is more of the same type of food? Now that would be a neat trick.

The food trick is very similar to the nicotine trick. The tobacco companies would have made very little money if a smoker had just one cigarette a day. How do they make them have more? Well they don't really have to do a great deal; the drug will do most of it for them.

ADDICTED TO AN ILLUSION

When nicotine leaves the body it creates an empty, insecure feeling, rather like a hunger for food. The feeling is so slight the smoker does not realize that the previous cigarette they had caused the feeling. They have another one and the empty, insecure feeling goes away. They no longer feel as low, as empty or as insecure as they did, and so end up believing there is a genuine pleasure in smoking. Yet all they are actually enjoying is the ending of an aggravation which was caused by the previous cigarette. All the tobacco industry then had to do was some product placement and advertising. Words such as 'smooth' and 'satisfaction' were used to describe cigarette smoking on advertisements. Every film and television hero was a smoker etc. As most people are aware, the body will always build up an immunity and tolerance to any drug and you therefore end up needing more and more to get the same effect. In the end a feeling of dissatisfaction is felt even when the addict is taking the drug. The nicotine companies found a way to create an *additional* hunger to a normal hunger. All addiction creates a hold which the addict believes is filled by the very substance which caused the hole in the first place. Junkie foods – foods which have had a great deal of their nutritional content removed and other chemicals added in their place – create a hole. Apples will not fill this hole initially; in the same way that an apple will not fill the hole nicotine has created for a smoker. This fools us into believing that fruits and vegetables and good wholesome foods don't satisfy and that junkie foods do. But this is the trick – this is the illusion. All that's happened is you have had an injection of your 'food fix' and some of the empty hole appears to have been filled. But the huge hole is only there because of the junkie foods in the first place. When we change our diet in the correct way, the hole disappears in no time at all and we feel genuinely satisfied.

Drug-like junkie foods and drinks are the real cause of the food and diet trap. They are designed to create *additional* hungers and feelings of *dissatisfaction* – the complete opposite of natural foods. The sad reality is that most people are suffering from malnutrition. In fact whenever you see someone who is overweight you can be almost certain they are suffering from this condition. When we think of malnutrition, we tend to see images of starving people in the developing world, so it's hard to imagine that someone who eats loads of food and has so much abundance of food around them is also suffering from it. But the fact is they are and it is vital you fully understand this.

WHAT IS MALNUTRITION?

The *Oxford English Dictionary* describes it as, **'A dietary condition resulting from the absence of some foods or the absence of essential elements necessary for health; insufficient nutrition'.** This is exactly what I was suffering from when I was over 30 lb (13 kg) overweight, and it is what every junkie food addict is suffering from whether they are overweight or not. They have a severe deficit of nutrients going into the body. Without nutrients feeding the cells, the body will of course be starving. It is no wonder many junkie food addicts feel hungry and dissatisfied a lot of the time: it's because they are. If the body doesn't get what it needs it stays hungry for nutrients. Hunger is not a pleasant feeling, it's an empty, insecure, dissatisfied feeling. What do you do when you feel hungry, empty and dissatisfied? **EAT!**

It is this simple: The less food you eat containing live nutrients, the hungrier you will become. The hungrier you become the more dissatisfied and incomplete you will feel. The more dissatisfied and incomplete you feel the more you eat to try and feel satisfied and complete.

This, in itself, of course is bad enough. However, an even greater problem we have are the *additional* hungers we experience on top of a genuine hunger for the right nutrients. These are caused by the additional chemicals often added to junkie-type foods designed to cause an even bigger hole. They are designed to cause an empty, insecure feeling, an identical feeling to a normal genuine hunger. Such feelings are the result of the withdrawal effects from certain junkie foods, or the effects of low blood sugar – which, again, are caused by the drug foods themselves.

These junkie foods really are a double whammy. Not only are they void of some genuine nutrients, they ultimately create a set of false hungers which feel exactly the same as a normal genuine hunger. And because they are sold as food, and not drugs, people remain none the wiser to the fact they are hooked. Instead, people who are caught in the food trap because of drug foods are called 'pigs', and are often ostracized and given no sympathy whatsoever. The people who are caught also believe it must be some flaw in their own character rather than a result of a very clever confidence trick – the food trick.

> ### it is the *false* physical hungers, along with the false advertising, that cause people to have mental and physical cravings for drug foods.

This is ultimately why people attempt to 'use' drug foods in much the same way drug addicts attempt to 'use' drugs: i.e. reaching for them in times of boredom, loneliness, or for comfort etc. What frustrates me most is that the people who make and distribute drug foods even have the front to advertise the fact that their product will not end a genuine hunger. They have the audacity to let us know that their 'food' will only seemingly satisfy a *false* mental and physical hunger. Our problem is that we don't question it because we believe it's our genuine choice and that we derive some genuine pleasure from it. A great example of this was an advert for a chocolate bar which claimed you could, 'Eat it in-between meals without ruining your appetite'. So what's the point of eating it then? I thought the whole point of eating was to satisfy your appetite, to end your hunger. With this advert they are blatantly telling us that their 'food' will not satisfy a genuine hunger. In other words it won't genuinely feed you. Another old ad that did this was the finger of fudge one. If you cannot recall, allow me: 'It's full of Cadbury good-ness and very small to eat, a finger of fudge is just enough until it's time to eat.' First of all what the hell do they mean by 'full of goodness'? Isn't it full of sugar? The second part says, 'it's just enough until it's time to eat.' In other words it's just enough to take the edge off the *false* hunger, but it won't ruin your *genuine* appetite.

The reason we are so easily fooled is not because we are stupid, but because such products *do* feed the false hungers; in the same way nico-tine feeds a smoker's hunger for nicotine and heroin feeds a heroin addict's hunger for heroin. When you end any kind of hunger you feel a sense of relief. A feeling of relief from any type of aggravation is pleas-urable and this is where the confidence trick really kicks in. The makers and advertisers of these so-called foods try to give the impression that there is a genuine pleasure in eating, even if you are not genuinely hungry. But it is a *false* sense of pleasure created by a *false* hunger and it's just a trick. On top of that you've got every diet and 'health' book giving the advice over and over again that you should simply, 'eat when you feel hungry'. But the point I am making is that the drug food eater has *additional* hungers and *is* hungry, but it is a false hunger created by the rubbish itself – they are effectively in a loop.

Until the junkie food addict realizes exactly what's going on, state-ments like 'eat only when you feel hungry' are ludicrous at best. Some-one like US born and bred Terriny Woods – who, at the age of just 15, weighed in at 41 stone 12 lb (over 260 kg) – was no doubt following the advice to eat only when hungry, but she was such a drug food addict and had built up an immunity to drug foods to such a degree that she probably felt the false hungers even when she was stuffing herself with drug foods in her desperation to relieve her false hungers. At this stage she would be in a *constant* state of withdrawal, would be hypoglycaemic and have a constant level of insulin in her blood (which, as I will explain in simple terms later, can cause a permanent state of dissatisfaction). And this condition was seemingly only lessened to some degree by more drug foods. She had created a monster of a hole and was simply desperately trying to fill it with the very things causing the hole in the first place. The more she tried the bigger the hole became … and the bigger it became the more desperate she became to fill this empty insecure feeling. The bigger the feeling, the larger the sense of relief when drug food hits the bloodstream and the bigger the sense of pleasure.

The more aggravations BiG FOOD creates, the MORE PLEASURE we appear to get from them, the BiGGER the Sacrifices we believe we are making when we stop and the HARDER we find the change.

This is why we feel such a sense of loss and missing out when we try to cut down or cut them from our diet completely. It's a trick – and requires a very open mind to see through it.

Eric Schlosser in his wonderful book *Fast Food Nation* wrote a small passage on gambling, which I feel works just as well for any form of addiction and works brilliantly to illustrate the food trick: 'It is the ultimate consumer technology, designed to manufacture not a tangible product, but something much more elusive: a brief sense of hope. That is what Las Vegas really sells, the most brilliant illusion of them all, a loss that feels like you're winning.'

That is also what **BiG FOOD** and **BiG DRiNK** is selling – the most brilliant illusion of them all, a loss that feels like you're winning. When you give yourself a 'lift' from drug-like foods it *feels* like you have just won, when in reality you have in fact lost – in many areas of your life.

'Nothing seems to satisfy like a Snickers'

This was another advertising slogan blatantly informing the drug food addict that nothing will satisfy their need like a drug food. Why? Because their need is a *false* one created by junkie foods in the first place. Let me explain in case this is starting to get confusing as this is probably one of the most important aspects of the book to grasp.

All the food in the world will never satisfy a smoker's physical and psychological need for nicotine. All the food in the world will never satisfy a heroin addict's physical and psychological need for heroin. Why? Because they are completely *separate* hungers created by the drug itself. Non-smokers and non-heroin addicts just do not have these hungers. This point is obvious when we are talking about what people clearly regard as drugs, but it is exactly the same with drug foods. And this is why it is essential to really open your mind and change the way you view these 'foods' – it is a vital part of freeing yourself of the diet trap for life.

All the natural food in the world will never satisfy a physical and/or psychological need for drug food. Why? Because it is a false physical and mental hunger that has fooled us all for generations. That is why you can seemingly satisfy your false need for junk without ruining your genuine appetite. It explains why even when I did eat fruit or salad it just didn't seem to satisfy me the same way as junk and drug food. And it also explains why I would sometimes feel stuffed but, at the same time, dissatisfied and still hungry. After all your stomach can only hold so much.

The excellent news is that the false hungers are very easy to get rid of and towards the end of the book I will discuss how to starve them to death, enjoy the process and set yourself free. First you need a full understanding of drug foods and false hungers. There are several products that create false hungers and I will cover each in turn. However, the biggest culprit of false hunger, the biggest drug food of them all and what really compels people to overeat and to eat as a response to emotion is a substance which, when it hits your bloodstream, has your body screaming ...

9

OH SUGAR!

Sugar not only needs a chapter to itself, but an entire book could be written on this subject. We do not have time for that and luckily you really do not need to know the entire history of the sugar industry to rid most it from your life. All that's required is full knowledge of exactly what happens when refined sugar enters your bloodstream and how it attaches itself emotionally to our minds, creating 'addiction'.

There is a danger this small chapter could get a little 'blah, blah, blahish', but as refined sugar is one of the biggest causes of food addiction and probably the largest contributor to many of the world's biggest killer diseases, it's worth paying full attention.

When natural food is eaten, it is first broken down in the mouth then passed into the stomach. Once there, it is further broken down and eventually passed into the intestines, where the energy and nutrients can slowly be absorbed. The body then has the job of getting rid of the waste through the usual outlets – bowels, bladder, lungs, skin, etc. White refined sugar however, (and that includes brown sugar), is *very* different. It goes straight through the stomach wall without being digested, giving an instant rush of glucose to the bloodstream. This causes your blood sugar levels to rise too high. You now have too much sugar in your blood and your 'PH balance' is out of sorts (this is not to be confused with your skin PH). Your blood PH level is very, very important. If it goes just a couple of points below or above what it should be you will die. Your body therefore has to do whatever it can to counteract your rocketing blood sugar levels and reinstate the body's normal balance. How does it do this? By using some of your body's bank account of the powerful hormone insulin.

The rush you feel when you eat 'simple sugars' is simply the rush of insulin entering the bloodstream

The insulin produced to deal with this high blood sugar causes your blood sugar to ultimately *fall*. When we feel the effects of low blood sugar what do we need? Food that can raise blood sugar rapidly – more refined sugar. The moment the insulin reaction has cleansed your bloodstream of this excess sugar, you will be running on empty – an empty feeling *created* by refined sugar. See the loop?

White refined sugar has no essential nutrients, vitamins, minerals, fats or amino acids. It simply contains 'simple sugars', which are extremely dangerous to the natural balance of the body. There is no need whatsoever for simple refined sugars in the diet of a human. The only reason for its inclusion is to:

A) Abnormally sweeten foods to pervert our natural taste buds
B) Extend shelf-life
C) Use as a cheap filler
D) Keep you coming back for more and more and more

It is a totally empty food that leaves you ultimately feeling empty. It is, however, used at every available opportunity by the junkie food industry.

SUGAR CAUSES LOW BLOOD SUGAR

If your sugar levels were properly balanced you would feel satisfied for longer and the hunger you feel would always be a genuine one. That simply is no good for **BiG SUGAR** – they need you to feel the effects of abnormal low blood sugar, they want your sugar levels to crash, they need you to feel unbalanced and empty. That way you will feel the need for a quick fix and thus the sugar industry is guaranteed repeat business like any other addiction led industry. This is because the *only* thing that appears to end the feeling is something which has more white refined sugar – the very thing that caused the problem in the first place. It's like treating the symptoms of a disease with the cause. White refined sugar causes *dis*-ease in the body, which in turn causes *dis*-ease in the mind.

Many people I see are under the misapprehension that they don't consume that much sugar. If they don't have it in their tea, coffee, or on their cereal, they assume there is little sugar in their diet. However, **BiG FOOD** relies on it and it is in virtually every processed food we consume. You can find refined sugar in bread, cereal, cakes, biscuits, nearly all soft drinks, cheese (yes some cheeses), virtually all ready meals, ice creams, burgers, sausages, and the list goes on and on and on. I also want to make clear that when I talk about white refined sugar I am not just talking about the sugar found in drinks, processed foods, chocolate, ketchup and so on. I am also talking about white refined carbohydrates. These include white rice, pasta, bread cereals and the like, all of which rapidly turn to glucose (sugar) in the bloodstream.

The fast food outlets – the ones who rake in well over £3 billion a year in the UK from junkie type foods, use white refined sugar in all forms to keep you coming back for more. They rely on its inclusion. Without white refined sugars, salt, and refined fats (more on these topics soon) they would nearly all go out of business overnight. Most would have literally nothing to sell.

I have mentioned that when you eat white refined bread, pasta, rice, flour etc. your sugar levels go up rapidly and more insulin is secreted to help counteract it. Any 'lift' you feel from a sugar or carbo 'hit' is very short lived and in no time you feel a drop as the body scrambles to balance its blood sugar levels. However, there is something else you need to be more than aware of, particularly if you are reading this book to lose excess fat. The insulin that has been produced by the pancreas to rectify your blood sugar is also known as 'the fat-*producing* hormone'. Its job is to transport the carbohydrate energy (which has been converted by the body into glucose) to the liver and muscle cells for short-term storage of energy. However, if there is too much glucose at once – which is inevitable when white refined foods are consumed – some of the excess glucose (energy) has to go into the long-term storage banks: in other words it is stored as FAT.

Let me simplify to make this insulin, low blood sugar thing very clear

Insulin is produced by the pancreas to counteract the excess glucose (or sugar) that floods the bloodstream when you consume white refined carbohydrates. Any over-spill from the high amounts of insulin necessary to tackle this onslaught are stored as fat. When the insulin levels start to come down, a signal is sent to the brain to inform it that sugar levels have now stabilized. Once sugar levels are stabilized, you feel satisfied. However, in no time at all, blood sugar levels fall as the food it was given was an *empty* fuel and one that is released into the blood much too quickly. When your sugar levels drop again to an uncomfortable level, you once again get an empty dissatisfied feeling. If you then try and satisfy this feeling with more simple empty junkie foods and drinks, the cycle will continue.

This loop is problematic enough and, along with the advertising and mind manipulation, is what keeps people hooked. However, just like a drug addict who needs more and more of their drug to try and feel satisfied as time goes on, so it is for the junkie food addict.

Here's why:

If the carbo/sugar addict attempts to satisfy his or her hunger by eating more white refined carbs (simple or complex), the insulin amounts released by the pancreas will be even *greater* and the feeling of satisfaction becomes even *less*. As stated, it is only when the insulin levels drop that the person feels satisfied. If you constantly consume these white refined 'foods' you end up *always* having a degree of insulin in your blood. This means never feeling truly satisfied and always feeling a slight void in your life. You become what is known as 'insulin resistant', meaning your body will need more insulin to maintain a normal blood sugar range than that of a person who is not insulin resistant. At the same time this process progressively lowers the level of serotonin in the brain. Serotonin is a neurotransmitter which helps to govern your mood. Too little of this essential brain chemical and depression sets in. This means a white refined carbohydrate works just like any other drug. It makes you feel low, both mentally and physically, but gives the impression that it picks you up – an ingenious aspect of the sugar food trick.

If you are reading this book in order to get a slim physique, then you need to realize that it's sugar, rather than fat, that is the main cause of your problem. This may be a bold statement, but it's true. Fat is much more satiating and doesn't leave us feeling empty. It is the empty feeling which creates the hole and the desperate need to try and fill it. It's the attempt to fill the ever-increasing hole which causes us to overeat and gain so much weight.

BIG SUGAR = MASSIVE FINANCIAL REWARDS

Once again however, when it comes to any aspect of BiG FOOD, BiG SUGAR aren't particularly interested in your health or your excess weight. While we all get fatter, so indeed do their profits. BiG SUGAR is BiG BUSINESS. Sugar is the second biggest traded commodity in the world and anything which potentially could get in the way of sales will feel the traders' might – even The World Health Organization. In 2003 it was reported by the *Guardian* newspaper that, 'The sugar industry in the US is threatening to bring the World Health Organization (WHO) to its knees by demanding that Congress end its funding unless the WHO scraps guidelines on healthy eating, due to be published on Wednesday. The threat is being described by WHO insiders as tantamount to blackmail and worse than any pressure exerted by the tobacco lobby'. This comes as no surprise to me as **BiG SUGAR** are just as powerful as **BiG TOBACCO** and has come under fire on more than one occasion for how it conducts some aspects of its business.

BiG SUGAR was furious at the guidelines laid out by WHO, which says that sugar should account for no more than 10 per cent of a healthy diet and on the attack it went. **BiG SUGAR** wants that figure to be 25 per cent. That's one quarter of your food consumption they want to be refined sugar – one quarter. Even 10 per cent is over the top when you think refined sugar is not necessary *at all* in terms of being essential to our diet.

'Taxpayers' dollars should not be used to support misguided, non-science-based reports which do not add to the health and well-being of Americans, much less the rest of the world,' said a letter put forward by **BiG SUGAR**. 'If necessary we will promote and encourage new laws which require future WHO funding to be provided only if the organization accepts that all reports must be supported by the preponderance of science.'

But a team of thirty independent experts had considered the scientific evidence laid out with regard to sugar and its conclusions were in line with the findings of twenty-three national reports. All of which have, on average, set targets of 10 per cent for added sugars.

BiG SUGAR's main argument, as unbelievable as it may sound, is that sugar isn't a 'bad' food. According to **BiG SUGAR** and the 'soft' drink industry, there is no such thing as a food that is bad for you. This is spin at its finest. I agree that if there is no choice whatsoever and you are perhaps in a developing country then yes no food is bad. When you do have a choice, as we do, then there clearly is such a thing as a bad food. Sugar, without question, is one of them. In fact to describe white refined sugar as a food should be against the Trade Descriptions Act.

Dr Riaz Khan, director general of the World Sugar Research Organization, said, 'The concept of "good food and bad food" displayed throughout "report 916" lacks scientific validity. It singles out single elements of the diet, such as sugar, meat, edible oils, and dairy products as being unhealthy. It is the most basic of nutritional principles that there are "good and bad diets", not "good and bad foods".' But how can that be? What does a bad diet consist of then? Fruit, veg, nuts, and seeds or one of refined sugar and refined fats? Surely it's 'bad foods' which make up a 'bad diet' – or have I gone nuts?

According to **BiG SUGAR**, sugar isn't bad for you at all. This reminds me of **BiG TOBACCO** swearing on national television and in front of US congress that 'nicotine is not addictive.' In a western world where **BiG TOBACCO** is becoming more and more ostracized, there is no question that **BiG SUGAR** is the new **TOBACCO** on the block. Disguised as 'food' and with none of the passive effects that **BiG TOBACCO** had to contend with, it will be much harder to prove the link between something as seemingly simple as 'sugar' and the massive rise in obesity, heart disease, and cancer. I can almost guarantee, and I hope, that in about thirty years from now some members of **BiG SUGAR** will be brought to book, just like those in **BiG TOBACCO**. I can also guarantee that a *direct* link from refined sugar to man's biggest killers will come out. **BiG SUGAR** can hide behind its 'scientific evidence' in the same way **BiG TOBACCO** 'proved' cigarettes were good for people once upon a time, but 'The Truth Will Out' as they say.

CANCER FEEDS ON SUGAR

Even today we know that cancer, as an example, loves sugar. The German biologist Otto Heinrich Warburg won the Nobel Prize in medicine for his discovery that metabolism of malignant tumours is largely dependent on glucose consumption. In other words – cancer feeds on sugar! White refined sugar has also been linked to the massive rise in obesity and type 2 diabetes, yet **BiG SUGAR** not only deny this adamantly but claim it's not even a bad food. When WHO suggested we should have no more than 10 per cent of our diet as 'added sugar', **BiG SUGAR** went into overdrive and threatened to use its weight to stop

WHO's funding. Please never underestimate the power of **BiG FOOD** and in particular **BiG SUGAR.**

> 'i'll buy a huge piece of meat, cook it up for dinner, and then right before it's done, i'll break down and have what i wanted for dinner in the first place – bread and jam ... all i ever really want is sugar.'

Andy Warhol, *New York* Magazine, 31 March 1975

In 1956, Surgeon-Captain TL Cleve, MRCP, formally Director of Medical Research of the Institute of Naval Medicine in the UK called sugar 'the saccharine disease' and said it was responsible for most of mankind's degenerative diseases. Dr Cleve and his associates noted:

'There is one common factor in all traditional healthy diets: the *absence* of sugar and all simple carbohydrates.'

Even Dr Frederick, the scientist who discovered insulin, tried his best to tell the world his discovery was not a cure at all and that the only way to prevent diabetes was to cut down on 'dangerous' sugar bingeing. He said, 'In the US, the incidence of diabetes has increased proportionately with the per capita consumption of sugar.'

Despite this there are still many in the medical industry who will still say diet plays little or no part in disease. In particular I hear so, so often that sugar and diabetes aren't connected.

WE NEED SUGAR – BUT OF THE RIGHT KIND!

The sugar industry hides behind the fact we need sugar as part of our diet. What they fail to tell us is yes, we need sugar in the form of good carbohydrates, but we don't need refined sugar – ever.

The human body was designed to get its energy from carbohydrates – but carbohydrates which are in their *natural* state, not ones that have been stripped of their life force (or 'refined' as they call it). I am talking here about natural fruits, vegetables, and whole grains such as brown rice. Our bodies were simply never designed to deal with a constant barrage of white, refined sugar and carbohydrates. The body will, of course, 'survive' for quite a while despite this abuse – but it's the quality of our *daily* lives that is being slowly destroyed and controlled by these products. When you eat natural, nothing-taken-out carbs, the body does what it was designed to do. It digests them and then it *gradually* releases their potential energy into your cells. This does not cause your sugar levels to go sky high and therefore the pancreas does not have to produce tons of insulin. The sugar found in fruit is fructose. The body cannot use fructose as it is, and needs to convert it into usable glucose. The time it takes to convert the fructose into glucose is essential in keeping the blood sugar levels correctly balanced. Plus, fruit sugar is a whole food. It contains all the enzymes (life force) the body needs for digestion, it is a pure 'live' food, it tastes wonderful and also contains fibre, which helps to 'sweep' the intestines clean and helps to prevent the sugar being absorbed too rapidly into the bloodstream. White refined sugar and carbohydrates do the complete opposite.

New Sugar On The Block

If white refined sugar wasn't bad enough, in the second half of the twentieth century came 'High Fructose Corn Syrup'. This is a mixture of 'fructose' and 'glucose'. The only place you will find this sugar is in man-made processed food. Although all fruit contains fructose, once this sugar has been removed from its normal home and mixed with glucose, it can no longer be handled by the insulin our bodies produce without causing some damage. High Fructose Corn Syrup (HFCS) is gold to BiG FOOD. It's cheap, is a great preservative and tastes sweet – bingo! How this hybrid sugar is allowed to be put in the food and drinks so many of us consume unsuspectingly is a mystery to one and all. The FDA (Food and Drug Administration) in the US and FSA (Food Standards Agency) here in the UK, have passed this substance as perfectly fine and dandy for human consumption. Always good to know they have our best interests at heart.

REFINED SUGAR – THE COCAINE OF THE FOOD WORLD

It's about time people started to realize that white refined sugar and hybrids such as HFCS are not just like a drug, but they act the same as any addictive drug. Sugar is a drug which, just like any other, makes the addict feel good with ... and empty without. However, unlike the other perfectly legal drugs like cigarettes, white refined sugar and carbohydrates don't even carry a government health warning – despite the fact that they are known by the medical profession to cause a multitude of diseases and have been heavily, and I do mean very heavily, linked to diabetes, hypertension in children and anti-social behaviour. Diabetes has more than tripled since 1958; right in line with the consumption of sugar – coincidence? A little over one hundred years ago only 1 per cent of the population had diabetes, now the figure is officially 1 in 12; unofficially it's a lot, lot more. There are many people who are unaware that they have what is known as type 2 diabetes (over 90 per cent of diabetics have this type: type 1 is where you inject yourself). As we now consume over a third of a pound of sugar each per day, the number of people suffering from this life-threatening condition can only rise. At present over 100 million people around the world have diabetes and that figure is projected to rise to a whopping 250 million by 2015. White refined sugar is also said to be responsible for the premature deaths of 3,000 British women every year due to heart disease.

This same white refined sugar is also the very substance found in so many low fat foods – which seems ironic given that white refined sugar causes insulin release and insulin is the *fat-producing* hormone. Yet over the past twenty to thirty years people have come to believe that their weight and/or health problem will be solved for life if they simply went ...

10

FAT FREE

I know that not everyone reading this book is doing so in order to lose weight, but there are so many people, fat or otherwise, who continue to buy 'fat free' and 'low fat' products in a bid for better health. I was guilty of this myself for years. However, what they, and I, failed to realize is the simple truth –

it's all a big pack of fat lies!

Not only do these products often contain more fat than is stated on the label but more importantly they are nearly always loaded with white refined sugar or a sugar hybrid of some kind. Unless I am missing something, doesn't the inclusion of refined sugar completely defeat the object of the exercise somewhat? Doesn't excess sugar turn into fat in most people?

To illustrate the whole nonsense of **'FAT FREE'** I could get a suitcase full of white refined sugar or hybrid and put a massive label on it reading, **'100 PER CENT FAT FREE'.** And the thing is I wouldn't be lying – the contents of the suitcase is totally 'fat free'. The fact that the majority of it would be converted into body fat and that you would be one more step closer to obese land and possibly injecting yourself with insulin, seems to be neither here nor there for the sugar loaded 'fat free' industry. After all, your health is not their real concern; they're after what's in your pocket. **BiG SUGAR** must have loved the whole 'fat free' obsession; it gave them an even greater market without any adverse publicity. Because we are so unbelievably conditioned to believe fat makes us fat, the sugar content of 'fat free' or 'low fat' products goes unnoticed. It's the headline grabbing 'Fat Free' on the label that deludes us into thinking it is in some way healthy and of course 'slimming'.

EATING FAT DOESN'T EQUAL EXCESS BODY FAT

Since the late 1970s the percentage of fat consumption per head has *decreased* by about 16 per cent in the UK– that's decreased, gone down, reduced. Yet just like in the US obesity has doubled since that time, with an increase in the average weight of 12 lb (5.5 kg). So we are fatter now than we were when we were consuming more fat. If eating fat was the underlying cause of the obesity epidemic, then surely the reduction in fat consumption would coincide with a reduction in the excess body fat of the nation. This is because it is not the fat so much but once again the sugar. It is worth knowing that the only foodstuffs whose consumption has increased in exact correlation to how fat we are getting is **WHiTE REFiNED SUGAR, SUGAR HYBRiDS AND CARBOHYDRATES.** This illustrates even further just how meaningless these 'low fat' and 'fat free' labels are, especially given that manufacturers tend to add more sugar in place of the fat.

The wording they use to lure people into buying these products is often pretty deceptive too. If you saw two packets of biscuits on a shelf, one is '80 per cent fat free' and the other contains 20 per cent fat, which one would you be more likely to buy? The truth is that so many more people would choose the apparent 'fat free' version, even though both packets contain exactly the same amount of fat. Or maybe they don't, the truth is you never really know the true fat content anyway. I had an expert on this particular subject explain that if you take the calorie blah blah and times it by the what-do-ya-call-it and then divide it by how many who-do-ya-ma-flips there are, the true fat content would be revealed. But once again 'we don't need to know'. All we need to know is that 'fat free' and 'low fat' is often a huge lie and most of the time it usually means that more white refined sugar and salt have been added to improve the taste. The salt content alone causes water retention, again adding weight and totally defeating said purpose. It also helps to push your blood pressure sky high. There really is nothing like a good low fat food to keep you slim and healthy. And the 'fat free' products I am talking about are literally *nothing* like a good low fat food.

POTATOES ARE FOR PIGS, CORN IS FOR CATTLE

While I am on the subject of 'low fat' or 'fat free' foods, here's another eye opener. Baked potatoes – the very product many turn to in order to lose weight – can cause your sugar levels to rise and a massive amount of insulin to be released. And, just to make sure by the end of the book you really know this stuff, don't forget insulin is the *fat-producing* hormone. Insulin in the bloodstream also prevents stored fat from being broken down – double whammy. Not only does it store fat, it also inhibits the fat it stores from being broken down. Am I saying don't eat potatoes? No. Am I saying that potatoes are as bad as a Mars Bar? No! Am I saying that potatoes contain no vitamins, minerals or essential fibre? No! All I'm saying is that if weight loss is a concern for you, no longer be deluded into thinking baked potatoes are the good slimming food we believe them to be. Remember, one great way to fatten a pig is to feed it potatoes, which is worth remembering the next time you are tucking into your big bag of Kettle chips or 'reduced fat' bag of 'baked' crisps. They're not as healthy or slimming as you think.

Popcorn is another apparent 'low fat' food. But once again corn can cause insulin levels to rise quite rapidly. Popcorn is usually covered in refined sugar too, so the insulin problem is compounded. The French have always said, 'Potatoes are for pigs and corn is for cattle'. This is because both help to fatten them up quickly. How many times have we avoided smearing butter on our potatoes or corn on the cob, yet it's often the corn and potatoes that have contributed to the weight gain, far more than the butter.

'If you can pinch more than an inch – you should go on a diet'

Do you remember the advert which implied that 'if you can pinch more than an inch', you should think about a diet of some kind? Do you remember what they were advertising? 'Special K'. A white refined carbohydrate breakfast. I believe the catchphrase may have caused more people to believe they had a weight problem than any other in history. In my opinion it caused many people to unnecessarily start dieting. And as we now know, dieting can potentially make people fat. What did they mean if you *can* pinch more than an inch? It should have been 'If you *can't* pinch more than an inch, then you're in big trouble.' A while ago my mother lost her husband and, as a result, had very little appetite. She reached the stage where she couldn't pinch more than an inch. This is not a sign of health: when the body reaches this level it can start to eat its own organs.

FAT PHOBIA

The Special K advert was a big part of the anti-fat campaign, which started in the Seventies, reached its peak in the Eighties, and is still going strong today. We have been bombarded with so much anti-fat propaganda, even from qualified government backed dieticians, for so many years we now believe there is something wrong with consuming even the essential fats needed for the body to function properly. Many people are literally 'fat phobic'. The amount of people I get in my seminars who still believe avocados and olives are fattening is amazing. I am not knocking them as I was conditioned to believe this nonsense too. It is true that they are full of fat, but they are full of good fats – fats which are essential to our health. The body cannot produce these fats by itself, which is why they are known as essential. It is vital we put fat into our body, but it is equally vital that it's the right kind. Never has one vital element of nutrition been so misunderstood by so many as fat.

The average child in the UK will consume 52 stone (330 kg) of *the wrong kind* of fat between the ages of 6 and 16. Can you imagine – 728 lb of the wrong fat going into the body over ten years? Is it any wonder children as young as eight are now showing signs of heart disease? Essential fats are not the problem, we need them – they are not described as essential for nothing. It's the stuff you find bacon and egg swimming around in on a Sunday morning that's the real problem along, of course, with the new twenty-first century hybrid fats. In fact I believe the two biggest threats to human health are hybrid and refined sugars and hybrid and refined fats. Hybrid fats, commonly known as 'Trans Fats' are far, far worse than saturated fats and they are lurking in more 'foods' than you can possibly imagine. So much so that in the summer of 2007 Trans Fats were banned in New York City and Philadelphia restaurants and throughout the food industry in Denmark. In the UK there is a move to ban Trans Fats from all foods, but it may well be a while before we see it removed completely. Even if it does get removed I can guarantee that whatever replaces it will be just as bad, but like Trans Fats, it will take years for the big fat truth to come out.

Why Are Trans Fats So Harmful?

A few decades ago a report showed a connection between animal fats and cardiovascular disease. This caused the huge rise in vegetable margarine as a healthy alternative to butter. Many claims have been made about margarines; the biggest being 'helps to lower cholesterol'. However, despite 'scientific evidence' showing it does help to lower cholesterol, it caused a rise in some countries of heart attacks. Israel has one of the lowest cholesterol levels in Western countries, but it also has one of the highest rates of heart attacks and obesity. Most margarines contain sunflower oil. This oil has seventy times the amount of omega-6s than omega 3s. You may well have heard of the essential fatty acids we require referred to as omega 3, 6, and 9. The *ratio* of these fats is essential to our health. For example, omega 3 and 6 should have a ratio of 1:1, not 1:70 as in the case of many margarines. Omega 6 is extremely inflammatory and must be balanced by omega 3. When you effectively 'boil' vegetable oil until it solidifies, you completely change the molecular structure and any reference to the word 'vegetable' should be followed with a visit from the Trade Description Agency.

Trans Fats have one redeeming feature for **BiG FOOD** – they don't go stale. This is why you will find them in cookies, cakes, crisps, flapjacks, croissants, pastries, and of course many 'vegetable margarines'. They are heavily used in any processed food they need to keep on the shelves for months. It is only due to financial reasons that these fats are used – they are not used for the goodness of your health but for the goodness of their bank accounts. Just like High Fructose Corn Syrup, both the Food Standards Agency and Food and Drug Administration cleared Trans Fats as 'safe' for human consumption – as always on the back of 'scientific evidence'. We always have to remember that just because something has been 'scientifically tested' or 'cleared' by a government body, it doesn't mean it is actually safe. I have done enough research over the many years I have been involved in this business to know that **BiG FOOD** has very deep pockets and many people can easily be influenced if the financial incentive is large enough. I am not suggesting that anyone in the FDA or FSA is corrupt. All I am saying is when it comes to making sure their high profit empty foods make it to the shelves, **BiG FOOD** has the power to 'prove' their product is safe. All the FSA and FDA do is look at the scientific evidence.

Hydrogenated or Trans Fats are completely alien to our systems, and encourage our bodies to store toxic fat residue. Research has shown that Trans Fats contribute to *many* more cardiovascular problems than saturated fats found in meat and butter. In fact there is now even evidence to show that saturated fat may not be harmful at all, let alone less harmful than Trans Fats. There is also increasing evidence to show that the link between saturated fat, cholesterol, and heart disease may not be there after all.

At least saturated fat can be found occurring naturally. After all even mother's milk is loaded with saturated fat and also cholesterol. If saturated fat and cholesterol is so bad why does nature provide the first food we have with them in? However, the debate about saturated fat may go on and on but Trans Fats are to be found nowhere in nature. They are completely unnatural and have also been linked to diabetes, heart disease and hardening of the arteries and veins. If you get nothing else from this book, do yourself a favour and never eat anything with Trans Fats or High Fructose Corn Syrup again. These are hybrids, completely unnatural and, in my humble opinion, are the biggest cause of degenerative disease in the world – even more so than tobacco.

You Must Eat Fat If You Want To Be Slim!

The right kinds of fat are not only essential to our health, but essential for freeing ourselves from the food and diet trap. If you go completely 'fat free' your body will be missing a vital component, you will be severely malnourished because of it and you will always feel hungrier than you should. The right kinds of fat help to regulate your appetite and keep you much more satisfied for longer. This stops the often dramatic and overwhelming craving for food people get when their bodies are missing a vital piece of nutrition. I now make sure that avocados are part of my daily diet. Avocados have the perfect balance of essential fats and are the only 'fruit' you can live on exclusively. They contain all the vital elements of human nutrition and have even made it into the *Guinness Book Of World Records* as 'The world's most nutritious fruit'. Unfortunately many diet clubs and misinformed dieticians and nutritionists made people scared to death of avocados, claiming because they contain fat they will make you fat – which is just total rubbish. I also eat plenty of seeds, nuts, and fish – all excellent sources of essential fats and all of which help to keep me satiated and regulate my appetite. The right fats also boost the immune system, govern our energy metabolism, are used as an emergency energy store and help to cushion the joints and protect the muscles. It even plays a part in our sex lives as we need fat to help make hormones like estrogen and testosterone. Fat also stimulates the brain, so it is hardly surprising that very low-fat diets have been linked with depression and other mental disorders. In short – we need fat.

Remember, just like the wrong kind of sugar, it's the *wrong kind* of fat that does the damage. If you keep putting in the wrong type of fats, your body will continue to crave the fat it really needs. In other words, the wrong fats create an even greater need for fat than necessary. The problem is when you first give yourself a 'wrong fat hit' you will feel better, but not for long. The body will soon realize that what it has been given is not the real stuff, and once again will send a signal to the brain saying 'I need more fat'. So you either use your willpower and control not to have any more (as you have been told all fat is bad) or you say 'Sod it – one doughnut won't hurt'. Either way, the body is, once again, lacking genuine nutrition and you are malnourished. This creates a feeling of dissatisfaction in the body, which naturally has a knock-on effect on the mind. Combine this with the emptiness and malnutrition refined sugar causes and you have the 'refined' fat and sugar cocktail that is the main cause of the food and diet trap.

The key here is to remove ourselves from what we have been conditioned to believe and embrace the right sugars and the right fats. It is also vital that you see behind **BiG FOOD** and their labelling tricks (more on that in a later chapter). Remember 'fat free' usually equals 'added sugar' and 'Sugar Free' usually means 'contains artificial sweeteners' (which also need a chapter alone – more later).

In summary, it is the wrong kinds of fat and the massive amounts of refined and hybrid sugars which cause malnutrition and 'false hungers' to form the basis of 'addiction'. There is nothing wrong with the right sugars (found in fruits, vegetables, and grains) or the right kinds of fats (found in fruits, vegetables, seeds, nuts, fish, and good quality 'grass fed' meats – which I'll talk about soon). So please never avoid fat, just avoid the **FAT FREE CON.**

As well as sugar, there is another white refined drug food hidden in many low fat, so-called healthier foods which people just don't seem to be too bothered about. In fact this life-shortening drug food is in virtually every processed food we buy, yet it is rarely seen as a major concern by the public. Most people are more concerned about losing weight and looking good to get hot and bothered about this substance. But it's about time we took a very realistic look at a killer substance that we are so badly hooked on that we even add tons more of the stuff to 'foods' that are already heavily laced with it. If feeling good, supreme health and long life are on your agenda then I strongly suggest you open your mind, take your head out of the sand and stop taking this subject with …

11

A PINCH OF SALT

If only it were a pinch then we really wouldn't have a problem. A pinch might be all you add to your food, but **BiG FOOD** loves the stuff and well over 200,000 tons of white refined salt is added to our food each year. It is worth pointing out from the start of this small chapter that white refined table salt, like refined sugars and fats, isn't necessary *at all* to a healthy human diet. **BiG FOOD** loves it as it once again helps shelf life and has an addictive quality.

Refined salt is one of the UK's single biggest contributors to disease. There have been many estimates over the years as to just how many people die prematurely because of excess salt consumption, ranging from 14,000 to 100,000 per year. It is almost impossible to know exact numbers, but it is undisputed that excess refined salt causes premature death. Too much salt increases the risk of high blood pressure, which in turn is linked to heart disease and stroke. With that in mind you would think legislation would be put forward forcing **BiG FOOD** to cut their 'hidden salt' in processed foods dramatically. However, instead of extremely tough laws preventing too much salt in processed foods we have 'recommendations' instead. If we had parking 'recommendations' rather than laws, I don't think anyone would take any notice. The Food

Standards Agency, who even have a 'salt reduction strategy', have recently said, 'We are all still eating too much salt. That is why it is so important that we check labels and choose the lowest salt options.' But instead of 'voluntary targets' for BiG FOOD on salt content and the onus being on Joe public to go through confusing labels and try to figure out just how much is in each portion, why don't they make it law? That way we could all simply buy food and know that someone in charge of making sure our diet is safe is looking after us. That way we could have some control over our salt intake.

The World Has Officially Gone Mental

But instead of making BiG FOOD pull their socks up, we have our over-paid councillors coming up with ingenious ideas to help us poor souls who clearly haven't a brain cell to rub together. There are many things that eat me, but the incredible misuse of our tax money is one of my biggest bugbears. This was illustrated in 2008 when Gateshead county council came up with the mind numbingly ridiculous idea to help people reduce their salt intake. Yes, just when you thought it was safe to pay your taxes, Gateshead councillors have been busy inventing a catering-sized salt pot with just five or nine holes in the lid, rather than the usual seventeen or eighteen. The theory is that people will cut down on their salt intake when they get fish and chips. When I heard this I assumed it was a joke, but apparently not. They called it, '... a novel and extremely simple solution'. But 'solution' to what? Surely all people will do is shake the pot for longer to get the required amount they want or add more when they get their take-away home. Also, this is only aimed at places like fish and chip shops, hardly a place which focuses on health. It's not the salt *we* add that is causing our arteries to block; it's the amount BiG FOOD adds.

ADDING IN-SALT TO INJURY

The reason for the big outcry to reduce our salt intake is because refined table salt contains highly toxic sodium – yes toxic. If there is too much of it overloading the body, the kidneys have to work their socks off to try to eliminate it. This in turn makes the heart work harder. And when the heart works harder, it pumps loads more blood through the kidneys – which means the end result is high blood pressure and high blood pressure equals strokes and heart attacks.

Despite this fact, **BiG FOOD** not only hides salt in food aimed at adults, but more sinisterly children. From the 'Happy Meal' to cereals aimed at children, hidden salt is often lurking undetected by the purchaser. The advertising of foods high in refined sugar, salt, and fat are also aimed at children. It's worth knowing that 96 per cent of American children recognize Mr Ronald McDonald. To put this in perspective, the only other fictitious character who is recognized more is Santa Claus. 'Get them hooked while they're young and create a lifelong customer', appears to be the directive of many in **BiG FOOD.** They seem unconcerned that children as young as four are already showing changes in their veins and arteries similar to those found in the early stages of hypertension, and that if they carry on using this substance throughout their lives they have a massive chance of either losing use of certain parts of their body through a stroke, or losing their life as a result of one of the UK's biggest killers – heart disease. An added 'extra' for **BiG FOOD** is that by adding salt it dehydrates people and makes them unnaturally thirsty. This leads to knock on sales of 'soft' drinks that are often owned by the very same companies adding the salt in the first place. If you are ever stranded at sea you are told above all else that no matter how thirsty you get you should never drink the water. Why? Because it will kill you quickly due to dehydration caused by the salt.

HIDDEN EXTRAS

Salt is in more foods than you realize. Bread, for example, is the biggest source of salt in the UK's diet. It's also in pastries, pizzas, cheese, cereals, cakes, burgers, pasta, rice, and so the list continues to almost all processed food on the shelves of most large supermarket chains. At this time around three quarters of the salt we consume is of the 'hidden' kind. An undercover *Dispatches* documentary found some of your lunchtime sandwiches contain a great deal more salt than you would think. The biggest culprit according to the documentary was the Subway 'Eat Fresh' chain with a twelve-inch Meatball Mariana containing 7.2 g (¼ oz) of salt, that's as much salt as you would find in eighteen packets of crisps – yes **EiGHTEEN BAGS OF CRiSPS!**

Each adult in the UK currently consumes, on average, 8.6 g (⅓ oz) of salt a day, which is about 44 per cent more than the recommended daily maximum of 6 g (⅕ oz). But even 6 g of added or hidden salt is completely unnecessary to our diet. This is because the exact amount of salt we require is in the foods nature provides for us. I know that many 'experts' tell us how we need salt, but I can only think that some experts are getting somewhat confused about the sodium and salt issue. Instead of saying refined salt is good for us, what they meant to say of course was, 'The body needs sodium, but *only* in its natural state – like the kind you find in foods such as fruits, green leafy vegetables, celery etc.'

At this point I can just hear you saying, 'But Jason, salt tastes so good, what would a boiled egg be like without the salt?' Okay I agree with that one, it takes a little adjusting to, but like sugar in tea and coffee once you do it a few times it actually tastes just as good. Unfortunately, refined salt isn't something we can't realistically expect to avoid entirely as it is found in just about all processed food. However, once you've changed your diet, as opposed to going on one, you will automatically be free from most of the hidden salt found in **BiG FOOD.** Remember the only reason **BiG FOOD** adds so much salt to their food is because it is a wonderful preservative (so much so that the Egyptians used to use it for storing dead bodies), it causes dehydration (so you drink more of their drinks), it's very cheap and can be addictive. It is the perfect ingredient for **BiG FOOD.** And while I'm on the subject of 'preserving', did you know that we now consume so much salt and other preservatives in our food that our bodies are no longer decomposing when we die? How wonderful.

THIS INFORMATION IS NOT ENOUGH FOR CHANGE

Many people reading this book will no doubt already know about how harmful refined fats, refined sugars and refined salt can be. However, simply knowing this information very rarely, if ever, enables people to change their diet in the long term.

I am more than aware of this as I was one of them. When I was overweight and suffering from many ailments, I may not have known all the bad things sugar does, but even if I had it wouldn't have stopped me. Why? Because I was in the 'food matrix' and was under the massive delusion that I loved my diet and there would be no pleasure in changing to 'rabbit food'. I simply thought 'life's too short'. I may have a shorter life, but at least it would be sweeter. I thought I may be fat but at least I am happy (which wasn't true at all, but we do try to convince ourselves and anyone who will listen).

At the same time we tend to use the infamous 'Uncle Fred' story to justify our apparent genuine 'choice' of diet. Everyone has one. You know the relative who ate rubbish, drank heavily and smoked yet was the picture of health till the day they passed. Have you noticed that the longer you tell the 'Uncle Fred' story, the older he became and the more junk he consumed. In the end, Uncle Fred drank a bottle of Scotch a day, ate nothing but fry-ups, smoked 100 cigarettes a day, lived till he was 650 and of course never had a day's illness in his entire life. Sadly, we not only end up believing anything we tell ourselves over and over again, but we regard Uncle Fred as some kind of genuine market research and ignore the enormous number of people who are having their lives cut short because of what they are putting inside their bodies.

FEAR KEEPS US TRAPPED

Addiction is only an irrational fear. It is the fear we cannot live the same way again without our particular drug or drug-like food and drinks. We fear we will never be able to cope or enjoy our lives the same way again without whatever foods or drinks we are hooked on. Despite addiction being an irrational fear, never underestimate the power of the emotional hook. It is very similar to a bad relationship. If you have ever had the misfortune of being in one, especially one of a mentally and physically abusive nature, you will recognize the hook. Despite being mentally and physically dependent, as in the case of all addiction to a greater or lesser extent, you feel trapped. One side is fearful of staying in the relationship and the other part fears life without. This is why many people whose health has deteriorated to the point where they have been told to literally change their diet or die, still continue to eat and drink themselves to death. Smokers know that cigarettes are likely to kill them, but still continue to smoke, even when they have had a leg amputated. Why? Because although people know they could die *someday* from smoking or eating rubbish, they also believe there is a genuine pleasure in doing it and they literally fear life more without it than with it.

Given the genuine choice, addicts of any kind want to stop taking their drug, but all drug addicts also want to continue taking their drug too. The nature of drug addiction is a mental tug-of-war caused by an illusionary belief about what the addict perceives they get from the drug. The same principle applies to certain food addiction. This tug-of-war in the mind cannot be removed by simply sticking a patch on, eliminating the wrong foods, taking slimming tablets, having your stomach stapled, or eating nothing but cabbage for three weeks or even trying to scare people off them. These approaches tend only to treat the physical symptoms of something that has a psychological cause. The problem can only be eliminated by removing the many years of brainwashing and conditioning and coming to a full understanding of the nature of drug foods and the 'diet trap'.

As I will repeatedly point out throughout this book, the real problem people have when attempting to change their diet is not physical. The physical feelings of emptiness that occur as a result of things like caffeine withdrawal or low blood sugar take just days to get over. In many cases, the feelings are so slight the vast majority don't even notice them anyway. How many times have you felt really hungry but for some reason you got involved with something else? In other words you changed your mental focus. You go for hours doing whatever it is that has taken your mind off the hunger, but what physical pain are you in? None whatsoever. Once you remember that you haven't eaten you will then eat. But the minute you go on a diet you are hungry all of the time – why? Because you are simply mentally hungry for the pleasure you believe you are missing out on. If we simplify the whole business of changing your diet, the only thing which causes us to suffer so much is not the physical element, but a self-imposed mental tantrum caused by the belief we have just had something we feel like we can't survive or enjoy our life without, taken from us. But what is so enjoyable about eating junkie and drug food? It's not something we really analyse, but exactly how do these empty fat and disease causing foods make us happy? What do they really do for us? What is the point in eating or drinking them? Why do we give **BiG FOOD** and **BiG DRiNK** our hard earned money simply to make ourselves ill, fat, and miserable? And what exactly will we be missing out on if we just decided to dump the majority of the rubbish from our lives?

It is time to explode the myth once and for all that when you change your brand of food you will be missing out on …

12

THE PLEASURE OF EATING JUNK

This chapter perhaps requires more of an open mind than most of the others. Like any illusion, it appears very real, so trying to convince people the vast majority of the pleasure they think they get from eating junk, is in fact non-existent.

This powerful illusion of pleasure is where the advertising, conditioning, and effects of drug-like junkie foods really come into play. Each combine very nicely to delude millions of intelligent people into thinking junk foods are simply wonderful and salads, fruit, vegetables, fish and whole grains are for very boring people with long hair who live up trees and have no life. **BiG FOOD** and their advertising agencies use whatever they believe is pleasurable and do their level best to link it to their food or drink. In just a thirty-second ad they have to make us believe we will not only get some extreme pleasure from eating or drinking whatever it is they are selling, but they also want to delude us that we can also avoid some emotional pain in the process. There is one major problem with this approach – it works. They are targeting our basic human driving forces – a desire for pleasure and a need to avoid pain. On top of this false advertising we have the 'foods' or 'drinks' themselves which do, without question, appear to give us pleasure and take away a degree of pain; thus giving the adverts some degree of credence. I say 'appear' to give pleasure because the pleasure is false based on the ending of a false physical and/or mental hunger caused by the 'foods' themselves and/or the emotional trick advertising.

THE JUNK FOOD CONFIDENCE TRICK

The real pleasure is the ending of that slight empty insecure feeling we know as hunger. When we end this aggravation we feel a sense of pleasure. How empty we feel will also determine how much pleasure we get from the food. When we are hungry the look of food and the smell makes us salivate. When we have had enough we often can't even look at the food any more. But what has actually changed? The food is still the same and so is the smell, so why don't you feel you would get any pleasure from it any more? The answer is simply because you no longer have an empty aggravation – you are no longer hungry. Unless you are hungry you simply cannot get the same level of pleasure from eating it. And the hungrier (or emptier) you feel, the greater the pleasure you do eventually feel when you fill it. This is the very essence of the confidence trick. By feeding you substances which are ultimately designed to cause greater hungers, those same substances also appear to give the most pleasure.

For example, if I am feeling abnormally empty due to my sugar levels crashing or a lack of the right fats (or both), there is no question that if I eat something containing simple sugars and refined fats I will feel a rush and that my empty feeling will temporarily be removed. The quick rush of sugar into my blood would cause my emptiness to be filled in seconds and because I have just ended an aggravation, I would feel a wonderful sense of pleasure. And because the aggravation is much greater when we have a sudden and abnormal drop in blood sugar, the sense of pleasure when we do load our body with junk is also greater. This is the genius of the food trick and **BiG FOOD**. The bigger the aggravation they cause the bigger the sense of pleasure when you relieve it. What also adds to the illusion is that if your sugar levels are way below normal and you try to lift them instantaneously with some broccoli or some fish, you have no chance. Genuine foods release their energy slowly to prevent any spikes in blood sugar, whereas drug-foods are designed to give you that hit.

What is essential for you to understand is that there is no 'hit' from drug foods, the pleasure you feel is simply the ending of an abnormal empty feeling often caused by what you ate previously. **BiG FOOD** have found an ingenious way to cause you not only to feel a greater sense of hunger, but have found a way to make you feel hungrier more. The more empty hunger you have the more pleasure you will feel when you try to end it. The more you try to end it with drug-like foods, the hungrier and emptier you will ultimately feel and the more false hungers you will create. You then spend most of your life either trying to exercise control not to try and fill the empty feeling and using tremendous amounts of willpower, discipline, and self-control. Or you say, 'life's too short' and eat more of the same. Each time you simply confirm the false belief that this type of food 'lifts' you and fills a void of some kind. I want to make it clear – the only void it appears to fill is the one it creates. **BiG FOOD** have created a situation where the vast majority of people in the UK are 'addicted' but don't really know it. Because it's not talked about, we all simply think we have no willpower or have flaws in our character, when the simple truth is we have simply fallen for one of the most ingenuous confidence tricks of the twenty-first century. The bigger the empty feeling these foods and drinks create, the larger the impression of a genuine high and the more we feel we are losing out if we stop. It is only the feeling of loss and the feeling of missing out that makes the process of changing one's diet difficult. If we can break down the illusion sufficiently so that you can clearly see the pleasure trick and realize there is, in reality, nothing to give up, then the process of change can be one of the easiest things you could ever do. **BiG FOOD** have simply created a way to make us believe we can have a greater pleasure, more often if we eat heavily processed food compared to if we were to eat natural food. It's a trick – and we need to see both the simplicity and the ingenious aspects of it.

SKI BOOTS

To illustrate it further I want to give a very simple analogy. Have you ever been skiing or snowboarding? When you finish on the slopes and head towards what is known as 'the wet room' you start to notice just how much your boots are hurting you. When you finally sit down and unclip them and then remove them, the feeling is one of the most pleasurable you can imagine. It can only be described as pure bliss. Many people get the same feeling if they have had a pair of uncomfortable shoes on all day and then remove them. The pleasure feeling can be quite magnificent. The point I am making is that just because you get an often immense feeling of pleasure when you take off a pair of ski boots, the pleasure is clearly only based on the removal of the aggravation you are suffering. The longer you have your ski boots on the *more* pleasure you will get when you eventually remove them. However, no matter how lonely, upset, angry, stressed or bored you are when you return from your skiing trip, you never think for one second that if you put your ski boots on and walked around in them for a few hours, you could give yourself a pleasure boost by removing them later on and so improve your day. If you did think such a thing then clearly therapy is where you need to be! We only believe it when it comes to 'the food trick' because it isn't obvious. It is very subtle illusion which has most people fooled. This is also why if you go *on* a diet as opposed to change it, all you are effectively doing is keeping your ski boots on for longer and so creating an even greater illusion of pleasure when you do manage to loosen them slightly.

The ending of any aggravation is pleasurable – but why deliberately cause the aggravation in the first place?

The ending of these false physical hungers is far from the only thing to create the illusion of genuine pleasure and short-term fulfilment. We have the **BiG FOOD** advertisers constantly creating a host of illusions on our TV screens to back up the physical illusion we already believe. They use all kinds of emotions to pull on your junkie food heart strings, but the biggest pleasure they use to peddle their wares is sex. Let's face facts – sex sells. **BiG DRUG FOOD** use it at every available opportunity. Just picture the very attractive lady lying in that beautiful claw-bath, water overflowing onto the floor of a huge luxurious bathroom. Slowly, seductively, sexually, eating a chocolate bar to the tune of 'Only the crumbliest, flakiest chocolate tastes like chocolate never tasted before'. Or what about the attractive woman taking a bite of a Bounty bar followed by an image of a tall, dark, handsome man smiling at her on a deserted beach (no doubt about to take her to 'paradise' and back). Ice cream makers have always been huge fans of linking sex with their product, just look at the Magnum and Häagen-Dazs ads. And while we are on the subject of pleasure, sex, and drug-like foods and drinks, let's not forget the Diet Coke man and his 11.30 a.m. Diet Coke break. I think the fact that they're using sex to sell this product is pretty undisputed. What the advert is saying is this: if you're a man and you drink Diet Coke you will look like the window cleaner in the ad and all women, just like those in the ad, will want to sleep with you. If you're a woman, it's saying if you drink Diet Coke you'll get to sleep with men who look like the hunky window cleaner. So it's totally true to life then.

These ads and hundreds of thousands like them use either sex or some type of emotional pleasure trigger to help sell these sugar loaded drug-like foods and drinks. But what on earth have any of the images we see in these type of ads got to do with the foods or drinks they're advertising? The substance being sold in the Diet Coke ad for example isn't the answer to obesity; in fact there are many reports that suggest drinks containing artificial sweeteners can actually cause people to *gain* weight (more on that later). Such drinks with the words 'diet' or 'light' are simply designed to make people *believe* they are doing something good for their health, when clearly they're not. But do we really ever believe it anyway? I used to go into a burger joint and order a flipple-dipple-whopple-dopper burger, mega fries, an apple pie and of course – a *Diet* Coke. Who was I kidding? Adverts like those for

Flake aren't selling a load of sugar and junk, they are trying to sell the lifestyle. They want you to think if you have a Flake you won't have a care in the world. While rationally we know it's all nonsense, they show it over and over again and 'bell' us to such an extent that often we make food decisions on a very subconscious level. As mentioned previously, what we often think is our genuine choice is actually a choice which has been very much made for us.

Pleasure You Can't Measure

Genuine pleasure is where you look forward with anticipation to what you are going to do, you love it while you are doing it and you love the feeling of fulfilment afterwards. In other words it satisfies your needs. Ending a *genuine* hunger with *genuine* food does precisely this if your need is for nutrients/fuel. That's why I now love my food, love feeling hungry and adore eating. I love the anticipation of good food, I love it while I am eating it and I love the feeling of total satisfaction afterwards. Conversely, the pleasure you experience when consuming drug-like foods and drinks is very often short lived. Many people like the anticipation, like it when they first start eating but usually feel bloated, fat, and guilty afterwards. This isn't genuine pleasure it's the short-term pleasure that all addiction seems to create. I used to smoke. I used to love the anticipation of having a cigarette, I used to like it when I first started smoking it but 99 percent of the time I would start to hate what I was doing even halfway through and I nearly always felt like crap afterwards. I experienced the same with certain junkie foods and the over consumption of them.

When it comes to the pleasure of drug-like foods it's all about image and about creating false physical hungers. Whatever the ad, they are selling a pleasurable situation, like having a hot bath in luxurious surroundings for example, and linking it to their product. And they are also selling a lifestyle. I just don't think the Flake ad would have had the same impact if the bath was one of those stuck in the corner of a very small bathroom in a council flat and the woman getting into it was 200 lb (90 kg) in weight. Is it possible that your image of the Flake would have been different if it were? How many would they have sold then? Imagine the window cleaner in the Diet Coke ad with a huge beer gut, builder's bum and a pair of bifocals on; all the women with bums the size of the Napa valley, dribbling over their birds-eye view of *his* amazing breasts. Once again do you think our image of these products would be different to what they are? Slightly.

HOOKED ON AN ILLUSION

These adverts are selling two illusions of pleasure. One is the image portrayed on screen; the other is the physical reaction you feel when you first put these drug-like foods into your body. The truth is, no matter how much these drug-like foods are dressed up, they never quite live up to our expectations. I always used to love the idea of eating rubbish foods, but the reality was never quite what I had in mind. This is because often what I had in my mind had actually been subconsciously planted there by some external image I had seen.

We are far from blameless when it comes to advertising either – we do it to ourselves. We often help the advertisers by creating images of wonderful situations in our minds, then we link some junk or drug food to it. Images such as vegging out watching a video with a tub of ice cream; eating a pizza while playing a board game with friends; or joining your friends for a dessert. But these situations are not enhanced by the foods.

Let me ask you a question. Have you ever been eating ice cream while watching a video and been happy at the same time? Yes, I should imagine is the answer. But have you also ever been watching a video while eating ice cream and been bored and miserable? Again I imagine the answer is yes. So what's changed? The ice cream is still the same, it's the particular video and how you are looking at your world that causes your feelings to change – not the ice cream. The situation is not suddenly transformed for the better because you've had some ice cream, very often it is transformed for the worse.

Drug-like foods and drinks do not make us genuinely happy – situations and certain people all help to make us happy. It's just that when people are forced to be without certain foods and drinks (i.e. when they're on a diet) they're miserable due to the belief they are genuinely missing out on something. The conclusion therefore is: miserable without and happier with. Many overweight people say, 'I like eating this way. I'm happy eating this way. I'm fat and I'm happy'. What they really mean is I am happier than when I'm on a diet. And, yes, they are, because diets can be living hell. But these people are still nowhere near as happy as someone who *isn't* experiencing the mental and physical false highs and genuine lows of being rooted in the food and diet trap.

IT'S NOT ABOUT THE TASTE EITHER

It is also easy to believe we consume certain foods simply because we love the taste and it's the taste alone that keeps us coming back for more and more. However, people really don't put up with the massive chance of heart attacks, strokes, diabetes, the constant mental and physical nightmare of being overweight simply because they like the taste of things. I used to have a compulsion to smoke cigarettes, but was the compulsion due to the wonderful taste of cigarettes? I never ate one of them. The only reason I smoked was because I was mentally hooked on what I thought a cigarette did for me and I was fearful of letting go. I felt insecure because of the cigarettes yet they appeared to make me feel more secure, giving the false impression that I couldn't live without them. We are more easily fooled with **FOOD** because unlike cigarettes, they do actually taste good. But no matter how good any food tastes, it is easy to have no desire to go near it when you strip it bare and see it for what it is.

For example, if I gave you a grilled steak and fries, which to you tasted absolutely delicious, and as you were eating them I told you the burger was made from dead cockroaches found on the kitchen floor, and the fries were in fact dried up crushed toenail clippings with added salt, would you carry on eating eat them? Clearly not and neither would

I. The point is no matter how wonderful the taste is, it would never be enough to override the knowledge you have learned about your burger and fries. I also love the taste of bananas, but if it was revealed that bananas caused obesity, heart disease, cancer, and psoriasis, it would be easy for me to stop eating them. I also love sardines, but again if a doctor told me they cause all kinds of medical problems, I wouldn't have any trouble never eating them again. Not only would I find it easy to stop eating them, but having been covered from head to foot in psoriasis and also overweight to go with it (nice), I would have loved the fact they have found the cause of my problem. However, when it comes to 'emotive' drug-like foods, the situation is different. This is why even when people know their diet is killing them, they still have a compulsion to eat and drink the foods which are slowly destroying them. Because they cannot rationalise why they continue to do it in spite of this knowledge, people have no choice other than to find reasons to justify their actions – not only to other people but also to themselves. One of the 'reasons' we use to try and justify our irrational actions is that we love the taste and can't resist it. But what I am trying to illustrate is that it is not the taste which compels us to carry on digging our graves with our teeth, in the same way it is not taste that encourages smokers to carry on smoking. There is an irrational emotional pull that keeps us trapped in the same way an irrational emotional pull keeps people in abusive relationships they would rather be free from. My definition of addiction is a simple one:

if The Thought Of Never Doing 'iT' Again Fills You With An Unnatural Fear You Are Hooked – if iT Doesn't You Aren't

I would be *disappointed* if I were told I couldn't eat bananas again, as I genuinely love them, but I wouldn't be *fearful*. The same would apply to sardines, apples, whole rice, fish. However, years ago if someone had said no more refined sugar, salt or fat at all for the rest of your life I would have felt fear. The fear I couldn't enjoy or cope with my life the same way without them. If you think about not having a certain food in your life and you suddenly feel your stomach falling through your pants – you are hooked. This hook has nothing whatsoever to do with taste and this really does require an open mind to see this aspect clearly.

Nature has designed things so that the hungrier we become the better all food will taste. **BiG FOOD** have cleverly played on this by creating additional intense hungers enhancing the flavour. On top of this we also need to understand that **BiG FOOD** employ 'flavourists'. These are companies who have the technology to make anything taste like anything. They can even make a table leg taste of chocolate if they wanted. Taste, like so many aspects of the drug-food industry, is a science in itself designed to confuse you even further.

> **There is real pleasure in ending a genuine hunger — this totally satisfies the mind and body. There is false, *short-term* illusory pleasure in trying to end a false physical and mental hunger, which in turn creates long-term pain.**

The short and long-term pain these types of food create becomes part of the trap. One of the first things I would do when I felt down or depressed was head straight for the fridge for a little 'pick me up'. But the more 'pick me ups' I ate the more down I would feel. The further 'down' I became the more I would try use 'food' to 'lift' me. I would carry on with what I call the ultimate 'Oh F*** it' mood. 'I've started so what the hell, I've done it now, I may as well just carry on.' But why did I head for the fridge in the first place? I wasn't genuinely physically hungry. I used to head for the fridge when I felt down for one reason – I honestly thought, whether consciously or subconsciously, that I could change the way I felt by eating some food. And all the advertisers are constantly perpetuating this belief. They really do give the impression that you can …

13

CHANGE YOUR MOOD BY EATING SOME FOOD

We are the only creatures on the planet who eat food to try to change the way we feel. This would be fine if it worked, but it clearly doesn't and as this is one of the major reasons people overeat, it is imperative we cover it.

If you try and feed any kind of emotion with any type of food you will, of course, create problems. This is because the body neither wants nor needs food at these times. Usually – depending obviously on the person – whatever you eat when you are not genuinely physically hungry will be stored as fat. I want to repeat that:

Whatever you eat when you are not *genuinely* physically hungry will be stored as fat

It was always meant to – it's the body's incredible survival mechanism kicking in. It assumes you are loading up on food, not because you are stressed or bored, but because you sense lean times ahead and have no choice. If there is going to be a shortage soon, the body wants to make certain it's going to survive and so stores the excess food in new, specially made, fat cells. This principle applies even if it's natural foods but, having said that, how many people reach for natural food when trying to feed an emotion? People often say they eat as a response to emotion, but what they really mean is that they eat *certain things* as a response to emotion. I mean when was the last time you heard anyone saying, 'I'm really p***ed off, sod it I'm going to treat myself to a bunch of grapes'? Not in this lifetime that's for sure!

People who eat to try to feed an emotion don't usually reach for grapes or strawberries; they reach for chocolate, cakes, fast foods, and ice cream. Why? Because these are drug-like foods and people turn to them in exactly the same way as a smoker turns to a cigarette in times of emotional void. But what people fail to realize is that a huge part of the empty insecure void feeling is caused by the very foods we are eating in an attempt to fill it.

Hunger is an empty insecure feeling. The hungrier we feel the larger the insecure feeling. This empty insecure void feeling is identical to normal emotional feelings we have such as fear, stress, boredom, and loneliness. If we are bored and we have an empty false hunger, the over-all boredom feeling appears greater. Because when we give ourselves a drug-food hit, it lessens the false empty hunger feeling. This in turn reduces the overall empty feeling and the illusion is created that we have somehow reduced a genuine emotional feeling. A person on the sugar rollercoaster will always feel more of a void than someone who isn't. This is why, come any emotional need, they will reach for a food hit. The overall feeling is reduced and it once again compounds the illusion that certain foods help certain emotions. The reality of course is that no food on earth can possibly help a genuine emotional need, which is why even after someone has 'indulged', they soon start to feel the same level of genuine emotion again. I say the same level, but after a binge they will feel even worse.

At the same time – in adverts, films, TV shows and in everyday life – we see other people feeding emotions with drug-like foods and drinks and so strongly believe there is something genuine in it. You don't see people like Rachel from *Friends* trying to comfort herself with a bowl of cherries, do you? No, she has a big bag of crisps or a tub of ice cream to help drown her sorrows. We think, 'if it helps Rachel, it'll help me'. Then we have advertisers bombarding us with a million different images showing how all we have to do is eat this particular food and we can change our mood.

The irony is that eating the wrong kind of food helps to cause the change in your mood

Many people are aware that food cannot change an emotion, yet they still reach for refined sugar and fat foods when feeling down. However, halfway through eating whatever it is they are using to try and 'feed' their emotion, they will feel even worse than they did, wonder why on earth they are doing it, and want to turn the clock back to the point just before they ate it. I know I did on many occasions. The problem is that initially – for the first couple of bites at least – these 'foods' do make us feel better than we did a moment previously. Why is this? Partly because we have just injected a dose of refined sugar and fat into our empty bloodstream, but also because we have told ourselves we will feel better with some food. If I told myself I would feel better if I had a beach-ball and I honestly believed it would be of benefit, then in the moment someone handed it to me, as strange as it may seem, I would actually feel better – for a second at least. It's a bit like the security blanket for a child; the blanket doesn't make them feel better, they just feel mentally low when it's taken away. The reason for this is a belief about what it represents. They clearly aren't suffering from 'genuine physical blanket withdrawal', yet they will have the same emotional trauma as someone on a diet or trying to stop smoking. This illustrates beautifully that it is not the physical aspect of most addiction that is the problem, contrary to popular belief, but simply an emotional mental tantrum. Remove the tantrum and the whole process becomes extremely easy.

I'M BORED

One of the most common excuses given for emotional eating is the one of boredom. I used to be the first to say this. But this excuse would never wash in the wild. Imagine you see a very large overweight squirrel stuffing nut after nut into its mouth and ask it 'Why are you doing that?' Now imagine it giving the answer 'I'm bored out of my head! I've been in the same park for years, seeing the same people every day. There's nothing else to do apart from eat. It fills the day.' What would you think? That's right, 'Stone me a talking squirrel!'

Seriously though, the point is this scenario sounds so stupid because you would never see a squirrel, or any other wild animal for that matter, eating for any reason other than hunger. If you could communicate and asked any wild animal why were they eating they would clearly reply, 'Because I'm hungry and I need to survive'. Ask the average human the same question and they can come up with a billion excuses, not genuine rational reasons. After all, the only rational reason is to end a genuine hunger.

I watched a documentary some time ago on attitudes to eating in different cultures. They asked one 12-year-old boy from the East, 'Why are you eating rice and vegetables?' He replied, 'Good for the heart, good for the mind and good for the soul'. Wow and he was only twelve. They then asked a 12-year-old kid from the States why he was eating a hamburger and fries: his reply was 'Hell man, it's 12 o'clock'.

I no longer care what the clock says. If I am not hungry why should I eat just because I have been conditioned to eat at certain times? If I go dancing for hours late at night I will sweat and build up an appetite, so I'll eat. I don't care who says you shouldn't eat at 3 a.m. If I am genuinely hungry at 3 a.m. I will eat.

In order to be slim for life we have to be honest with ourselves. If you are sitting indoors by yourself and you're bored out of your head, the situation will not alter if you have a chocolate bar in your hand – you will still be bored. When I was a child and I was bored, my mother would never say 'Oh, go and stuff your face, that will solve your boredom', she would say, 'go and do something'. Why did this always work? Because boredom is caused by an emptiness in your life, a momentary void while you think of something to do. Boredom itself is not the cause of why people overeat or eat the wrong types of foods. Neither is stress, loneliness or depression. The cause is the belief that you can dispel negative emotions with food. Without that belief you won't eat when you bored, stressed, lonely or depressed. For the same reason you would probably never take heroin when you're stressed or bored. For not only do you know it would not solve the problem, you are well aware it would result in a living nightmare. The fact is many people are going through a living nightmare every day because of drug-like foods.

If you are bored it is not a sign you are low on chocolate or that you have a burger, fries, and cake deficiency. It simply means you need to do something. Instead of eating you need to look for something that will genuinely fill these moments.

BACK TO FRONT

The truth is not only do these foods fail to do what we think on the emotional front, but they do the complete opposite. They are often the very reason why you feel bored, tired, stressed and in the mood where you can't be bothered to do anything. The irony is we attempt to use this type of food to improve our mood, yet often our mood is a direct result of the food itself. When I used to smoke I would say, 'I smoke because I'm stressed' – it never dawned on me that I was stressed because I smoked.

The point is this – refined sugars, salt, and fats affect the central nervous system causing feelings of irritability, restlessness, low blood sugar, and emptiness. It puts stress on every organ in the body and helps to speed up the ageing process. The wrong type of fats clog up the arteries, cause blood cells to literally stick together and they starve the body of its life force – oxygen. There is no question that this will affect the way you feel on a daily basis. Just look at the many children you see in the supermarket screaming for their next sugar fix and tell me drug foods don't affect human behaviour. And let's not forget the effect of the 'E' numbers that are added to so many processed foods.

ARE YOU ON ONE MATEY?

Ever heard the expression 'Are you on one matey?' Well, it's a question often asked in clubs in reference to the drug Ecstasy – commonly known as just 'E'. But these aren't the 'E's I'm interested in. I'm talking about the many 'E' numbers found in products masquerading as 'foods'. These apparently harmless additives are anything but. The next time you see a child, or adult for that matter, acting hyper or strangely it may be worth asking them, 'Are you on one matey?' But which one? E102 perhaps, otherwise known as tartrazine, which is used in breadcrumbs to coat things like fish fingers and the like and has been closely linked to asthma and hyperactivity. Or how about E110 (Sunset Yellow FCF), a beautiful colouring used in many children's drinks, which has been linked to asthma and also eczema. Then it could be E220, which is no less than sulphur dioxide; or the little beauty E252 (potassium nitrate) which is no less than a fertilizer. Oh and let's not forget that they could be on ethylene bisdithiocarbamate, a fungicide used on potatoes and one which causes tumours and birth defects in laboratory animals. Is it possible that putting these things into the human body along with the sugars and salts, may affect the way we think and behave? It's not just possible – iT'S A FACT.

One deputy head teacher, Cherry Lazenby, completely banned sweets and fizzy drinks during break times at school because the children were becoming difficult to control and teach.

She said: 'Immediately after morning break and lunchtimes there is a difference in the children's behaviour. They are hyper, noisy, rowdy, and can't sit still or concentrate.' She goes on to say, 'Surveys have revealed that many pupils eat vast quantities of food with a high sugar content and with additives known to contribute to hyperactivity'. But again you don't need surveys or scientific research, just have a look you around at people's behaviour.

ANOTHER DOSE OF HYPERACTIVE DRUG FOOD

Yet despite growing evidence, people still don't seem willing to see the clear link between certain foods and behaviour. Children with ADHD (Attention Deficit Hyperactive Disorder), for instance, are being given drugs like Ritalin to try and calm them down – the problem is nothing to do with that can of soda, chocolate, crisps, E numbers etc. it appears, no, the child is clearly low on Ritalin. This drug is described as the 'chemical cosh' because of its ability to 'calm' hyper children. But it is said by many parents to simply turn their kids into zombies. You could inject some anaesthetic into the kids and get pretty much the same effect – but what does it do to treat the *cause*? I am not saying that all ADHD is caused by **BiG FOOD**, but there is just no question that when you consume foods that create all kinds of problems for the natural balance of the body it is going to have an impact on the natural balance of the mind. Why, in the twenty-first century, is the first 'answer' to any problem still to go the drug route? If I were sceptical I would say, **MONEY!** After all, you simply cannot patent fruits and vegetables.

There is no question that what we put into our bodies has an effect on every aspect of mental and physical health. The human body is a perfectly balanced, finely tuned machine which requires certain fuels to function correctly. You simply cannot keep pouring the wrong fuel in for years on end and not expect it to have a major impact on how we look, feel, and think. Despite the very obvious link between what we consume and our mental and physical health there are still many in the medical profession who adamantly deny any connection between what we eat and disease. We often hear that 'alternative' medicine and practitioners can be 'dangerous' with regard to some advice they give out. While this can be true with some, I believe what is more dangerous is people in the medical profession – the very people we trust and take what they say as read – refusing to accept that the food and drinks we consume are one of the biggest contributors to all degenerative disease. How can anyone with a degree of common sense not see that what we ingest will affect our entire biochemistry, including our behaviour. The amount of children being diagnosed with ADHD has gone into free fall and drugs are being given out like Smarties.

I would love to write an entire book just on children, food, and drugs, but we don't have time. The point of this chapter is to illustrate that you cannot feed an emotion with food and the illusion of short-term emotional change is just that – an illusion. In order to break totally free there are many more illusions and untruths we need to explode. How to break free comes later in the book and once you have the right mental instructions you will be amazed at not only how easy it can be, but you will be kicking yourself you didn't see it for yourself years ago.

Let us continue our journey with perhaps the most reached-for drug-like food in times of emotional need. It is arguably one of the most falsely advertised drug-like foods out there – a product that people have been totally conditioned to believe will change the way they feel: a real mood food. This one may not apply to you, but read the next chapter nonetheless as it illustrates many vital points. However, I have been in this business for years and no other junkie food seems to create as much emotive response as this one. If you want true freedom it's time to say …

14

CHOCS AWAY!

Now there are people who eat chocolate here and there, and there are those whose life seems to revolve around it. If you are a true die-hard choc-head then this little chapter may not cut the nougat. For a much more in-depth look at chocolate and the industry in general, get hold of a copy of my other book, *The Simple Way To Stop Eating Chocolate*. However, I will do my level best to make you see the light here.

Before we get into all the conditioning, advertising, and misinformation that surrounds **BiG CHOCOLATE**, let's just look at what it is. Chocolate, as we know it, does not naturally grow on trees, it is a man-made substance. People sometimes argue that cocoa (one of the main ingredients of chocolate) is natural, but you could carry that way of thinking as far as you like – after all heroin is natural and so too is tobacco. What I am saying is that the combination of cocoa, sugar, fat, milk, and chemicals is not natural.

Have you ever actually tasted unsweetened cocoa? Take my word for it, it tastes revolting. What makes it taste so disgusting is a naturally occurring drug-like substance found in cocoa called theobromine. Although this chemical is found in all chocolate, the darker the chocolate the more it will contain. Theobromine, like any substance which has addictive qualities, can cause an unnatural desire or need for more. This is often why when you think about having 'just the one' chocolate you will often continue to eat more, even if you start to feel bloated and sick.

Theobromine tastes incredibly bitter, so how on earth did they ever get so many people to eat it? It is true that there are a few people who like raw unsweetened cocoa, but they are few and far between. The vast majority find the taste incredibly bitter. The only way to make it palatable is to add in plenty of the cocaine of the food world – refined sugar. The sugar not only gives a hit of pure glucose to the bloodstream, but it also covers the bitter taste of the theobromine. When you eat mass-produced chocolate you are effectively getting two addictive drug-like substances in one – theobromine and refined sugar. However, these two aren't the only poisonous drug-like substances found in mass market chocolate. Trans Fats and HFCS (High Fructose Corn Syrup) have also found their way into some over the years. Then you have skimmed milk powder, fat-reduced cocoa milk, more fat, malt extract, full cream milk powder, refined salt, lactose, whey powder, egg white, milk protein, flavouring, biscuit, yeast, crisped cereal, colourings (E171, E120, E101, E160, E133), glazing agents, butter fat, lecithin – plus many more I have undoubtedly missed. These ingredients came from the wrapper of just one mass-market chocolate bar.

I have already mentioned Trans Fats, or 'hydrogenated oil' as it is often listed as, in the 'fat' chapter. However, I cannot repeat enough how harmful this type of fat can be. It is banned in some parts of the world and not surprisingly as it can be deadly. When hydrogenated fat enters your system it literally eats holes in your blood vessels. You may not see 'hydrogenated fat/oil' on the label of some mass-market chocolate bars – instead they may put the less threatening, 'trans-fatty acids' or 'partially hydrogenated', but if the name seems less threatening it doesn't make the fat any less so.

For years the harmful effects of this type of oil have been common knowledge to the people in the know. Hydrogenated oil or 'Trans Fats' can easily create a build-up of LDL cholesterol (the bad one), the small LDL molecules squeezing beneath the blood vessel linings, narrowing the passageways with a layer of 'plaque'. The process of hydrogenating fats creates molecules which are forced into shapes that were never designed to fit in the human body and they have been found to be a major cause of heart disease and cancer. In fact, just so we know what we're dealing with here, this kind of fat is so harmful that US government experts have declared 'there is no safe level of consumption'. In light of this Mars and Nestlé made newspaper headlines in 2003 when they announced to the British people they were removing 'Trans Fats' from some of their chocolate bars. But, please don't be deluded into thinking that whatever replacement fat they have in mind will be health in a wrapper. Always remember it took many years before Trans Fats were seen in their true light, so don't be surprised if the replacement fat hits the headlines at some point in the future.

Then, of course, we have the milk products. One chocolate bar manufacturer even bragged 'A pint and a half of pure cream milk goes into every bar'. A few years ago I would have thought that was good, but that was in the days when I thought for some reason we had the same digestive system as a calf. Am I now suggesting that milk is a drug-like food? No. But it is not the extremely healthy food we have been totally conditioned to believe it is, which I will cover in full very soon. There are also reports of other nasties in chocolate. A leading homeopathic practitioner was overheard at a seminar saying, 'Keeping cockroaches at bay is such a problem in some chocolate factories that by law there can be up to 6 per cent of crushed cockroaches in all chocolates. They sometimes fall unnoticed into the mixtures.' Now this has the distinct ring of urban myth about it, as it is completely untrue and chocolate factories are in reality some of the cleanest places on earth. However, just the thought is enough to put some people off.

AD CHOC

As well as the detrimental addictive ingredients within mass-market chocolate, we have the massive amount of advertising dedicated to promoting chocolate as a mood enhancer and often even a 'health' food. They have managed to create a set of 'bells' for virtually any occasion. Chocolate is seen as the ultimate treat and the ultimate mood food.

'A Mars a day helps you work, rest, and play'

This is one of the most well known slogans for chocolate and it has been so drummed into us for so many years we don't question the absurdity of it. How can a mass market chocolate bar containing refined sugar, fats, salt and other rubbish, help anyone to work, rest, and play? Aren't they contradictions of one another anyway? How can the same food help to act as a stimulant (work or play) and as a relaxant (rest)? I found out recently that someone actually took Mars to court over their 'it helps you work, rest, and play' slogan. Guess what? Mars won – I'd love to know how they proved their slogan to be true.

Virtually every chocolate bar ad is either aimed at children (get them hooked while they're young), or has an emotion linked to it – a way of supposedly helping you out in times of emptiness. A Bounty Bar will supposedly take you to paradise; a Twix will apparently help you escape 'the norm' (that little grey git). You can take time out with a chocolate bar that is actually named Time Out. You can also have a break with a Kit Kat or give yourself a boost with a bar called Boost, or you can be a real man with a Yorkie Bar. When I now see these ads it makes me wonder why I didn't see just how stupid they were.

The sheer audacity of some of the chocolate ads never ceases to amaze me. I remember years ago watching an ad for an Aero bar that featured a woman sitting behind a desk, clearly bored out of her head. Looking for something to do to ease her boredom she reaches for an Aero. As soon as she takes a bite her whole face lights up, sparks fly from her mouth and a gospel choir comes out of nowhere. Everyone's clapping, smiling, happy, and singing the tune of 'Why can't all chocolate feel this way?'. Because of course that is precisely what happens when you eat an Aero bar isn't it? In reality, the woman would be sitting behind her desk bored out of her head, reach for the Aero and while eating would still be totally bored out of her head. Why? Because her problem is not caused by a lack of chocolate, therefore it will not be solved with some. She has a good job deficiency. The advertisers, however, are creating a bell on a subconscious level – and it works.

The truth is this approach has worked so well for chocolate that most people give this stuff to their friends and loved ones as a way of saying 'Thank You' or 'I Love You'. Think of the Cadbury's Roses advert. It's all about people doing nice things for people and getting rewarded with this particular box of chocolates. They show this over and over again along with a catchy tune 'Thank you very much for doing the dishes, thank you very much, thank you very, very, very much'. In the end when you think of a good way of saying thank you, you will think of their product. They have managed to get people to say thank you with a product which is known to be addictive, clogs the arteries, makes people feel mentally low and contributes massively to weight gain. Thank you very much indeed.

Chocolate is now linked to so many days and times of the year: Mother's day, Father's day, Valentine's day – any day, in fact, seems like a good day. Easter to most people now simply means chocolate eggs. When I was a child, up until about the age of ten or eleven, there would always be a stocking full of delicious, wonderful-tasting fruit and nuts on the end of my bed on Christmas morning. I cannot recall exactly what year it changed, but it soon became the norm to have a stocking stuffed with chocolate. So strong is the conditioning with this stuff that some people even give it to sick people while they are lying in hospital. There are others who go as far as to believe chocolate is better than sex, if you truly believe that there is only one thing you need to do – change your partner!

I read an article with disbelief recently in which a psychologist said, 'Eating chocolate has a calming effect and helps us deal with stress'.

Her theory is based on her observation that 'people tend to feel calmer after eating chocolate and high fat meals. It is suspected that it is chocolate's combination of sweet creamy texture and high fat that makes it irresistible'. First of all, who feels calmer? Those who are suffering the irritable effects of low blood sugar? Just a thought. And what about the high stimulants contained within chocolate – are they suggesting that a stimulant relaxes you?

COMPLETELY POTTY

Even famous children's stories are not immune to the pervasive idea that chocolate is some kind of mood enhancing food. *Charlie And The Chocolate Factory* is an obvious case but it is certainly not an isolated one. In the third Harry Potter book we see chocolate being used as a comforter; literally an aid to help you get back to normal after all your happiness has been sucked away by the evil 'Dementors'. I know this is only a story, but why couldn't the author have used some bright, delicious fruit instead? We all come into contact with our own versions of Dementors every day and the people who make chocolate want you to think that if someone or something drains your happiness it can all be solved with a bar or box of fat-, sugar-, and theobromine-loaded chocolate.

The truth is that you really are on a hiding to nothing with mass market chocolate. The minute you have some, you either have to have more or you have to use your control to stop yourself eating more. Either way you tend to be onto a loser.

I agree that what's deemed as good quality dark chocolate is often different, but **BiG CHOCOLATE** is my main focus here and that's the heavily sugared chocolate bars and boxes. It's worth knowing know that even when you see 60 per cent cocoa bars, it can still mean 30 per cent sugar and even if you do get 'good quality' high cocoa dark chocolate it means a higher concentration of theobromine – the stimulant which, when given to dogs, has the potential to kill them. (Please never give dark chocolate to your dog!) With dark chocolate though, despite the high theobromine content, because it is so rich, rarely do people have the same compulsion to eat as much as they do with high sugared mass market chocolate.

Many people consciously realize that you cannot eat food to change your mood and that food cannot feed you emotionally. However, one of the biggest arguments is that unlike smoking, eating is extremely sociable. It is almost impossible to argue against the fact that it is very sociable to eat genuine food and end a genuine hunger with genuine people. But it is not sociable to eat drug-like foods with people just to try to be sociable, and anyone who genuinely believes that it is, is totally …

15

OUT TO LUNCH

If you are going to have a dessert at a restaurant, what is the first thing you tend to do? Usually you ask anybody else if they wish to 'join you'. If everyone declines, you will use whatever persuasive powers you have in order to tempt as many people as you can to have some. You become a sales person for **BiG DRUG FOOD.** 'Oh go on. You only live once. They do a mouth-watering hot fudge cake covered in fresh cream. What do you think? Changed your mind?' Sometimes those people who are incredibly desperate for someone to join them will verbally try to bully someone into joining them. 'Oh what's wrong with you, you boring git. You used to be fun. Stop being so unsociable, lighten up'. But at what point do people stop being sociable just because they aren't shoving sugar and fat down their throat? How do people stop being fun? All they are saying is that they don't want some refined fat and sugar.

The reason why people say such things is simply due to the fact that we all, on some level, feel odd eating rubbish foods alone. After all, you don't get this nonsense with peaches or sardines do you? To be 'sociable' is, 'to act in a sociable manner, mix socially with others'. But by simply *not* shoving sugar and fat in your mouth, how does that make you all of a sudden unsociable? How can it make someone unsociable if they are still out at dinner with friends and still chatting?

When you change your diet it doesn't mean for one second you stop going out for meals with friends or hold dinner parties. That's the mind-set of someone who goes 'on a diet', not someone who successfully 'changes their diet'.

Personally, I love going out for meals, especially with a group of people. Often a whole evening can be centred around the food, as it is in many different cultures. There are many cultures that take hours and hours over a meal. Guests are served small courses and gradually feed themselves in-between having a great social experience. But being sociable and ending a hunger are two separate entities. If you happen to be genuinely physically hungry and you go to dinner with a group of nice and fun people, then you have two pleasures at once. You satisfy a genuine physical hunger, which makes you feel wonderful, plus you are with your friends and therefore satisfying your need for interaction and fun.

If, however, the people you are sitting next to happen to be Mr and Mrs Dull who have come all the way from Dullsville for your lack of entertainment tonight, then all the sticky dessert in the world isn't going to make any difference – they will still be dull. Refined sugar and fat does not make an evening, it's the people and the interaction that do.

The irony is that people who are caught in the food and diet trap spend most of their time being unsociable because of their concerns about food. I used to avoid 'doing lunch' at times because I was trying to control my intake of food. Being fat and paranoid about my body also meant I would avoid social events such as swimming, going to the beach with friends and dancing. I was just too tired and too lethargic and often suffered from the 'I can't be bothered' syndrome. When you are on virtually any kind of diet you are completely unsociable and when you do eat you feel so lethargic you can't be bothered to be sociable.

You will be more sociable when you feel more alive, fitter, and healthier. Your confidence will return to such a degree that you'll wonder how you ever managed to get by before; your nervous system will be functioning properly; your sugar levels will be balanced – and there'll be no more false hungers. You'll have more energy and you'll never feel deprived as you will have *genuine* freedom of choice.

On the physical side, it is incredibly easy to either shift those unwanted bulges and/or tap into a new lease of genuine energy. The truth is no one is fat – just toxic. If you carry excess weight you simply have stored poison around your body. Your body can do one of only two things with toxins: store them or get rid of them – it cannot use them. If the body does not have enough energy to get rid of them it will store them. And where does it tend to store excess waste for most people? **FAT CELLS.** It takes energy to shift excess weight and clean you out. Your body at this time simply doesn't have the energy to do this. It spends most of its energy and time trying to digest, use, and store the junkie foods you are putting into your system.

As mentioned at the start of this book I read many, many books on health and nutrition, all explaining the physical side of things very well. The problem was they contradicted one another and not one single book I read ever mentioned the tremendous physical and psychological benefits of …

16

FAST FOOD

Yes, fast food is the secret key to health, a slim body, clear skin, longevity, and tremendous amounts of pure energy. I forgive you if you think I have lost leave of my senses, I must stress that your idea of fast food and mine will be completely different at this stage.

The problem is that when I say 'fast food' the first thing that springs to mind for most people are drug-like foods such as: KFC, Pizza Hut, McDonald's, Burger King etc. That is because we talk about how fast the food gets to us. And **BiG FAST FOOD** are certainly very good at getting the food to us **ASAP.** In the 1980s McDonald's ran an advertising campaign claiming if you stopped your car at traffic lights it gave you enough time to pick up a 'meal' from their 'restaurant' and be back in the car before the lights had changed. Now that is fast – *super fast.* However, what most people don't realize is that the minute this stuff hits your stomach and digestive tract it ceases to be fast.

BiG 'FAST' FOOD *slowly* clogs up your arteries with refined fat; *slowly* fills your bloodstream with insulin as a response to excess refined sugar; *slowly* overworks every organ in your body; *slowly* drains you of genuine energy; *slowly* but very surely stores fat; *slowly* speeds up the ageing process; *slowly* uses up valuable nerve energy; *slowly* causes your red blood cells to stick together and *slowly* starves the cells in your body. This is not *fast* food.

The only thing this type of fast food does quickly is to rapidly raise blood sugar levels. It often boosts them to such an uncomfortable and abnormal level that your body has to use up some of its insulin bank account – fast. As the insulin quickly transports the excess sugars in the blood to various storage areas in the body, you soon start to feel the effects of *low blood sugar*. How do we try to solve that little problem? And so the loop goes on and on.

Nearly all of the **BiG FAST FOOD** chains are peddling drug-like foods. Like any drug the body builds up an immunity and tolerance to the drug which means the person needs more and more to get the same 'effect'. This is why people may start with just one cigarette a week and before they know where they are they are soon on twenty a day. The same applies with drug-like foods. This is why over the years we have seen **FAST FOOD** portions getting bigger and bigger to even the now famous **SUPER SIZE.** The bigger the portions the bigger the need and the spiral, like any drug spiral, continues to grow. **BiG TOBACCO** have rightly had a hammering over the years for peddling their wares under false pretences. **BiG FAST FOOD** have yet to have the hammering they deserve, but with the wrong kinds of food killing more people than all drugs on the planet combined, I feel we will be seeing lawsuits similar to those aimed at **BiG TOBACCO.** The argument of course, as it was with cigarettes, is, 'people know the facts and if they continue to choose to overeat on junk food then it's their choice'. But as I will continue to point out throughout this book, genuine choice goes out of the window when we are talking about addiction of any kind.

HALF TON HOSPITAL

There is a hospital in the US known as Half Ton Hospital. You may have already guessed it is home to people with severe weight issues, usually to the tune of over 50 stone (317 kg) in weight. This hospital illustrates the level of addiction to **BiG FAST FOOD** more than any other. Despite the fact these people are removed from their houses with mini cranes and are knocking on death's door, they still continue to eat **BiG FOOD**. One man, who was lying in the hospital weighing in at 52 stone (330 kg), used his bedside phone to call Pizza Hut for a delivery to his bed. This isn't a man who simply likes the taste of pizza, it's a clear addiction. The 'food' he is ordering is not genuine food, it's **DRUG FOOD** and it is killing this man both physically and mentally.

A Channel 4 programme entitled *Half Ton Woman*, followed the story of Renee Williams, who was at the time 'the world's largest woman' – she was nearly 70 stone (444 kg). 'When you don't have that thing in your head that tells you you're full, it's disgusting the amount of food you can eat', she said. But the thing in her head which is not telling her she is full, is in fact the thing in her body. It is the lack of genuine nutrients making the body scream for food and the drug-like compulsion of excess refined sugars and fats. Unfortunately she passed away, but her frustration of not feeling genuinely full fast enough is felt, to a greater or lesser degree, by many millions. The main cause of her problem was not her genes, but **BiG FAST FOOD**. These companies, just like **BiG TOBACCO**, should be brought to book. Renee Williams didn't choose to continue to eat the food that was killing her, she was heavily addicted to highly addictive 'food'. If she had genuine freedom of choice, she would have chosen to eat nothing but fruit and vegetables until she was well.

COMA FOOD

Clearly not everyone who is overweight consumes **BiG FAST DRUG FOOD**. In fact, it is safe to say there are many who would never venture into a place like McDonald's even if it was the last place to eat on earth. However, they do consume **BiG FOOD,** and often plenty of it. The effects of malnutrition and the drug-like reaction from what could be described as *mild* drug food found in many 'normal' foods, compels most people to consume more food than they ever actually need. The average person will consume over 75 tons (75,000 kg) of food in their lifetime – that's

75 tons of food! It is worth knowing that it requires more energy to digest, extract the nutrients and dispose of the wastes of the wrong kind of foods than anything else you will do. Burdening our stomachs and digestive systems with too much food on a consistent basis puts a strain on every organ and leaves no energy or time for the removal of toxicity (including excess fat) in the body. Too much food is also the biggest cause of premature death in the western world and many people completely underestimate the effect excess food consumption has on their health.

It is essential to fully understand that nothing will even come close to the amount of energy you will use up trying to deal with excess food. To add some perspective to this, even running the marathon will not take up the same level of nerve energy as having to deal with excess food consumption. I realize that sounds unbelievable, but think about it. Running a marathon is tough. Actually after running the New York marathon in 2007, I can say 'tough' doesn't even come close – 26 miles (42 km) of sheer endurance, endeavour, and incredible mental focus. If you interview someone after they have run the marathon they are of course very tired and very short of breath, but the point I wish to make is they are still awake. However, try interviewing someone after they have finished a large Christmas dinner, always a bit tricky because most people have usually 'nodded off'.

Do you know why people fall asleep after a big meal? There is so much processed food going into the body at once that it simply doesn't have the nerve energy to cope. It then looks for every available resource of energy in order to try and break down the junk, extract whatever it can from it, get rid of whatever it can and then store what it can't get rid of (usually in fat cells). In short –

The body does not have enough energy to keep you alive and awake at the same time

This means that if you fall asleep after a big meal you are effectively in a coma. That is what happens when your body has to cut off eyesight, hearing, and consciousness in order to try and muster the energy to deal with the nightmare amount of *different* processed foods that have dropped into the stomach all at once. The human body was never designed to deal with so many different processed foods; it requires natural live foods. I think you don't need a degree in nutrition to realize that if a digestive system which was designed to cope with high water content foods like fruits and vegetables, had to deal with huge amounts of heavily processed foods, it would struggle. You need to understand that when you overeat to the extent you have that sleepy bloated feeling, your system goes into a 'red alert' situation. The stomach desperately tries to break it all down before passing it onto the 30 ft (9 m) worth of very bendy intestinal tract. After something as heavy as the usual Christmas dinner the body will provide just enough energy for you to open your eyes, turn the pages of your TV guide and press the buttons on the remote control. But that's all the energy you're getting as it still has to deal with all the many courses of slow food you have just consumed.

I realize that Christmas dinner is a once-a-year thing, but it does help to illustrate the point. If we think about it, it's not just Christmas dinner that makes us tired and sluggish. I often used to get very tired after eating a big meal in the evening, but I put it down to a hard day catching up with me and not the huge amounts of incredibly difficult-to-digest food I had consumed. But what excuse did I have for falling asleep after Sunday lunch? Was it because I was having a tough day then? The day had hardly started. The reason I felt tired after a Sunday or Christmas lunch was because the food I had eaten was very hard for my *already* tired and battered digestive system to deal with, and so it took the energy it needed from other departments. You need to realize that every single department in the entire body will suffer in the long run if you keep doing this. To use an analogy, if one person in a company is having to do the workload of two or three, and at the same time does not even have the correct tools to work with (i.e. live nutrients in this case), they will not be able to cope for very long and soon the whole company suffers. With all the will in the world if you have too much work for the time allocated it cannot be done and you will have to leave the work to one side (fat cells usually) in the hope that there will be some 'let up' so you can deal with it later. Your body is the same. The question is when will later be?

How's Your Health Account?

The human body will do anything it can to survive regardless of how we abuse it. But no matter how incredible the machine, if you keep abusing on a consistent basis, the chances are it will give up on you. Every time you consume junkie type foods you are dipping into your health account. Like any account, the more we withdraw, the poorer we become. The only place we are ever truly rich is in the area of health; if you are rich financially but poor physically, you are ultimately poor. This is why it is so important to flush your mind of all the misinformation you have been subjected to about food and health, and take control of your own body and be in full control of your account. Unlike a money bank account, it is not always easy to see what's truly happening. Many people look fine on the outside, but are crumbling within. What springs to mind is the seemingly 'healthy' and fit-looking 40-year-old who dies of a heart attack on the tennis court. Looks are deceiving. I wonder how old his heart really was? He was forty but his heart might have done ninety years' worth of work.

If you really want a level of health and vitality you never dreamed possible, and the body of your dreams, you need to give your body a rest from this constant **BiG FOOD** abuse. What's needed is a brand new 'work-force' to come in and clean the rubbish out. The body was simply never designed to cope with the barrage of slow, hard-to-digest food that we consume on a daily basis. I am not saying that it cannot cope with this amount of food to some degree, because clearly it does. If the body is genuinely hungry it will digest almost anything – but only a certain amount of anything. However, if it is starved of life, and at the same time is asked to do more and more work with little or no tools, it will slowly crumble and everything you do will feel equivalent to climbing a mountain.

True Fast Food

As I mentioned at the start of this chapter, the human body was specifically designed with fast food in mind, and again I don't mean burgers and KFC. I mean foods that are *fast* for our systems to digest, fast for our systems to assimilate (taking what it needs for human function and growth) and fast for the system to eliminate. I am talking about real, genuine fast food – a set of foods that will quickly inject nutrients into every cell in your body, giving it a brand new workforce that is specifically designed to clear out excess fat and waste. A set of foods that contain massive amounts of what our body thrives on – water, which flushes out waste matter and keeps oxygen flowing in the system. Genuine foods that contain their own digestive enzymes, foods which keep you slim, and looking and feeling fantastic.

I will give you plenty of examples of genuine fast foods soon and I will explain what part they should play in a modern twenty-first century world. I will repeat that when you finish this book you will have the genuine choice to eat and drink what you want. This isn't about eating nothing but vegetables and tofu! In order to be slim and healthy for life also means being realistic and flexible for life. There will not be any food you can't have when you finish this book, but I am imagining there may be many you don't want to have.

However, before I arm you with a way of thinking that will set you free and enable you to change your diet and so slim in an extraordinarily easy way, there are a few more food myths we have to cover. Over the years we have been told many foods are good for us and some are bad. But what happens when the foods we have been told, often by officials, are not only good for us but vital for our survival, turn out to be not so good after all? There is one particular food which springs to mind that we have been completely brainwashed into believing is vital for our survival, but one which many don't realize can be ...

17

A MEATY PROBLEM

Meat – a problem? 'But it's full of iron, protein, vitamins, and minerals', you might say. 'It's the bedrock of any decent meal; it's what keeps us strong, healthy and bouncing with energy. What would Christmas or Sunday dinner be without the "bird" or a joint of meat? What about barbecues? What about pork crackling, rib-eye steak and, oh my God, what about bacon sarnies?'

The truth is, if you were to eliminate meat you would probably be a great deal healthier, you would most probably have more energy and you could still enjoy social occasions. However, and I wish to be very clear here, you don't have to stop eating meat altogether in order to be healthy. If the meat is of good quality (and you will know what that really means after this small chapter) you can easily continue to eat some meat after you read this book and still be healthy. However, there are a few things you may like to know about meat if your goal is a healthy and slim body.

Like most of the subjects in the book, an open mind is required here. Some people have such deep-rooted beliefs, often installed since early childhood, that they are unwilling to entertain the idea that meat could possibly be a bad thing. I fully understand this as I was one of them myself. For a few years I worked in a butcher's shop, my uncle's to be precise, but I was never a butcher (my uncle would be the first to agree with that). As you can imagine I had a pretty strong belief that meat was simply the best thing you could eat. I was constantly surrounded with posters which read 'Protein, vitamins, minerals, iron *and* two veg', 'Meat To Live', 'Lamb for Lovers' and the like. All this, of course, backed up everything my teachers, family, and even my doctor had told me ever since I could communicate. It seems we have all been somewhat hoodwinked for many years about the subject of meat. We have been conditioned to believe that unless you eat meat you will not get enough protein, be lacking in vitamin B12 and be weak and feeble. I would like to dispel a few of the myths, especially the ones about meat providing strength and energy.

Have you seen the size of an elephant? Would you say they are strong? They aren't just strong, they are *the* strongest land animal in the world. Have you any idea the amount of meat they eat to maintain the massive strength they have? None. That's a zero! Elephants don't eat any meat whatsoever and yet are one of the most powerful animals on earth. Even what are regarded by many as our closest living relatives, the great apes, only eat meat in emergencies and once again they are hardly built like Kate Moss. They are three times as heavy and thirty times as strong as the average human and yet their diet consists mainly of nature's fast food – fruit. Please also understand that the digestive system of an ape is still virtually identical to ours. If they do have to eat meat in order to stay alive – they eat it *raw* (this means it still contains enzymes and these help with digestion, assimilation, and disposal). You don't see a group of silverbacks cooking up a t-bone on the barbie now do you? So now you might be thinking 'raw – err how disgusting, we would never do that.' Exactly, that's the point. For most of us the thought of eating raw meat is disgusting – we have to cook it in order to try and make it edible. Even before it's cooked many meats have to be 'hung' for many days to try and make them tender in order to make them even remotely palatable for humans. If you tried to hang meat for a week in the wild someone would soon nick it!

Not only is the meat we eat not fresh; it is often very old. Any enzymes that may be left in it we totally destroy by cooking it. Please remember that when you cook anything above 118°F (48°C) – a temperature that is too low even to register on most cookers – you kill it. We were told for years that we should cook food in order to destroy all of the harmful bacteria and, yes, when you cook some foods, this is what you do. But what else do you think you might be killing at the same time? Most of the live nutrients. You simply can't destroy one without destroying the other. When I was growing up I had to live with my aunt for a year. She used to start cooking the Sunday dinner at about 9 a.m.! By the time the meal was served there was more nutrition left on the kitchen walls and ceiling than was left in the food. I now understand why food smells so good when it's cooking – it's all the goodness coming out.

Am I suggesting you eat raw meat? No. In order to make it remotely edible we do have to cook it (though some people do eat steak virtually raw). Am I suggesting you eat no meat at all? Again no, not unless you choose not to. What I will suggest, however, is that you follow a few guidelines. When natural omnivores eat meat, they do not eat it at the same time as other difficult-to-digest foods, and they don't eat it that often. They also do not have an already beaten-up digestive system and they eat tons of high-water-content 'live' foods that are packed with enzymes and energy. All of this enables them easily and comfortably to deal with the small amount of meat they do consume. It follows then that our bodies can easily cope with 'some' meat and there is no question, if we eat 'good quality' meat, we can also gain some good nutrition from it. The point I wish to get across is that although we *want* to have meat from time to time, despite what we have been completely brainwashed to believe, we don't *need* it for our survival.

A VERY SLOW FOOD

In terms of digestion, however, excess meat consumption really can be a problem. Meat is what I describe as a very slow food. It takes a great deal of nerve energy to digest and use the stuff. I have said that in order to shift stored fat and increase energy levels, you have to 'free up' energy in the body and at the same time supply oxygen and nutrients to your cells. Red meat, in particular, takes a great deal of time to digest, it is very slow to leave the stomach, very slow at getting through the intestinal tract and very slow to be eliminated. Red meat can be so hard for an already-tired system to fully eliminate that often it never fully leaves the body. This is not simply hearsay. It was reported that when the actor John Wayne died of colon cancer they found 14 lb (6.3 kg) of rotting flesh in his colon due to excess meat consumption. I am unsure how true that story is, but my father died of colon cancer and they found a similar amount in his colon after he died. It has been said that the average regular red meat eater will end up with anything from 2–16 lb (1–7 kg) of decaying flesh in their colon by the time they are 50.

When Ivan Pavlov, the famous 'bell' man, researched how long certain foods took to be digested he discovered that meat stays in the stomach for an average of four hours when it is eaten alone. This time is apparently more than doubled if you add a load of potato and Yorkshire pudding at the same time (more about combining foods in a moment). Now when I first heard that I thought 'so what?' Well it turns out that most fruit, salad, and vegetables only stays in the stomach for about 30–45 minutes, true fast food. Freshly extracted juice only take about 15 minutes. The reason meat is there for so long is because the body has to work hard trying to digest it before it passes through the intestines which takes another 20 hours. It finds the task difficult because we only have a tenth of the hydrochloric acid of natural carnivores. Hydrochloric acid is the acid the body uses to break down the toxins in meat. It seems fairly obvious that humans were not meant to deal with meat on a regular basis as we have such a small amount of the acid needed to digest meat properly. At the same time the saliva we produce is alkaline, yet the saliva of all carnivores is acid. We also have an incredibly long intestinal tract, while all meat eating animals in the wild have very short intestines. This enables the meat to pass through quickly to avoid putrefaction. Nature designed food for every creature to be as fast as possible. Meat is broken down a lot quicker if it's eaten at the same time as some high-water-content, nutrient-packed salad, vegetables or some fruits. The nutrients and enzymes help to digest it and the high water content helps to transport it through the body.

THE MEATY TRUTH

The truth is that meat is so far from what we would naturally eat that we even have to rename the stuff in order for most of us to eat it. When I worked at the butcher's shop, if someone came in and asked what I recommended for a barbecue I never said 'How about some pigs' heads that have been crushed, boned and minced with some added water, chemicals, rusk and encased in small tubes of pigs' intestines'. Somehow I don't think I would have sold too many if I had! No, I would say, 'How about some sausages'. Children have no idea what they are eating. Ask the average child where their bacon sandwich came from they will say Sainsbury's or Tesco. Somehow I don't think they would get as much joy if, while they were watching the film *Babe*, we broke the hard truth to them. Even the hard Gordon Ramsay (**YES CHEF!**) could barely bring himself to kill the pigs he reared at home on his *F Word* programme. His children weren't exactly ecstatic about it either. The same emotional dilemma doesn't seem to apply to yanking a 'living' apple from a tree, or even killing a fish for that matter (for most anyway).

MYSTERY FOOD

It wouldn't be so bad if we were eating organic 'grass fed' whole meats, but often the meat we are eating is not only not organic or whole but it's part of what I call the 'mystery' food group. Chicken burgers, beef burgers, chicken Kiev, chicken nuggets, sausages, hot-dogs etc. are all examples of mystery foods – meaning it's a complete mystery what's really in them. What you think you are getting is often not meat at all but a load of synthetic, man-made, chemically-bound 'foodstuffs' – a small percentage of which might actually be some meat. I mean, a hot-dog, what the hell is in it?

And don't be fooled by the many fast food outlets that boast about their burgers being 100 per cent pure beef. By 100 per cent pure beef they mean 100 per cent pure cow. Which includes the colon, the intestines, the liver, the kidneys, the spleen – just about everything in fact. In many cases it's not the meat from one cow either, it's a combination of hundreds of herds from many different farms. My advice is to skip the frozen meat meals like chicken Kiev and stick to organically produced 'grass fed' whole meats. At least that way you know it is chicken, or turkey, or whatever. When it is encased in breadcrumbs or a pig's intestine it becomes a 'mystery food'.

Please also note that organic white meats are nowhere near as acidic to the body as red meat and the body has a much easier time dealing with them, so if you want some organic chicken with steamed veg and a water-rich, nutrient-packed salad it will not interfere with your success – in fact it's an extremely healthy meal. The general rule if you are still going to consume meat is: nothing from a cow or pig where possible and make sure you know what the animal ate.

JUNK FOOD FOR COWS AND CHICKENS MEANS JUNK FOR US

I think as far back as the 1950s meat was a different animal, so to speak, to what we have today. The chickens and cows of yesteryear were fed on natural grasses and their nutrition was at least balanced and then passed to us. However, the vast majority of the meats consumed today are from herds which are on a junk food diet themselves. The only reason **BiG FOOD** give the chickens which are bred for human consumption a junk food diet is profit. A naturally grown chicken usually takes about seven months to reach its full size; in many parts of the world a commercially grown chicken can reach its full size in just seven *weeks*. The inclusion of hormones like estradiol and zeranol designed to fatten them up faster has been banned from the EU, but there are many aspects of **BiG FOOD** I don't fully trust and imports can sometimes escape such rules. One thing for sure though is that even in the EU, the food your average chicken and cow is getting is not nutritionally balanced and is causing more health problems for humans than people realize.

The loss of green pastures to battery practices and the demand for cheap meat, lead to chickens and cows being fed on mainly corn, soy, and wheat. You may think, 'so what?' Well the reason this is so detrimental is due to the balance of essential fatty acids. They are called 'essential' because the body can't make them and must get them from food. In the Fifties meat and milk used to have a good 1:1 ratio of omega 3 and omega 6. However, because of a diet of corn, soy, and wheat, the ratio can be as bad as 1:40. That is forty times more omega 6 than 3. It is worth knowing that omega 6, unless balanced on a one to one basis with omega 3, is extremely inflammatory. Omega 6 also stimulates the production of fatty cells, whereas omega 3 limits the production of fat cells. The balance and quality of omega-3s and omega-6s in our bodies stems directly from the food we eat. The conclusion therefore is if you are going to eat meat make sure you know what it is and what it has been fed on. Not all 'free range' are 'grass fed'. Grass fed is what you need for a good balance of essential fats. Having said that, you really don't need to eat meat at all to get good quality fats and if you decided to skip meat altogether you wouldn't need to worry what on earth they had been fed on.

CARNIVORES? OMNIVORES? HERBIVORES?

There has been a lot of argument about whether we were designed to eat meat or not. After reading the evidence on both sides, and believe me I've read loads of it, I have once again used the best resource I know to come up with my own conclusion – common sense. All I know is that if I was in the wild and had the choice between picking a banana from a tree next to me or chasing down an animal, I'd choose the banana. It's much easier than catching, killing, and cutting up an animal. But if I was hungry and there wasn't any fruit available, and all that was left were some animals roaming around, then watch out 'Babe' – I'm coming to get ya! We would eat anything rather than starve and in times of genuine hunger your body can easily cope with meat.

So in terms of whether you can eat meat or not the answer is clear – yes we can. In terms of whether we actually need it to live the answer is also very clear – no we don't. The meat industry, along with various government agencies, have managed to convince seemingly everyone that unless we get tons of protein we will die. They have also managed to convince us that meat is the best source of this much-needed protein. Massive advertising campaigns like the 'Meat to Live' one constantly back up this huge myth we've been taught since birth – so let's lay this one to rest once and for all.

WE JUST DON'T NEED THAT MUCH PROTEIN

Think about it. In the first six months of life we literally double in body weight. At no other point in our life does this happen in such a short amount of time (although it can often feel as though it does). We need more protein during the first few years of our life than at any other time. And the reason – the body is growing nails, hair, bones, tissues, etc. It needs a good source of protein for this – namely mother's milk. Here's the thing, mother's milk contains a maximum of 2.2 per cent protein. Also, protein is not built from protein anyway – it is built from amino acids. The reason we eat cows is because apparently their protein is very similar to ours – which seems like a very good argument for eating your next door neighbour! And what is all the fear about not getting enough protein anyway? Where did this fear come from? Have you ever met anyone with a protein deficiency? No, me neither. But I have met loads of people suffering the effects of too much protein. It is up to you to use your common sense, but if you are in any doubt just ask yourself, where do cows get their protein from?

'Are you telling me i have to eat grass to get my protein?'

Clearly not, I'm saying it seems that whatever food was specifically meant for each species has exactly the correct amount of protein – despite what the 'experts' may tell us. The closest living relative to us is said to be the Bonobo chimpanzee. It is thought this species is closer to us genetically than it is to any other chimpanzee on earth. Our digestive systems are virtually identical and our DNA is 98 per cent the same. They eat nothing but fruit and green leafy vegetation, yet they are very strong and powerful. I am not suggesting that we need to do this for a second, nor am I suggesting that just because the Bonobo eats certain things then it proves we should too. I am just pointing out that once again we have been handed a load of nonsense by a heavily subsidised meat industry when it comes to the protein and meat issue.

Let's be very clear – our bodies were designed to deal with meat, but not all the time and not at least without the help of nutrient-packed, water-rich live food to help it along. If you have meat once, twice, even three times a week it will cause you no problems whatsoever and you will still easily and comfortably arrive safe in the land of the slim – especially if you change your brand to white meat. In fact, if that's all you're having, it will probably be of benefit to you. Equally, not having meat will also cause you no problems whatsoever. The question of meat comes down to not whether you can, but whether you really want to.

Personally I have been a vegetarian, a vegan, and someone who eats meat. I didn't eat any meat once for over four years. I now do not restrict myself to any label. When I do eat meat, I make sure it's white, organic where possible and more importantly 'grass fed'. The idea is to understand the effect meat can have on your system, and then to be flexible and free to eat it intelligently. My main choice of animal protein and a good ratio of essential fatty acids is fish. If I am classed as any type of 'arian' it would now be a 'pescitarian', which means I don't really eat meat but I do eat fish.

The body can deal with fish a lot, and I mean a hell of a lot, easier than even white meat. Fish is a great source of the essential fats we need, along with the essential amino acids which are the building blocks of protein. Although you can easily get these fats from avocados and nuts, and amino acids from pulses, grains, and nuts, I sometimes just like a piece of hot cooked fish on a bed of water-rich, live salad – especially if I'm eating in a restaurant. Because of the omega 3 fatty acids contained within most fish, fish is also perfect as an anti-inflammatory food, great for skin conditions as an example.

Personally I've never understood people who claim they are vegetarian and yet eat fish. Apparently there are even people who claim to be veggie and justify it by saying, 'I don't eat meat apart from chicken and fish'. That's like saying I don't smoke apart from pipes and cigars.

Many people think that if they stopped eating meat they would miss the wonderful taste of it, but remember the chapter on 'changing your diet'. You will learn to enjoy the taste of anything you have on a regular basis and most people already like at least some kinds of fish. And anyway, meat has never really tasted that good and has always been a bit dull. Why do you think we add salt, pickle, ketchup and the like? With foods that we are biologically adapted to eat we don't need to add stuff to improve the taste, and we also do not need to rename them. You don't have to rename an apple, a pear or a banana to make it mentally acceptable, and you certainly don't need to add ketchup or pickle to a pineapple to 'improve' the taste. But remember –

You do not have to stop eating meat altogether to be slim and healthy

– so if you don't want to stop eating meat altogether: **DON'T.** If you enjoy your turkey or chicken at Christmas then have it. If you want a Sunday roast – enjoy. If you like a nice bit of chicken on the barbie – feel free to tuck in. In fact, if you are ever in the position where you have a choice between a plate full of white pasta and some meat and veg, go with the meat and veg every time (as you will see very soon). Good quality whole meats are not the real enemy here – it's the mystery food 'meats' and drug foods that you've got to look out for. Whole meats are only a problem when we burden our system with too much at the cost of everything else. In fact, if you look around there are many vegetarians who are overweight and incredibly unhealthy. The main reason for this is that most people who stop eating meat still haven't got it quite right – they simply substitute meat with an even more toxic junk food. Although they call themselves vegetarians they really are more like …

18

'DAIRY'-ARIANS

'Dairy what?' Dairyarians. I wouldn't look it up as I made up the word. The point is I know many people who stop eating meat but then massively increase their intake of dairy products. I know many vegetarians who would end up not eating at all if they also had to drop dairy products. It seems it's cheese with everything if you are a veggie. The main problem is that many people go vegetarian for either reasons of health or for animal rights issues. What they fail to realize is they fall flat on both fronts, as you will see as I expose the apparent health food for what it is.

The dairy industry, along with many governments, has literally been 'milking' us for years. Not only did they manage at one time to make milk compulsory in schools, but even today doctors, dieticians and a host of other 'experts' still insist that milk is one of the best natural foods we can consume and if we don't our bones and teeth will crumble. I have just one thing to say about most of what we have been taught about milk and dairy products:

Complete Bull

Have you seen the teeth of a great ape? Do you know how much milk they drink? None. Great apes also have big, strong and very healthy bones and osteoporosis is completely unknown. It is not just great apes who don't have problems with their bones or teeth despite not drinking any milk, but when you think about it, not one single adult mammal drinks milk after they are weaned – except us. Somehow the dairy industry along with powerful backing from many governments, have managed to convince us we need dairy or we will perish. They have managed to do this despite the fact that not even cows drink milk. Calves do, but cows *never* drink milk. That is because it is completely unnatural for any mammal to drink milk of any kind after they are weaned. It is even more unnatural (after weaning age) to drink the milk of a completely different species.

If you are thinking that cats and dogs drink milk, please bear in mind who controls what they eat. Cats and dogs are now suffering many of the diseases we have and many are now very fat indeed. If humans were meant to have any kind of milk it should of course be from our own mother – not the mother of a calf. But mother's milk either dries up or it becomes very uncomfortable for the mother to continue, hence we, like all mammals, should be weaned off milk at an early age. You can try and get some mother's milk now if you like. But be warned – you'll get arrested and disowned!

The milk of a cow is clearly meant for its own kind and I don't care how many people with nutritional qualifications coming out of their backside say otherwise. It is meant for a mammal that has a digestive system with four stomachs; one which weighs an average of 200 lb (90 kg) at birth and 2,000 lb (900 kg) just two years later. If you want that kind of weight gain then all you need to do is eat loads of dairy. Also don't forget that the vast majority of milk and dairy we consume now are from cows that are fed a junk diet. This leads to the ratio of omega 3s and omega 6s being way off the 1:1 it should be. This then in turn leads to our milk and dairy being potentially incredibly inflammatory and even more fattening than it would have been fifty years ago. In an age where we are perhaps consuming more milk than ever, it may be worth paying more attention to where the dairy you do consume comes from.

Such is the belief that the milk of a cow is good for a human, very rarely if ever, do we put any ailments down to this 'health' food. For example, I was badly asthmatic for many years and wouldn't go anywhere without my inhalers. I had both the blue and brown versions and was taking puffs on them at least eight times a day. Within just four weeks of eliminating all dairy from my diet I no longer had asthma and I haven't had it since. I must stress that if you have asthma your problem will *not* necessarily be solved by avoiding milk or becoming a vegan. However, given the inflammatory and mucus forming nature of today's dairy you can be almost certain that in most cases it will be drastically improved. You will hear from many in the medical profession that any link between dairy and asthma is complete nonsense spouted by 'alternative' practitioners who don't know what they are talking about. This is extremely frustrating as many in the medical profession are in a much better position than most to influence people in the right way. To say diet plays no part in disease (as many in the medical profession do) is lunacy at best. And to say there is no evidence to say milk affects asthma is incredibly naïve.

Milk and dairy products are known to be mucus forming. This isn't hearsay, it is as clear as it gets. When you have mucus it becomes harder to breath – this isn't rocket science and you don't need a PHD in medicine to see just maybe it could affect disorders such as asthma. The reason why so many people have such intolerance to milk is simple – because we shouldn't be drinking it. The mucus build-up is somewhat of an 'action signal'. It is the body's way of saying, 'I am having difficulty dealing with this rubbish, if possible, please don't do it again'. But how on earth are we meant to recognize and act on these clear signals when we have been told by experts that milk is good for us? We often put the many health problems that today's milk can potentially cause down to other factors, while we continue to drink and eat products made from the mucus and fattening product.

Why Milk Can Potentially Be Harmful

Milk contains a protein called casein; it also, as you are no doubt aware, contains calcium. The casein and calcium are chemically bound together. In order for the protein to be used efficiently and the calcium to be utilized properly the body requires certain digestive enzymes to separate them. These enzymes are called rennin and lactase. Here's the problem – if you are human and are over the age of three (and if you aren't, well done for learning to read so early on) you will no longer have these enzymes (some humans do continue to produce lactase, but the majority don't). Do you think there might be an obvious reason why our bodies stop producing the enzymes that break down milk properly after the age we are meant to be weaned?

LINING YOUR STOMACH WITH GLUE

It's tough enough for the body to deal with human milk after weaning age, but at least this was meant for an animal with one stomach – us. This is why goat's milk is better for humans than cow's milk – they also only have one stomach. But just because it's better doesn't mean it's good. Once again, this milk was meant for 'kids', not the goat and not for us either. Both goat's milk and cow's milk contain a much higher amount of the protein casein than human milk and it's this stuff which is a major problem for our digestive system. Cow's milk contains over 300 times more casein than human milk. 'So what' I hear you say 'isn't casein protein? The more the better surely'. It is worth knowing that casein is used as a base of one of the strongest wood glues known to mankind. Casein literally sticks to the walls of the stomach and lining of the intestines. The mad thing is we know this but we just don't think about it. How many times have you heard people say, 'I'm going to have a few beers tonight, but before I do I'm going to line my stomach with milk'? And that really is what's happening – you're lining your stomach and intestines with a glue-like substance.

I know this subject often causes controversy and I have had many heated debates with people who are unwilling to let go of their deep-rooted beliefs about this subject. But it really is hard to argue with plain common sense and my common sense clearly tells me that the milk of a cow is meant for a calf – not a human being. If you were driving along the road and saw a well dressed man kneeling down sucking on a cow's udder would you think, 'how natural', or would you call the authorities? It is simply not normal for adult humans to drink the milk of a cow and it is quite amazing to think how we all have been conditioned to such an extent that people who don't think it's normal are the ones who are described as mental.

CHEESED OFF

While we're on the subject, let's not forget that milk is used to make numerous different products, from Yorkshire puddings, biscuits, cakes, chocolate, and muffins to the most obvious one – cheese. At this stage I usually hear cries of 'don't take away my cheese!'. This cry I fully understand as let's face facts, cheese can taste pretty damn good. However, please remember you do not have to become a vegan to gain freedom from the food and diet trap. I just wish to look at cheese from a different perspective in order for you to gauge the amount you will allow into your system on a weekly basis.

I personally like the odd bit of cheddar, but blue cheese very rarely passes my lips. Do you know how blue cheese is made? They get some solidified cow's milk, put holes in it and leave it until mould sets in the holes and settles. Let me say that again, the blue in most 'blue cheese' is mould! If you saw the same stuff on your bread you would never eat it. So why on earth are we eating mould? Is it because of the taste? Most children hate blue cheese and spit it out on first contact. We simply 'acquire' a taste for blue cheese by having it on a regular basis. And why do we persevere to even get to the stage where we like it? Well I believe we often get caught up with a lot of the pretentious nonsense that surrounds so many foods, especially cheese. Someone eating a Cheddar sandwich, drinking a can of beer, with a fag hanging out of their mouths, is seen as being different to someone with a piece of stilton, biscuits, a glass of white wine, and a 'fine' cigar – yet they're consuming more or less similar things, alcohol, nicotine, and dairy. In fact the person with the blue cheese is eating added mould. It seems strange that the more something has gone off the more 'sophisticated' it becomes and the more we seem willing to pay for it.

'But Jason, if i do choose to remove most meat from my diet and drastically reduce or eliminate dairy products, where will i get my protein and calcium — and what about vitamin B12?'

The above seems like a reasonable question, but only because of the conditioning and misinformation we have been subjected to since birth. An elephant wouldn't worry about where it's getting its protein or vitamin B12 and it certainly doesn't concern itself with the amount of calcium its getting. I was once a vegan for a few years, but I didn't waste away. I really don't care about vitamin B12 and neither should you. Once again it falls in the ever-increasing category of – *we don't need to know*.

It always seems very strange to me that people start to get concerned about whether they are getting enough vitamins, minerals, protein, and calcium *after* they change their diet. When they are eating virtually nothing but McDonald's, ice cream, processed and totally de-natured foods, they don't seem that worried. But the minute you talk about having fresh fruit, veg and freshly extracted juice, they start to worry: why? Because the meat and dairy industries have perpetuated fears for many years that are totally unfounded – like the one about not getting enough calcium. I know I have repeatedly said that we really do not need to concern ourselves with the likes of calcium, but in order to put your unfounded fears to rest there are a few things you should know.

THE CALCIUM CON

The main use of calcium is to help neutralize acid in the body. This means that every time you put something acid forming in your body you rob your body's bank account of calcium. Our bank balance is mainly stored in our bones and teeth. Luckily we have quite a hefty bank account but, once again, if you keep withdrawing without making deposits you will go bankrupt. And when the body files for calcium bankruptcy the consequence is brittle bones and loss of teeth. In fact osteoporosis (brittle bone disease) is now a common condition – and it's common because of what we are putting into our bodies. However, if what they say about dairy products and calcium is true, this should not be happening. Our intake of dairy products has gone up drastically over the past thirty years, yet so has the rate of osteoporosis.

The fact is most people have got it back to front. They are so busy worrying about where they are going to get more calcium from that they don't think about what's depleting their current store. As usual we are so busy treating the symptom we don't look for the cause. Every time you drink coffee, cola or alcohol, smoke a cigarette, or eat a fast-food burger your body has to use its calcium stores to help neutralize the acid effect they have on the body. The question is not where do I get my calcium, but rather how can I prevent the scavengers coming in and taking it all? The irony is further compounded when you think that the modern day cow's milk can create an incredibly acidic reaction, causing calcium to be pulled *out* of the body.

Milk products are used in massive quantities by many of the fast food giants. The most obvious place they use it is in milk shakes, but it is also found in their pastries, biscuits, doughnuts, chocolate sauces, ice creams, and the slices of plastic-looking worryingly yellow cheese you find in your cheeseburger. And we try and wash this down with a thick, glue-like milkshake … if we can get it up the straw. Milk is also used in the new Fast Food giants of the twenty-first century – Starbucks and Co. Every Latte is mainly milk, not coffee. And I fear it will be a long time before you find grass fed cow's milk at your local hip and trendy coffee bar.

Having said all of this, dairy produce, just like meat, does not need to be eliminated from the diet completely in order to have excellent health and a slim body. If you do have dairy though, do your best to make sure it's of the best quality it can be. Grass fed herds are best and organic where possible.

It is what you do *most* of the time that determines your health; the body will easily cope with a bit of dairy and the whole point of this book is to give you the freedom of genuine food choice and freedom from a diet mentality. Your body will of course gain some nutrition from dairy, but I just wanted to open your mind to the fact it is not the all-singing and all-dancing health food we have been hammered into believing it is. Also be careful of just how much you are consuming but might not be aware.

A large part of **BiG FOOD** is **BiG DAiRY** and **BiG MEAT.** Both of which have managed to persuade us that we cannot survive without them and have persuaded governments to keep subsidizing. It is even more amazing that meat and dairy are so heavily defended when there is ever increasing evidence which links their intake to many diseases, including some cancers.

I realize there may be many vegetarians reading this book who are now perhaps realizing they are in fact more like dairyarians and as such are doing their health and energy levels no favours at all. I know many vegetarians who are in fact dairyarians, but these people went veggie for two reasons – health and animal welfare. The problem is, as I mentioned at the start, they fall flat on both counts. If it's for health then they are certainly not better off substituting milk products for meat products. Given the choice between a veggie cheese-ridden lasagne and some chicken and steamed veg – go for the meat every time. And as for animal welfare (which I realize is a totally different subject), they certainly haven't done anything to help the cause as dairy herds often go through much, much worse torture than those reared for slaughter only.

Now that you are aware of the pitfalls of being a dairyarian you're probably thinking of a substitute food. If you are, please be careful not to make the next big mistake – that of turning into a 'starcharian'. This is a person who, you guessed it, eats tons of bread, rice, potatoes, corn, and pasta at the cost of most other things. In terms of getting slim, healthy, and tapping into a level of energy you haven't felt in years, you are better off eating some good quality meat, a little dairy produce every now and then and saying ...

19

PASTA LA VISTA BABY

If anyone from Italy is reading this I can forgive you for wanting to throw the book against the wall. Even if you aren't Italian, you may well be thinking that pasta is full of fibre and essential carbohydrates and it's a perfectly healthy food. In which case, you may be wondering why we need to say goodbye to pasta.

Well actually you don't need to say goodbye to pasta at all, you just need to perhaps change the kind of pasta you have and the amount. The mistake people tend to make when they cut down on meat and dairy produce, is to drastically increase their intake of white refined carbs, which, as you now realize, in terms of health, energy, addiction, and weight gain, are a nightmare. I cannot repeat enough how harmful – both in terms of mental addiction and physical abuse – these white refined foods are. It is not just white refined sugar that causes massive mental and physical problems, it's *any* white refined carbohydrate. They are the insulin-producing, fat-causing, energy-robbing, stomach-bloating, paste-forming, empty drug-like foods that help to keep people rooted in the food and diet trap.

Good riddance to white rubbish

This does not mean you cannot have complex carbohydrates and still be healthy, it just means the answer is to switch to the 'whole' varieties of these foods. That way you can still have your pasta and bread but in a form that will not do you as much harm as the white versions. I say as much harm, as even the 'whole' varieties aren't all what they seem when bought from **BiG FOOD.** You need to understand that even something like 'wholemeal bread' is not always as healthy as the label suggests. In some varieties of wholemeal bread you can find things like hydrogenated vegetable oils, sugar (yes sugar), salt (and plenty of it), plus various other ingredients not really conducive with human consumption. They are also, like pasta, loaded with wheat. Despite wheat being given a 'good health' image it's yet another food that isn't all it's cracked up to be. Many people are now what's called, 'wheat intolerant' and 'wheat free' foods are rapidly finding their way onto many supermarket shelves. One of the biggest problems with wheat, especially for those looking to drop the excess pounds, is water retention. To be fair you hardly need to be a scientist to have already worked this out. Have you ever noticed how your stomach sticks out after eating a load of pasta or bread? That's primarily the wheat. You don't get this so much when you eat rice do you? This is why I'm a big fan of wholegrain rice and less of a fan of wholemeal bread and pasta. Again, don't get me wrong, these wholemeal versions are in a completely different league to their white cousins and I'm not saying they're bad foods, I'm just saying if you want that elusive flat stomach, if you do eat them – go easy on the wheat.

Closer To The Grain

Wholemeal and wholegrain versions of all complex carbohydrates satisfy your hunger for longer as their energy is released steadily, unlike the 'up and crash' cycle you get with the 'refined' white versions. The body also requires fibre, and wholegrain rice and good quality bread can be the next best thing to fruit and veg for helping to 'sweep' the intestines. The fibre also helps to slow the rate at which the complex carbs are converted to glucose, making most wholegrain products low GI (if your into your Glycaemic Index levels). Plus, of course, this way of eating is for the rest of your life, so it's important to feel free around all food. The trick is to have a full understanding of the foods available to us and know exactly which type to have, as well as how much our bodies can 'get away with' and still stay slim and have optimum health.

WATCH OUT FOR THE YEAST 'PARASITES'

Most of the breads we buy also contain a lot of yeast and many people consume far too much due to their addiction to white carbs – another excellent reason for changing brands. Over consumption can eventually cause an overgrowth of yeast in the gut (otherwise known as candida albicans), which in turn causes even further cravings. Imagine a colony of yeast parasites living in the body. The more you feed them, the more they breed. The more they breed, the more yeast they crave to try and satisfy their insatiable appetite. Have you ever noticed that green hairy mould you get on old bread? Well now imagine an overgrowth of virtually the same mould inside your body with living parasites buried within. That is candida albicans – lovely. All white refined sugar products help to feed the little blighters, as does the sugar found in milk.

Please understand again that a certain amount of both yeast and wheat is fine and some people reading this book will not have these 'parasites'. But at the same time there will be many people who do and those who do often suffer from bloating and fatigue directly after eating white refined pasta, bread and the like. If you have an unusual craving for bread and/or pasta you can be almost certain it's not you who wants it, it's the yeast, wheat, and sugar parasites within. The answer is to realize it's not a genuine hunger and starve the little blighters to death. It is also worth pointing out that white refined flour when mixed with water creates a paste that would be worthy of any roll of wallpaper!

Your body is over 70 per cent water and when you ingest flour it becomes like thick paste in your bloodstream, often sticking to the walls of your arteries. Potato crisps also have this effect.

CARBO-DE-HYDRATE

Carbohydrates are designed to supply energy, vitamins, minerals, essential fats, amino acids (building blocks for protein), fibre, and water. With that in mind it seems rather odd that things like flour and wheat are described as 'hydrates'. Carbohydrate actually comes from the fact that carbs such as fruits and veggies are very high in water, which is essential for the body. Even a banana is made up of over 84 per cent water. Remember, carbohydrates are designed to supply energy *and* water. However, the complex carbs we eat, even of the wholegrain kind, are lacking the water content we require for easy digestion and removal of wastes. This is why I often refer to them as just carbs, as the 'hydrate' part is not strictly appropriate. This is why when I do have carbs I make sure the hydrate part comes from water-rich foods like green salads and vegetable juices.

I do still eat bread, although it now tends to be wholemeal pitta bread or some toasted rye bread or pumpernickel. I usually warm the pittas and stuff with loads of water-rich, nutrient-packed fast foods – creamy avocados, fresh tomatoes, alfalfa sprouts, cucumber, olives, lemon juice etc. I also love to toast some rye bread and spread some avocado and simply add some black pepper and lemon juice – gorgeous. I also have stone-ground, buckwheat, and wholemeal breads. The key word is 'whole'. White refined is 'empty' food – anything that was ever good about the grain has been totally removed, rendering it dead and, as you by now should realize, potentially dangerous. So when buying any grains you need to look for the closest to the original whole versions as possible – *whole* oats, *whole*meal bread, *whole*grain brown rice, whole, whole, whole. Unlike the extremely heavily processed white variety, whole complex carbs can actually help to regulate insulin, stabilize blood-sugar levels and keep things moving – if you know what I mean.

Many whole carbs, especially rice, also contain some valuable nutrients which are easily utilised by the body. So as you can see I'm not suggesting for one second you say goodbye to pasta, bread, rice, and oats – just change the type and amount you have. If you do choose to eliminate these carbs, even the whole varieties, once again you will not perish. Bread, just like meat and milk, is another food we have been totally conditioned into thinking we must have or we will suffer a nutritional deficiency. Even if you decided to drop bread and pasta completely from your life, you really wouldn't be any worse off. Actually, I know many people who have simply removed bread and pasta from their diet and their excess weight fell off while their energy went up. I don't know anyone who didn't feel a great deal healthier when the pasta and bread were banished from their diet.

Once again, the question is not whether you can have white refined pasta, bread, and rice – after all you are an adult and you can do what you want – but whether you really want to. Personally I have no desire to flood my body with a fat-producing, energy-stealing, empty non-food – especially when there are millions of high-fibre, nutrient-packed, energy-releasing foods on offer. Just because I don't eat white pasta and bread doesn't mean I am being restricted or deprived. It was when I was eating foods of that nature that my mind and body was constantly being deprived.

As you can now see, meat, dairy produce, and refined carbs all create their own challenges for the body to overcome, but the body can deal with small amounts of pretty much anything.

So there is no need to stop having dinner parties, eating carbs, fish or even lean white meat and there is no need to start eating nothing but grass! Don't panic – you will see clearly by the end of this book that you will be free to eat and drink whatever you wish, whenever you wish – this is all about freedom.

One of the main reasons why many people are lacking in energy and remain fat is because when they do eat these slow, clogging foods, they don't eat them one by one or with any high-water-content natural food. The big mistake is that they pile them all in at exactly the same time, course after course, seemingly without worry or care as to what happens after they swallow it all. As you now know, each one of these foods affects the body to a greater or lesser degree when eaten alone, but put them all together and **BOOM!** – you've just concocted a potentially very …

20

LETHAL COMBINATION

What do Dr William Hay and Ivan Pavlov have in common? They are both scientists who have carried out in-depth studies into the time it takes certain foods and combinations of foods to be digested by the body. If you are one of these people who has been on the diet rollercoaster for years you have by now probably done your own scientific studies into this subject. Whether you have or not, please pay attention to this chapter as you will learn everything you need to know about the effects of what is well known in the food and diet world as 'food combining'.

I have already mentioned in 'A Meaty Problem' that our friend Mr Pavlov found that it takes four hours for meat to leave the stomach and a further 20 hours for it to get through the intestinal tract. What I touched on, but have waited until now to expand on, was that the minute you add other heavily processed foods into the stomach at the same time, the overall length of time it takes the body to digest it can more than double. In terms of freeing up energy for weight loss and health this can be very detrimental. Here's why.

When you eat concentrated protein (meat, milk, cheese, fish, eggs, etc.) your body produces acid-based digestive juices to help break it down. However, when you put a concentrated starch food (potato, bread, pasta, rice, corn, cereal, oats, rye, etc.) into the body it produces alkaline-based digestive juices. 'So what' say you, 'it's all sounding a bit blah, blah, blahish'. Well it's actually worth knowing this bit of blah, blah, blah. Do you remember chemistry lessons at school? Remember what happens when you mix acid and alkaline substances together? They neutralize each other – i.e. they cancel each other out. Now because the human body is so efficient, and because the two juices are actually produced in different parts of the digestive tract, the acid and alkaline juices don't completely cancel each other out in this situation (although there are still many 'expert' combining teachers who are convinced they do). However, there is no question that the body has to work a hell of a lot harder to try and break down two concentrated foods at the same time, especially when each require their own specific digestive juice. In fact, the job is made so much harder that the time it takes the stomach alone to deal with this heavy workload will be more than doubled.

Ivan Pavlov recorded that if foods that require different digestive juices are eaten at the same time, it can take anywhere from 8–14 hours for those foods to leave the stomach. To put this in perspective, food should never be in the stomach for longer than 3–4 hours. If it remains there for longer because it is part of a badly combined meal, then putrefaction and fermentation occurs. Meat putrefies and starches like potatoes ferment. Now throw in a cow glue; a highly sugared, theobromine-laced dessert (more carbs and protein); a few alcoholic drinks (carbs plus all kinds of other things) and a couple of cups of coffee – while your body is still dealing with meat and potatoes – and you've just put yourself into a slow food coma. Or in our language, we've just nodded off after our Sunday lunch or Christmas dinner.

The other person I mentioned who studied what is now known as 'food combining' is Dr William Hay. As any self-respecting dieter will know, he created the famous Hay Diet. For those who have not only heard of it, but have tried it, please let me put your mind at rest by saying:

This is not a food combining diet

In fact, this is not any kind of diet – it is freedom from ever having to diet again. I'm only mentioning what happens when certain foods hit the stomach to give you an added physical tool to aid in your journey to the land of the slim and healthy.

The Hay Diet was the first in a long line of diets based on the principle that proteins are fine when eaten alone, as are carbs – but never the twain shall meet. In fact this is the whole philosophy behind the famous UK slimming club, Slimming World. Slimming World has changed a great deal over the years and many people have had incredible success using the combining principles it was based on. Although Slimming World has changed a great deal from its early days, the main premise for years was that you don't just have separate protein and carb meals, you have completely separate days. They had what was known as a Red day and a Green day. Red days were where you could eat your proteins and Green days were for carbs. The theory was, and is, obviously based on the findings of Hay and Pavlov, and, because the body is only dealing with one concentrated food at a time, it works – well to a degree anyway. I say to a degree because rarely does just separating your carbs and proteins result in the long-term success people are looking for. The main reason is because many people who embark on, say, the Hay Diet, or are members of a diet club which teaches the same principles, usually still have a diet *mentality* and are often still struggling with other foods and not feeding their body what it needs to get healthy. Usually the only change they make is not mixing proteins and complex carbohydrates.

The difference for you is that by the time you finish this book you will not have a diet mentality, which means you can easily use food combining as a great physical weapon against fat and ill health whenever you choose to. That means when you want to and where it fits into your life, not constantly so that it dominates your life and you become obsessive about it. In fact, when fully understood and used properly, this combining food in the correct way makes an amazing difference to how you feel and really helps to free up valuable nerve energy for weight loss. The difference can be a whooping 5–9 hours of extra energy if you combine sensibly, which is why on the physical side of things it's a great tool to have. But in order for it to be an effective tool and one you can use in everyday life in order to have lifelong success, you need to know the full facts. And once again there are a few myths that need exploding about this combining stuff.

CHINESE WHISPER

If you whisper a truth to someone and ask them to pass the information on, by the time it reaches just the tenth person the facts will have already changed. Exactly the same thing has happened with this combining thing. Very few people have read the original works of Hay or Pavlov. What the vast majority of people have done is read or heard the headlines and not the full story. Anybody who knows anything about combining tends to believe and purport that you should *never* mix proteins and carbs together no matter what. These are what I call the 'headliners' – people who become so extremely obsessive about not mixing proteins and carbs together that they appear to have convinced themselves they will internally combust if they have a cheese sandwich! I'm not kidding either – I know because on one of my many diets I used to be one of them.

What you need is the full food combining story and not just the headlines. That way you can, as I do now, feel totally relaxed about it and use it to your advantage whenever you wish.

Once again common sense needs to come into play here. If protein and carbs should never be mixed no matter what, why do people in the East – who according to Hay principles 'badly combine' all the time – tend to be much healthier and much slimmer than their Western counterparts. (Sadly, things are now changing on this front thanks to BiG FOOD moving in.) Also, if the never mix proteins and carbs rule is correct then it means that nature herself has got it wrong. After all, she combines proteins and carbs in most of her foods, even mother's milk. So how can this be if our friends Hay and Pavlov were correct?

The answer is in the *ratio* of carbs and proteins. In nature, although some proteins will also have carbs, the carbohydrate content will always be low. And in the East they apply the same principles as nature herself when it comes to combining protein and carbs – one or the other always dominates in their dishes. They tend to have lots of rice, plenty of veg and little strips of pork, chicken, duck or fish.

Our problem is the result of eating huge portions of equal amounts of protein and carbs at the same time – usually clumps of meat and loads of potatoes. And when we do, the undisputed fact is that it will take double the time to leave the stomach than if they were eaten separately or in the correct ratio. The correct ratio means that if you want a couple of potatoes with your fish and salad, fine. If you are having a water-rich chicken salad and you want a few chips on the side – have them (yes chips). The key is not to waste too much energy on digestion. There is a vital reason for this –

it takes vital nerve energy to lose weight and gain health

I cannot repeat this point enough and this is why one of the biggest changes you need to make is from slow food to fast.

I could spend the next fifty pages on this combining thing, but it would all get a bit blah, blah blahish (if it hasn't already) and I don't want to bang on unnecessarily. The fact is if you have understood the above, then you now know enough to use combining as a helpful tool to get you to the land of the slim and healthy. As I have said, the main problem is that many people who follow the Hay and Pavlov school of thought often let this combining stuff rule their entire life. In other words they're not free to eat, which is the whole point of this book. And, as I've said, it's often the only change they make. So initially they will have some weight loss as the body has more energy, but it still won't be enough without a full understanding of the food trap – they will still never feel free or be free. And it's no good simply separating your carbs and proteins if you are still consuming tons of drug foods and drinks and at the same time are still not getting enough vital nutrients. What's the point of a 'Green day' if all you're consuming is tons of white pasta, biscuits, refined sugar, and bread. They might all take the same amount of time in the stomach, so therefore are 'correctly combined', but so what. People who have Green days like this (which ironically can contain no green at all) are not going to achieve the kind of success they're looking for, especially if the pasta and bread are white and refined. And while I'm back on that subject please be aware that **BiG FOOD** have no scruples and will deliberately try to delude you into thinking you are eating healthily when you're not. One of the biggest tricks is literally to dye white refined bread with caramel to make it brown. I want to make it clear –

'Brown' bread is just white bread that has been dyed, 'brown' bread is not wholemeal bread — 'brown' bread is a con

And this isn't the only con. Don't be fooled by things like 'brown' sugar either, it's simply white refined sugar that has been dyed – usually with caramel. They just dye it brown to make us think we are getting something healthy. This kind of almost subconscious false advertising really gets on my goat. If you look around they do this type of thing with so many different foods. By adding certain colours to packaging or selective 'buzz' words they attempt, often very successfully, to make us believe that what we are buying is a very healthy food. How they are still allowed so blatantly to mislead the public is a mystery. Before you can free yourself completely from the food trap and change your eating habits for life all of the trickery must be dispelled entirely. So before I get on to explaining how to get into the right frame of mind and exactly how to implement and actively make the change, there are a few more things you should be aware of. The price of not knowing is certain members of **BiG FOOD** continuing to control the way you think and raising their glasses as they continue to wish us all a very …

21

CON – APPETITE

Mainstream advertising on TV and radio and product placement in films conning us into believing certain drug-like foods will change our emotions for the better is bad enough. But perhaps even more sinister is the blatant, subconscious advertising that goes on by **BiG FOOD** in the packaging and advertising of certain foods, claiming health benefits. I am talking here about certain buzzwords and colours they use that act like an instant 'bell' to make us believe we are buying something that is good for us and our children. And the reason why we think that certain foods, which when looked at properly are actually junk, are good for us is not because we are stupid, but because they manage to twist things in such a way that our first impression of the food is 'healthy'. You never get a second chance to make a first impression, as they say, and **BiG FOOD** and their advertising work force are more than aware of this.

Some of the biggest buzzwords you need to look out for are GM free, natural, and organic. The minute we see these words we believe the product is healthy. Yet many times they are totally meaningless. Let's look at 'GM free' for a second. GM stands for genetically modified. Many people in the UK became very wary of GM foods in the late Nineties because of the massive amount of bad press they were receiving – Prince Charles famously voiced his concerns about them and they were widely referred to as 'Frankenstein' foods. This led to many food manufacturers and outlets doing their utmost to inform us that their foods were GM free. This unfortunately gave the very false impression that if something was GM free, it was good for you. Everyone was so busy worrying about GM that they seemed oblivious to the fact that they were still eating foods that were far from healthy.

One of the major UK newspapers even ran a full colour article giving list after list of GM free foods. They also had a colour scheme to make it easier to see which foods were GM free, which ones contained only a little GM and which contained a lot. The colours they used also helped to confuse people about what is healthy or not. One of the main colours used by so many food manufacturers to fool us into believing we are buying a good food is green. Green is now linked in our minds with health; so much so that all they have to do is add a bit of green to packaging and we become instantly fooled.

In this article on GM foods the colour they used to indicate foods and food outlets that were totally GM free was none other than our natural friend – green. Red was used for places or foods that used a lot of GM and amber for a bit here and there. What seemed a touch mind-blowing to me was that 'restaurants' like McDonald's and KFC were listed in the green column! This indicated that they were totally GM free. This may be the case, but so what, does it really matter? All this means is that the drug-like foods they sell were not genetically modified, but they have still been totally *modified* from their original state. The sugar started life as part of natural sugar cane; is the stripped, refined version not simply a modified version that will potentially cause health problems? The milkshake certainly didn't start life looking like that and if you think about it I don't think there is one single thing that is in its natural state (except of course the new range of McDonald's 'salads'). So as far as I'm concerned I don't care if they're GM free – they are not white refined sugar free; refined bread free; dairy free; meat free; high-blood-pressure producing, water-retentive salt free; or mystery-food free.

The fact that they are GM free is completely irrelevant to whether they are healthy or not – so don't be fooled. Also bear in mind that EU rules say a product can have 1 per cent GM ingredients without having to declare it anyway. GM only means something when talking about natural foods, but then even that word gets bandied about so much we now are unsure as to what that even means.

IT'S ALL NATURAL – BUT THEN SO ARE YOUR CAR TYRES

'It's all natural' or 'Made with only the finest *natural* ingredients' etc., etc. Let's lay this bogie to rest once and for all. If it ultimately came from this planet they are allowed to print 'all natural' on the label if they want to. This seems okay on first hearing but if we really think about the statement it means anything that has ever been made must have ultimately come from this planet. Which means that your car tyres, the chair you are sitting on and your clothes are all natural – but it doesn't mean they would be good to eat, even if you painted the chair green! Even the boys and girls at Red Bull have managed to use this word in a recent advertisement for their latest drink Red Bull Cola. The heading on the advert reads: Strong and Natural. On their website it reads 'natural caffeine from natural coffee beans'. In that case couldn't I sell 'opium cola' and advertise it as '100 per cent natural' and use a strap line 'natural opium from natural opium plants'? The word natural can be used on almost anything and **BiG FOOD** love to use it wherever they can. A true natural food is any food which hasn't been interfered with by humans. These include fresh fruits, vegetables, seeds, and nuts. You can then extend this onto meat and fish, as the only form of processing tends to be simply cooking. You cannot have a 'natural' cola any more than you can have a 'natural' muffin, bag of crisps or cheesecake. You can no doubt get natural cocaine and natural heroin – natural isn't always good!

IT'S ORGANIC, SO IT MUST BE GOOD

The organic bandwagon is running at full speed and is being fuelled yet again by a lot of nonsense. Let's cut the crap and spill the organic beans on the way this word often misleads. Just because a food has the word 'organic' printed on it, **IT DOESN'T MEAN IT'S GOOD FOR YOU.** Next time you go to your local supermarket just have a look at the amount of drug-like foods with the word 'organic' plastered all over them. You can now even get organic sugar-loaded mass produced chocolate. There are also organic cakes, organic biscuits, organic crisps, organic tinned sauces, and even organic white refined sugar, bread, rice, and pasta.

Can you see how if the words organic and chocolate are used in the same sentence your brain can be deluded into thinking organic chocolate is actually healthy chocolate? And the same goes for virtually any food – if it happens to be made from ingredients which don't contain artificial pesticides, then the word organic can be plastered all over it. But again it doesn't mean it's good, healthy food. It makes no difference if the sugar cane grew without the need for artificial pesticides; it has still been refined and as such is a drug-like food which causes many problems.

An organically-grown orange is obviously better than an orange which has been grown with artificial pesticides, but if you then take that orange, cook it, add tons of white refined flour and sugar to it then bond it altogether with some glue-like cow's milk it becomes completely irrelevant that the orange started its life 'organic'. The process has stripped away anything that was ever good or 'organic'. The orange is now well and truly dead. So if you are going to buy processed, sugar-ridden rubbish, save your money and forget the word 'organic'.

The words organic or GM free are only significant when we are talking about fresh fruit, vegetables, meat, dairy products, whole grains, and fish. Although there are many arguments at the moment as to whether organic foods really are better for you or not, I would always recommend organic fresh produce over the rest. Common sense once again tells me that a fresh food that contains added man-made chemicals is bound to be nutritionally inferior to one that does-n't. However, this does not mean that 'normal' fruit and veg are not worth buying if they are not organic – far from it. Please always bear in mind that even with some of the artificial pesticides, fresh fruit and veg are still in a completely different league to drug-like foods and will always supply the body with plenty of water, nutrients, and the natural sugars it needs. So if you cannot afford organic produce or it's unavailable – don't worry. This is also where juicing can help as most of the pesticides end up in the 'pulp' (the bit left behind) and not in the juice. Once again, to help illustrate my point you can of course no doubt buy organic cocaine and heroin.

'Contains real fruit'

I love this one. Labels on crap food giving the already deceived public the impression that because it contains 'real fruit', it must be good for them. Everyone knows that fruit is without question nature's finest food. It is the most nutritious, the sweetest and the most visually stimulating food on the planet. This is why **BiG FOOD** use it as often as they can to fool us and our children we are doing something good. By simply link-ing whatever totally de-natured product they are trying to sell to the amazing health-giving properties of fresh fruit they persuade us that their product will provide these benefits. I think nature should sue for some kind of plagiarism.

What many people do not realize is that once you expose fruit to oxygen it begins to oxidize – or go off. The live nutrients begin to die the minute they are exposed to air. You will have seen this yourself when you have taken a bite of an apple and witnessed how quickly it turns brown – this is the fruit dying. Once dead it is about as much use to the body as the latest state of the art widescreen TV would be to Stevie Wonder. So whenever you see a tin full of something which contains 'real' fruit – you are guaranteed that the fruit is now a shadow of its former self. Not only have a great deal of the life-giving properties of the fruit long gone, but in order to preserve it you can be sure they have added something which has now turned a perfectly natural food into a quite unnatural version of what it once was.

The makers of breakfast cereals are perhaps the biggest culprits of this. Many adverts show beautiful colourful images of fruits falling from the sky into a bowl of cereal. They then add a catchy slogan, something like 'as part of a healthy diet' plus the inevitable and misleading, 'May help to keep your heart healthy'. Notice the word 'may'. 'May' doesn't mean anything. Nor does 'could', 'possibly', or any of the other rubbish they come out with. I may also win the lottery; well I could do if I possibly had the numbers. Then you have **BiG FOOD** whose primary aim when it comes to most cereals and sweets is to lure children into buying their particular brand. If they can convince parents at the same time that they contain some goodness, bingo! **BiG FOOD** have the front to give the impression to children and parents that things like Starburst and other sweets are in some way good because they show pictures of bright and colourful fruits on their adverts. I want to make this point very clear, unless the fruit is fresh, ripe, and whole or the juice freshly extracted, most of the life-giving properties of the fruit are now gone. Why we get so excited about a cereal claiming it contains 'real mango' I will never know. Why not simply eat some mango? – the whole thing contains 'real mango'!

'No artificial colours or flavourings'

Once again this gives the impression it's good, but surely we shouldn't be adding artificial colours in the first place. Not only that but the claim is meaningless as it is often put on products which don't have them anyway, such as pasta or tinned fish. And when they do add colour or flavour to foods they once again try to fool us they are healthy by stating they are 'natural colours' or 'natural flavourings'. And while I'm on the subject, you need to be aware that flavourings and colourings are huge, and I do mean huge, business. The 'flavourists' (yes that's their official title) can make anything taste and smell like anything. That's why so many synthetic lumps of greasy vegetable spreads taste and smell of real butter. Do you know what actually distinguishes a natural flavouring from an artificial one? Well believe it or not the only difference is that a 'natural' flavour is a flavour that's been concocted using an out-of-date technology. What that means is natural and artificial flavours sometimes contain exactly the same chemicals, they're just produced through different methods. The world has officially gone nuts.

FAT FREE – LOW FAT – REDUCED FAT

The biggest con of them all though has got to be 'fat free' and 'low fat'. **BiG FOOD** don't like these labels, they **LOVE** them. Each time they print **FAT FREE** or **LOW FAT** they are effectively printing money. A few years back Mars brought out an apparently 'healthier' chocolate bar – Mars Flyte low fat chocolate bar. Their slogan: 'Pleasure without the guilt – take flight'. Now I am not into calories and they do fall into the 'we don't need to know category', but in terms of the con it is worth knowing that a Cadbury's Flake has 180 calories and yet the no-guilt Flyte has 196. And when it comes to reducing fat, remember that extra sugar is often added instead – so we're back at the old problem of excess sugar being converted into fat anyway. Peta Cottee of the National Food Alliance sums it up when she states, 'There is no legal definition of what low fat means and shoppers are lulled into a false sense of security when they see these descriptions on labels … Phrases like fat-free are highlighted without it being revealed how much extra sugar may be added to their product'.

Then you have 'reduced fat' versions of the same foods. Reduced Fat is not the same as Low Fat. The definition of Low Fat is a food which contains 3 g (0.1 oz) of fat or less per serving, and 30 per cent or less of total calories. Which is all nonsense anyway as a) it's confusing to most and b) Low Fat usually means more sugar which is converted to fat anyway. Reduced Fat, on the other hand, refers to foods which claim to contain at least 25 per cent less fat than the original version. This does not mean for a millisecond that the reduced fat version is low fat at all.

If the original content of some reduced fat muffins was 20 g (¾ oz) and the fat has been reduced to 15 g (½ oz), it is still five times higher than the 3 g (0.1 oz) per serving that officially qualifies as low fat.

'LIGHT'

Then you have words such as 'light' written all over food that is laced with white refined sugar – the very substance which helps to make people fat. They have pulled the same stroke with cigarettes too. The word 'light' is used on cigarette packets to give the impression that they are healthier, but once again it's all bull. The most annoying and unforgiving part about **BiG FOOD** using words like 'light' or 'fat free' on certain food products is that, just like the tobacco companies in the early Seventies, they are fully aware these products are not going to help people lose weight and get healthy. Not only is it not going to help them, but nine times out of ten it will exacerbate the problem. For research for the book I purchased a great deal of different foods and drinks which appear healthy but on further inspection are anything but. In front of me now I have a carton of 'Purple Grape *light* Juice Drink.' Also on the front in large type is 'approved by H.E.A.R.T UK The Cholesterol Charity.' 'Reduced sugar' and 'a source of antioxidants' have also made front-of-carton billing. You would think from a quick glance on a supermarket shelf you have picked up something very healthy for you and your kids. On further inspection of the carton however you will see that this drink is not only made from concentrate, but it has refined sugar and artificial sweeteners. Aren't grapes sweet enough? Why do you need sugar *and* sweeteners?

ENRICHED WITH ...

Then you have the 'enriched with vitamins and minerals', the 'added calcium' and the 'fortified with ...' labels. Once again you can't just add processed, totally de-natured vitamins and calcium and expect them to make a drug food good – because they just won't. The biggest beef I have with them is that they imply they are doing you a favour by adding these things and enriching your food. Don't forget the only reason why it was poor to begin with was because of them and the only thing they are enriching is their bank accounts.

It seems strange to me that it is perfectly legal to buy 'organic', 'GM free', 'no artificial colour', 'fat-free' white refined pasta. This all combines to give the very false impression that you are buying a health food. But who cares if it's organic, GM free or has no artificial colourings? **iT'S STiLL A WHiTE REFiNED DRUG-LiKE FOOD.** Can you imagine if the tobacco companies started to sell organically-grown, GM free, no artificial colouring, vitamin-enriched, all-natural, fat-free, low-calorie, light, added calcium, and fortified with vitamin C cigarettes? Would it make any difference? No, because they would still contain nicotine, which is the drug that compels people to have more and more, and keeps them enslaved as well as over four thousand other chemicals. And exactly the same principle applies to drug-like foods. The white refined sugars, carbs, and refined fats are like the nicotine of the food world.

BiG FOOD are using 'enriched' or 'fortified with ...' more and more – in an attempt to make us believe they are on our side and care about our health. Even Diet Coke has decided to 'fortify' its drink with vitamins and minerals. I can only assume this must be some kind of wind up! Why are we 'enriching' and 'fortifying' in the first place? Why do these labels even exist? How have we reached the point where we think we see the labels themselves as natural? **BiG FOOD** wouldn't need to enrich our foods if they didn't deplete them to begin with.

WHEAT FREE

I am also amazed at the use of some labels, which have simply nothing to do with the product being advertised. For example, I recently saw an oat flapjack with a label saying 'Wheat Free'. On the surface all sounds good, but *of course* it's wheat free ... it's made of oats! That would be the same as sticking a label on an apple saying, 'Free of any artificial flavours, colours and preservatives' or 'Totally Wheat Free'. Just because a label appears to be sending a message of 'health' or one of doing you some kind of favour, it doesn't mean it actually is.

FAIR TRADE

More and more we are becoming aware of the unfair practices in **BiG FOOD.** The first time I saw a label on a bunch of bananas stating they were 'Fair Trade' simply alerted me to the fact the others must be Un Fair. I think we should buy fair trade whenever we can, but again please don't think just because a food or drink is fair trade it is necessarily good for us. If, for example, some fair trade cocoa has been mixed with tons of white refined sugar, refined fats and milk from a junk food cow, it doesn't mean it's good.

I'd Rather Not Have A Bowl Of Coco Pops

As I have mentioned breakfast cereals are **BiG BUSiNESS** for **BiG FOOD** and adding a little cocoa is a wonderful lure for children. Parents are constantly looking at labels, especially when they are buying food for their children. Unfortunately the average parent used to have to do their best to decipher the 'Nutritional Information' on the side of the packet. In twenty-first century Britain, however, the FSA (Food Standards Agency) have introduced The Traffic Light system. This is meant to enable us to see what is healthy at a glance at the front of each packet of food. You have a list of calories, sugar, fat, saturates, and salt. Under each heading you have a percentage so you can see at a glance the percentage of an adult's guideline daily amount. Each nutrition stamp is, as you may have guessed, colour coded. I have in front of me a box of Kellogg's Coco Pops and I am looking at the front nutritional stamp compared with the ingredients list on the side. On the front the colour used on the stamp is a light blue. Light blue doesn't alert you to any kind of danger. The top percentage per 30 g (1 oz) serving is sugar at 10 g (⅓ oz). That's one third of each portion dedicated to refined sugar. That's one third of the box. Yet underneath where it says 10 g there is an 11 per cent sign. The 11 per cent represents the percentage of an adult's guideline daily amount. At first glance it looks like it's 11 per cent per portion, when in reality it's 33.3 per cent. Are they also suggesting that it is okay to have nearly ten bowls of coco pops in a day to meet your sugar needs? This is the point, not all sugars are created equally and the refined sugars you find in **BiG FOOD** are not a healthy way to meet your sugar requirements. When you turn to the side of the packet you can then read the full list, although with today's busy world what parent will bother given they have the 'nutritional stamp' on the front? The full list is as follows:

Rice, Sugar, Chocolate (6 per cent) (Sugar Cocoa Mass), Fat Reduced Cocoa Powder, Calcium Carbonate, Salt, Glucose-fructose Syrup, Barley Malt Flavouring, Flavouring, Niacin, Iron, Vitamin B6, Riboflavin (B2), Thiamin (B1), Folic Acid, Vitamin B12.

Notice the vitamins and minerals at the end of the long list. The fact it contains a small amount of vitamins and minerals means they can use this on the main body of packaging to give the impression what you are buying for your little loved ones is healthy in some way. On the back of the box we have, *'Kellogg's cereals are a great way to get carbohydrates. As well as the goodness of tasty grains, they also give you a source of iron and B vitamins, which help to release energy. Swimming is great fun, so make sure you have the right fuel for the pool'* Notice they say, 'a source of iron and B vitamins'. They don't say a *good* source, just a source. Opium is also a source of sugar. They have also managed to get the 'goodness' on the main body of packaging with reference to the rice used, even though it's heavily refined and covered in sugar. Talking of sugar, not only is it the second ingredient, but also the third in the form of Sugar Cocoa Mass and number eight with Glucose-Fructose syrup – yet another refined hybrid sugar. This is just one packet of one food, if we spent time trying to analyse every processed food we would be there forever.

There is only one way to distinguish good food from bad and that is the label. Not what's on the label, but the label itself. People often ask me, 'what am I looking for on the label', to which the answer is simple – the label! (The point being that if a foodstuff has to have a label in the first place then it's not the most nutritious food.) It is true that by the time you read this book new regulations will be in place, which will prevent certain foods from making health claims. Unfortunately this won't stop **BiG FOOD. BiG FOOD** have **BiG POCKETS** and **BiG POCKETS** can get you as much scientific backing as you like to back up any 'health' claims you wish to make. I challenged an advert by Flora in 2008. The ad read, 'No Food Lowers Cholesterol More'. My argument was that unless every single food has been tested for its cholesterol lowering abilities the advertisers cannot make this claim. After all, it does state that no food lowers cholesterol more. However, the reply I got back from the ASA (Advertising Standards Agency) rejected my claim. The ASA argued that next to the claim that no food lowers cholesterol more it stated, 'The UK's No. 1 cholesterol lowering brand*'. The ASA said, 'The asterisk refers to small print that states, "Based on Nielson value sales data for leading cholesterol lowering brands MAT 01.12.07.".' Firstly who ever reads beyond the headlines of adverts to study the small print? And secondly, where did all these 'cholesterol lowering' processed foods come from? It seems everyone is out to help you lower your cholesterol levels, despite the fact it is still not fully understood exactly what part low cholesterol levels plays on heart disease. Please get hold of a book called *The Great Cholesterol Con* by Dr Malcolm Kendrick to see how messed up this whole cholesterol situation is. Doesn't it seem strange that the ASA would come down on me like a tonne of bricks if I ran an advert saying, 'Fruit and Vegetables – No Food Group Helps To Lower Cholesterol More' yet it is perfectly fine for **BiG FOOD** to do so with a processed food? It is actually against the law to make any health claim with regard to a particular condition about fresh fruit and vegetables. Yes it is against the law! I also challenged the other statement on the same advert, 'Flora Loves Your Heart' due to my belief that they are suggesting you can look after your heart by having this heavily processed spread. I didn't see anyway they could possible make such a claim, especially when the medical jury is still very much out on whether there is any link between cholesterol levels and heart disease. The ASA once again rejected my complaint simply on the grounds they investigated a similar claim a few years ago and rejected that one. They sent me the details of that claim and it is even more mind-blowing than the rejection I received, you almost won't believe it when I tell you.

A few years back Flora ran an advertisement which showed two corn cobs, one had a knob of Flora on it. The text under the first one stated 'Healthy'. Text under the second, Flora covered cob, stated 'Healthier'. They had a sub heading 'it's true, not all fats are bad. Adding a knob of Flora to your food* really is healthier because it's rich in heart healthy oils omega 3 and 6 and low in bad saturated fats'. The small print stated '*As part of a healthy diet'. Firstly I have an issue with 'low in bad saturated fats' when mother's milk is loaded with saturated fat and once again the medical jury, despite the media converge, is still out on this. The main issue though is the obvious one – how can adding a processed food make a natural food healthier? Well according to the document from the ASA it is, '… because Flora spreads were a dietary source of PUFA's (good fats), as well as a source of vitamins A, B, D, and E, adding a knob of Flora spread to a vegetable, as part of a healthy diet, was healthier than a vegetable on its own'. I can now say without doubt the world has gone bonkers! This means you could argue that if you drank new Diet Coke Plus (the one which has been fortified with vitamin B3, vitamin B12, and vitamin C) while eating a banana, it would be healthier, as part of a healthy diet (don't forget that one), than if you had a banana by itself. After all, as well as the goodness of the banana you are getting vitamins B3, B12, and C. In fact, I think you could take this even further and suggest that adding chocolate to a vegetable would make it healthier, as part of a healthy diet, due to the fact it contains certain antioxidants the vegetable doesn't.

All I am saying is look how **BiG FOOD** and **BiG DRiNK** play the advertising game. Look for the small print and be aware that although people like Flora haven't done anything illegal, it is worth using your common sense. My overriding common sense tells me that adding a man-made processed spread to a vegetable created by nature will not 'improve' the vegetable.

THE NO-LABEL ORGANIC DIET©

One of the easiest ways to almost guarantee the best diet on earth is to simply skip as many label foods as possible. Think about it, we all drive ourselves nuts wondering what to eat and obsessing over labels, but why don't we simply skip the labels. If around 70 to 80 per cent of our diet was made up of 'No Label' – especially if also organic, free range, grass fed, or whatever is relevant to the particular no label food – we wouldn't need to worry about labels at all. Our systems can deal with a certain amount of rubbish, so if some does slip through, the 70 to 80 per cent No Label diet will counteract it. This way we won't ever have to worry about our diet again.

When I say 'No Label' I am not talking 'Mystery Food'. It seems crazy that there are so many rules governing what you need to put on labels and yet what I deem as 'Mystery Foods' don't require a label at all. If a burger is sold in a packet, it needs a label, if it is sold by a man in a cart it doesn't. Crackers! So although theme park and concert food, like hot dogs and burgers are No Label – clearly they aren't what I am talking about. Fruits, vegetables, nuts, seeds, meat, fish, and whole grains – none of which require a label. The only sign you need on the no label foods are the ones which tell you the source. If we were in the 1950s no stamps or signs would be needed at all. But in a twenty-first century world where we have our fruits and vegetables covered in pesticides, fungicides, and herbicides and where the animals we eat are fed a diet of junk, it is essential, where we can, to look out for the 'organic', 'locally grown', 'grass fed' etc., etc., when buying No Label foods.

The statement simply to eat 'No Label' foods would be all that were needed – and this book would have been just two pages – if we weren't dealing with addiction and mind manipulation by **BiG FOOD.** As it is we are, and in order to gain true freedom you will need to fully understand Food Freedom mentality. This will be with you soon, but it is essential each element of **BiG FOOD** is stripped bare. With that in mind it is not just food which gets the 'let's hoodwink the public' treatment. A major part of the 'food' industry's revenue comes not from what people eat, but from what they drink. And they use all the same false advertising, misleading labels, and physical drug-like substances to trap you. It is time to raise our glasses to what is anything but a ...

22

LIQUID ASSET

I think that anyone who is reading this book is already aware that our bodies need water and plenty of it. The planet is, after all, made up of over 70 per cent of the stuff and so too are our bodies. The foods ideally designed for human consumption should contain at least 70 per cent water. Even a banana, which you would imagine contains very little water, does in fact contain over 80 per cent. In fact there is not one single fruit or vegetable meant for human consumption that contains less than 80 per cent water. The pure water contained in fruit and vegetables can be described as a true 'liquid asset'. It is not only pure and organic water but it also has the added advantage of being genuinely 'enriched' with live nutrients. This live liquid replenishes your body's health accounts, making it feel light and flowing with energy, and much, much less susceptible to disease.

However, the majority of liquid we consume is a far cry from the pure nutrient packed water you find in nature's finest. From Red Bull to Coke, we are consuming millions of litres of liquids which are slowly contributing to disease, speeding up the ageing process and keeping us fat – including 'diet drinks' (as you will find out very soon).

The advertising for what I describe as **BiG DRUG DRiNKS** is even bigger than that for **BiG DRUG FOODS.** They are, of course, bound to make more money out of drug drinks as they not only create withdrawal symptoms and low blood sugar, but they are also designed to cause dehydration. On top of this, as they don't fill the stomach, there is no cut-off point. All of this means it's very easy for them to convince us that it is, once again, our genuine choice to drink these substances. These drinks, like alcohol, are cleverly designed to cause the dehydration you believe you are getting rid of with the drug drink. At the same time, if you are in a constant state of withdrawal (from caffeine for example) or your sugar levels are beginning to crash because of your white sugar addiction, then you are certainly going to feel a sense of instant satisfaction and instant pleasure – first from the liquid, then from the partial ending of the caffeine withdrawal and finally, from bringing your sugar levels back up. The combination of all of this gives the very strong feeling of pleasure. But again, as with any drug, the pleasure is simply the ending of a set of aggravations – mental and physical – which has been caused by the drug itself. In this case you have three aggravations in one, all seemingly being satisfied with an instant fix of the drug drink. So the relief the body feels will be quite immense, which gives you an instant feeling of pleasure, an instant rush that makes you believe you are choosing to drink this muck. But I cannot repeat this point enough, it's not a genuine pleasure, it is a false one and is the equivalent of carrying around a heavy boulder just to get the pleasure of putting it down every now and then. In such circumstances you would feel better, but why pick it up in the first place?

The problem is that you have been carrying around the boulder for so long you can't even feel it any more. You now believe this is a normal way to feel, you think it's just life and the usual stresses and strains that are dragging you down – not the added boulder. And because nearly everyone you meet feels the same, you believe it must be normal. But it's not normal – you are waking up with a drug food and drug drink hangover every single day. How do you solve this problem? An instant drug food and drug drink *lift*. These foods and drinks appear to be your best friends: life's knocking you down, but at least you can always rely on your coffee and muffins (or whatever) to help pick you up. But the more you try and lift yourself up with these types of drinks or foods the hangover will always get just that little bit worse. When it does you either have to use willpower, discipline or self-control not to increase your intake, or give in to it and increase the dose. But you are still using the very things that are causing you to feel like crap on a consistent basis. This is why people have such difficulty changing their eating and drinking habits – they feel as though they're losing a friend and hence experience a sense of loss. That sense of loss is often just too much to bear and results in a feeling of emptiness. What do most people turn to when they feel empty and alone? A friend. If you believe that these drug foods and drinks are your friends and will actually solve the way you are feeling you will 'give in' and the whole cycle starts again. That is why people struggle when they try to quit certain drug foods or drug drinks. It's not the withdrawal from the drug that is the problem, but the *belief* that you get something from them and you are losing something. We need first to remove the belief, *then* get rid of the drug-like foods and drinks. The way to remove the false belief is to strip it bare and expose BIG FOOD and BIG DRINK for what they are.

THE BATTLE OF BIG DRINKS

The two major players in the drug drink war are Pepsi and Coke and these two have been battling for years to get the biggest market share in this extremely lucrative market. Advert after advert, one product placement after another, celebrity endorsement after celebrity endorsement, they will seemingly do anything and say anything in order to get your business. The main market share is once again children and teenagers; one in eight of whom are now consuming twenty-two cans of cola each week – yes **TWENTY-TWO CANS!** As a nation we get through eight to ten thousand million litres of 'soft' drinks every year, and that number is constantly on the increase. I often wonder though how much Coke, Pepsi or any other 'soft' drink they would sell if by law they had to do some 'truthful' advertising?

'Buy Coke. Just one can contains 6—7 teaspoons of white refined sugar — almost guaranteed to 'hook you' on its own. And in case it doesn't, we've added highly addictive caffeine with the sole purpose of making it habit-forming. And let's not forget the phosphoric acid — something so toxic and dangerous that if you put enamel into it, it would dissolve it. if that's not enough, we've made sure that the acid effect on your body will rob calcium from your bones and teeth, while the sugar will cause tons of the fat-producing hormone insulin to be secreted — which is guaranteed to overwork your pancreas. Plus the added white refined sugar will coat your teeth like nothing else and the beautiful tasty phosphoric acid will help to dissolve them. So please, as our slogan has read for years — HAVE A COKE AND A SMILE ...

... if you are still able to that is.

I wish to make myself clear here and explain I am not simply talking about Coke, I am talking about virtually all 'soft' drinks. They are all pretty much loaded with refined sugar and caffeine. If Coke had no competition they wouldn't even need to advertise. A few fixes of this drug-like drink and they've got you, usually for a very long time. The only reason why they all advertise their drug drinks over and over again is because they all contain the same addictive and health-destroying crap, but if they can convince you their brand is 'cooler' or tastier you will switch – and that's all they want.

Coke – 'No added preservatives or artificial flavours – never had, never will'

Whereas my advert was clearly made up for Coke, the above tag line, believe it or not, is genuine. It is, at time of rewriting this book, Coke's most recent advertising campaign. I never thought I would ever see the day where Coke would use language in their advert giving the impression it is healthy in some way. The advert suggests that because Coke has remained true to the one 122-year-old secret recipe invented by Dr. John Pemberton it contains no modern preservatives or flavouring. The advert also has the tag line at the end, 'Never had, never will'. This is meant to reassure us all that they will keep true and even in the future will not introduce unnatural ingredients. But unless I am way out on a limb here – isn't refined sugar a preservative? It may not be a 'new' preservative, but it is one never the less. As for no artificial flavours, there is not a great deal between 'artificial flavours' and 'natural flavours'. They are both created by people in laboratories called 'flavourists' and both have exactly the same ingredients. It's all about the *source* of the ingredients rather than the ingredients themselves. How on earth can you have a product that contains up to seven teaspoons of white refined sugar (or high fructose corn syrup), phosphoric acid, caramel colour, and caffeine possibly use an advert stating, 'no added preservatives or artificial flavours' and give the impression it is healthy in some way? It is even more unbelievable when a recent study has shown the following:

TWO CANS OF FiZZY DRiNKS A DAY CAN DOUBLE YOUR RiSK OF DEVELOPiNG ONE OF THE MOST FATAL TYPES OF CANCER

A study published in the *American Journal of Clinical Nutrition* showed that drinking two or more fizzy drinks each day was linked to a **90 PER CENT** extra risk of pancreatic cancer compared with people who never drank them. The researchers found the risk of developing the disease was related to the amount of sugar in the diet. They said the most at risk were those who drank high quantities of fizzy or syrup based drinks twice or more a day, who had a 90 per cent raised risk of developing the cancer. Those who added sugar to food and drinks at least five times a day ran a 70 per cent extra risk compared with those who didn't. Dr Susanna Larsson, of the department of environmental medicine at the Karolinska Institute, Stockholm, said higher sugar intake was probably responsible. 'We think it's to do with insulin. If you eat and drink more sugary food it increases your blood sugar levels which affects the amount of work the pancreas has to do. It could stimulate growth of the pancreas and this could lead to cancer.'

I cannot emphasize enough the importance of getting white refined sugar and carbs out of your diet. Only 2 per cent of people diagnosed with pancreatic cancer survive more than five years.

AIDS RECOVERY

Then there's Lucozade which, when I was growing up, was marketed for sick people. If anyone was ill the first thing you bought them was a big bottle of Lucozade. They managed to convince an entire population that if you were ill it would be of benefit to drink some Lucozade. Their slogan even seemed to back-up what they were saying and in turn our beliefs about it: 'Lucozade Aids Recovery'. Some doctors were even recommending this to their already sick patients. This stuff is loaded with refined sugar (or Glucose Syrup) flavourings, preservatives, colours, and even caffeine. How on earth it 'aids recovery' is a mystery. Lucozade has a whole new image in the twenty-first century and have latched onto the ever growing 'sport' and 'energy' drinks market. BIG DRINK have really jumped onto this one and have launched a new breed of 'stimulating', 'vitalizing', 'boosting', 'energy-giving' drinks. These drinks actually claim to 'increase physical endurance', 'improve and increase concentration and reaction speed', 'lift you' and 'give you an energy rush'. There is only one thing I have to say about them:

Total bull (usually of the red kind)

I think the most famous 'energy boosting' drink has to be Red Bull. Apparently 'It gives you wings', their words not mine. How Red Bull is meant to give you wings is a mystery. It's not only Red Bull, there are plenty of companies that have joined the 'boost' drink lucrative market. You have 'Power Horse', 'Dynamite' and a few others like them claiming similar nonsense. They were always onto a sure bet too with these kinds of drinks as most of their customers are waking up every day with a degree of drug food or drug drink hangover (or a combination of the two). The more wiped out people feel, the more 'energy boosting' drinks they sell: their need for 'wings', a lift in other words, becomes greater by the day. Red Bull and the like contain a lot, and I mean a lot, of caffeine – more than Coke that's for sure and ingredients which were enough to make the French ban the drink altogether in early 2004. The ban was overturned in 2008 but Red Bull is still prohibited in some countries. Red Bull recommends people drink no more than two cans per day, probably due to the very high caffeine content. However, as it is obviously unregulated, this recommendation goes unheeded by many and as a result there have been several reports of **ARBR** (Adverse Red Bull Reactions). American pop singer and actor Jesse McCartney had a health scare from consuming too much Red Bull which drastically lowered his iron count to single digits. He was put on supplements and **ordered to stop drinking Red Bull by his doctor.**

The real question when it comes to the almost overnight creation and need for instant energy drinks is: why are we all of a sudden feeling so low we constantly feel the need for an artificial boost? What has happened? It seems the more new 'energy' foods and drinks that come onto the market, the more tired we are all becoming. Is it not obvious that these false stimulants ultimately cause energy *lows* in the same way it has been proved that many headache tablets, with continued use, actually cause headaches in the long run. The need for any drug is caused by the drug itself, drug foods and drinks are no different. As I will continue to repeat they are designed to create a hole where there never was one while at the same time give the impression they are the only thing which can fill it.

IT'S ISOTONIC

Another energy drink, Lucozade Sport, claims: 'In tests against water, athletes using Lucozade Sport drinks are proven to improve their sporting performance by 33 per cent. Why? Sport scientists have proved that depletion of carbohydrate energy stores and fluid impair performance. Lucozade Sport is isotonic – it's specially formulated to be in balance with your body's own fluid. It quickly delivers a boost of carbohydrate energy to the working muscles and supplies fluid fast, which together help to maximize performance and endurance.'

Here's the thing – so does fruit! I could make exactly the same claim about fruit, as it would enable you to go on longer than water alone – but then you don't need to be Inspector Morse to work that one out do you? Look at what they actually say, 'Sports scientists have proved that depletion of carbohydrate energy stores and fluid impair performance'. Do you think they worked that one out by themselves? **OF COURSE IT WOULD**, as we'd then lack two of our basic requirements – water and carbs (fuel). If you replace them you will of course improve performance and endurance. If you are an athlete be assured there's simply no better form of carb energy than humble fruit – just ask Tim Henman. Like drug foods, drug drinks sometimes do the complete opposite to what we are led to believe they will.

Red Bull and isotonic sports drinks are not the only new players in the drug drink game, and they are far from being the only ones to promote their product as in some way good for you.

SUNNY DE-FRIGHT

When I first wrote this book some eight years ago now, my exposure of Sunny Delight was quite new. People were shocked to read that what they thought was a perfectly good 'fruit juice' was in reality full of sugar and artificial chemicals and very little fruit juice. I remember when it first came out, one minute nothing and then almost overnight large bottles of Sunny Delight were in just about every supermarket. Not just in them but rows upon rows of Sunny Delight were taking up very expensive chiller cabinet space.

Sunny Delight, when it first came out, showed a big bright sun and of course the words Sunny Delight. In the corner it read: 'The great taste of 4 fruits with 5 vitamins. Vitamins A–B (1&6) C–E enriched beverage.'

Given this wording, and the fact the stuff is displayed in the 'fruit juice' fridges, most people were convinced that what they're buying was a very healthy, vitamin-packed fruit juice. They were in fact buying a bottle of highly-sugared, chemical-laced liquid which contained at the time just 5 per cent fruit juice.

The thing which really angered me about this particular product was that the advertising was not only aimed at children, but the marketers deliberately set out to convince parents that they were buying a 'healthy' juice drink for their kids. Parents who tell their kids that Coke and Pepsi are a 'no-no' were letting them have Sunny Delight with impunity – some still are.

Things have changed since then and Sunny Delight is no longer Sunny Delight, it's simply Sunny D. They have either **'NO ADDED SUGAR'** or 'Less Sugar' printed on the label and things like, 'we're **RE-iNVENT-iNG!'**. They even have a 'Sunny D Parents Advisory Group' in their bid to do the right thing, and add 'Help us do more!' on the labels too. While it is true that Sunny D is much better than it was, please remember that the original still has added sugar and the sugar free version has artificial sweeteners. They brag on the ingredients list at the side that they have 15 per cent fruit juice from concentrate and have, 'more than you think …' written next to it. But when I see a juice drink I assume most of it is made up of fruit juice, so 15 per cent is not more than I thought at all. Trying to find Sunny D isn't as easy as it was. Competition for the fruit juice and smoothie market is massive and space is more precious than ever. I also think the bad press Sunny D got didn't help with who will stock it. I was in Sainsbury's yesterday trying to buy some for research; I couldn't find it and asked an assistant. This was his exact reply, 'Sunny D? I don't think we sell it any more. Isn't that the stuff that turns you orange?' Clearly it doesn't, but it's hard to come back from that kind of bad press. Sunny D is better than a Coke for sure, but that doesn't mean it's better than 100 per cent pure fruit juice.

BiG DRiNK will literally stop at nothing to get your money and keep you as a customer for life – regardless of the cost to your body or sanity. Their problem is that the stuff they are pushing rots teeth, helps to weaken bones and – more importantly for most people – makes them fat. And customers were beginning to recognize this. So what did companies like Coke and Pepsi do? They brought out diet versions of their highly toxic drug drinks in an attempt to make people believe that if they switch to the diet brands it would help them lose weight. It worked, millions believed it – I was one of them.

These diet drinks are deliberately marketed to give you the impression they are in some way healthy and, of course, their main aim is to make you believe they will help you to lose weight. The truth is you have about as much chance of getting healthy and losing weight with the help of these products as getting run over by a number 12 bus going up the side of Ben Nevis with Ronald Reagan at the wheel!

The sad fact is they conditioned and hooked us so much on 'normal' Coke and Pepsi that we thought it was good when they came out with a non-fattening alternative. However, the nightmare substances to be found in the diet versions, combined with the fact we believe them to be non-fattening, means we end up drinking more of them than the 'real' stuff anyway. Of all the substances I talk about, one of the very worst is to be found in virtually all diet drinks. It's one which I believe is reason enough to give yourself a true …

23

DIET COKE BREAK

Ah yes, Diet Coke, the drink which – and please listen carefully – 'Can help you lose weight as part of a calorie controlled diet'. Guess what, reading a newspaper can also help you lose weight – as part of a calorie controlled diet! I want to make it clear – anything that is toxic to the body is not going to make it healthy nor is it going to help it to lose weight healthily. How they get away with this type of clap-trap is a complete mystery. It becomes even more of a mystery when you hear of the many health problems which have been linked to diet drinks and foods.

There is only one reason why people drink diet drinks – they are 'sugar free' and as such the hope is it will stop them getting fat. But there is now strong evidence to suggest these diet drinks and foods actually contribute to weight gain. Let me say that again –

There is strong evidence to suggest that diet foods and drinks can actually make you fat

The one ingredient common to all these 'sugar-free' drinks and foods is the chemical aspartame, also known as E951 and better known under the brand names of Nutrasweet and Canderel. Aspartame was discovered accidentally by the chemist James Schlatter back in 1969. He was testing a new chemical as a possible anti-ulcer drug when some of the liquid went on his hand. When he licked it he discovered a gold mine – it tasted incredibly sweet. Aspartame is reportedly over two to four hundred times sweeter than sugar yet contains virtually no calories – pure gold for **BiG FOOD** and **BiG DRiNK!** He just knew he was onto a massive financial winner.

It took over sixteen years for US drug giant Searle (his company) to win FDA approval for the sweetener. In 1981 an internal memo from three FDA scientists advised *against* the approval of aspartame. Yet in exactly the same year Ronald Reagan, then president, fired the FDA commissioner and a Dr Arthur Hull Hayes inherited the job. Just three months later aspartame was passed for limited use and within two years was allowed in drinks. The floodgates were open and many countries followed suit. These days aspartame is found in just about every 'sugar free' food and drink you can think of. It's even found its way into sugar free gum, baby foods, and chewable vitamin tablets.

So why was the FDA so against it for so long? Because aspartame has been linked to ninety-two different symptoms including headaches, skin problems, poor vision, depression, carbohydrate cravings, panic attacks, irregular heart rhythms, behavioural problems, seizures and most worrying of all – brain tumours. One senior FDA toxicologist said,

> **'At least one test has established beyond any reasonable doubt that aspartame is capable of producing brain tumours in animals'**

Your brain is normally protected by something called the blood-brain barrier; a safety net that usually prevents harmful substances passing from the blood to the brain. The problem is that aspartame is believed by some to damage the hypothalamus – the area of the brain responsible for regulating the emotional control system, the hormonal and reproductive systems, *appetite*, immunity, and memory. It is worth noting that this area of the brain is not protected by the blood-brain barrier – hence the possible link to brain tumours. This could also explain why headaches are a common complaint for some aspartame users. The surgeon general, head of the public health service in the US, said they believe aspartame usage to be a major contributing factor to the 22 million Americans who suffer from mental disorders.

Dr Hyman Roberts for the Palm Beach Institute for Medical Research in Florida, initially welcomed aspartame: 'When it was introduced, I recommended it to diabetic patients because it contained no sugar, calories, cholesterol or sodium. I thought it was a godsend.' But he had second thoughts after more and more patients developed problems such as chronic headaches, impaired vision, and panic attacks. He soon narrowed down the culprit to aspartame. Around 1,200 patients reported an adverse reaction to this nightmare substance, the most common being headaches. Dr Roberts added, 'I have also had numerous diabetic patients whose condition has been exacerbated by aspartame, including eye and nerve problems. However, when they were taken off aspartame they improved dramatically'. His findings are supported by those of Dr Russell Blaylock, a Missouri neurosurgeon who has what he sees as conclusive proof that aspartame causes terrible changes in behaviour. He says, 'My advice is if you are consuming products containing aspartame, stop using them for three weeks and see for yourself the dramatic difference in the way you feel'.

I believe the main problem is that far from solving weight problems – which with the word 'diet' written all over it claims to do and is usually the only reason people buy the stuff – it is suggested by many that it actually *causes* overeating. Here's why. Aspartame seems to impede the production of the chemical serotonin and a lack of serotonin is not only widely believed to cause depression and mood disorders, but is also linked to such eating disorders as binge eating. This kind of defeats the whole object of diet drinks somewhat don't you think? Dr Ralph Walton, professor at the department of psychiatry at Northeast Ohio University's College of Medicine, believes the calorie-saving advantage of aspartame is totally thwarted because it makes people prone to binge eating. He even says, 'If you feed a laboratory animal aspartame, you wind up with an obese animal'. His advice to those trying to slim is pretty clear:

**'... if you are trying to lose weight,
you should stay away from aspartame'.**

He is not alone either. Betty Martini, a leading US food safety campaigner, is equally scathing. 'We see literally thousands of cases of people who have been taking aspartame for a long time, and they are always overweight. Aspartame actually makes you crave carbohydrates so that you gain weight'.

Aspartame also dehydrates the body, creating a greater need for fluid. You can physically only drink a certain amount of water before the body tells you it's had enough, but with diet drinks you can consume one after another and still feel thirsty.

As you can see there are plenty of reasons to avoid anything with aspartame. But, as always, be your own scientist. If you have drunk diet drinks for years and are still fat what more proof do you need? If you are drinking diet drinks and keep getting headaches – **LISTEN TO YOUR BODY.** Diet drinks are just as bad as the original version, if not worse, so once again **BIG DRINK** is having a laugh at our expense. The original sugar loaded versions contribute heavily to making us fat, by making them addictive and bombarding us with misleading advertising, and then sell us billions of cans of the diet versions a year, which can make us binge eat, crave carbs, dehydrate our bodies and still keep us fat! Diet Tango's old slogan perhaps sums it up: 'you need it cos you're weak' – how's that for saying up yours? That's like a cigarette company saying you need cigarettes because you're weak, but you become weak because of cigarettes and you need them because you're hooked. And the same goes for sugar, caffeine, and aspartame.

I remember once doing an event in the Canary Islands and witnessing first hand just how highly addictive diet drinks can be. One young lady was on at least 2 litres (3½ pints) of diet coke a day. Just being without her diet Coke for a day led to her behaviour changing for the worse (similar to a smoker who has been without their cigarettes). It reached such a level of desperation that at 3 a.m. she went out hunting for a bottle. This isn't hearsay, I witnessed her physically shaking with my own eyes and her drastic mood swing.

If nothing else, even if you don't make any other change, do yourself and your kids a huge favour by breaking free from aspartame or *any* other artificial 'sweetener'. When I first wrote this book hardly anyone was aware of the possible harm aspartame can cause for some. Eight years on and more and more people are getting the message. **BiG FOOD** are getting wind of this and many are producing new scientific evidence which 'proves' aspartame is okay and people like me are simply paranoid alternative health practitioners. Or they are starting to use different artificial sweeteners. Whatever sweet surprise coming around the corner you can bet your life it will cause some hiccup to the fine balance of the workings of the human body. It's this simple:

SUGAR FREE = ARTiFiCiAL SWEETENER

If you see 'Sugar Free' written on the packaging of anything 99 per cent of the time you can be sure it contains some kind of artificial sweetener. It is very important you remember that:

FAT FREE = LOADED WiTH SUGAR
SUGAR FREE = LOADED WiTH ARTiFiCiAL SWEETENER
NO ARTiFiCiAL SWEETENER = LOADED WiTH SUGAR

BiG DRiNK use so many label tricks and if you care about your one and only body and the health of your family, it is essential you start to see what these labels really mean. Diet Coke are to the diet drinks market what McDonald's are to the fast food industry. Because they are at the top they are the ones who usually get shot first. However, once again it is not just Diet Coke, it is pretty much any diet drink. Diet Pepsi, Diet Lilt, Diet Tango and so the list will go on and on. There is even a Sugar

Free Red Bull now – which only illustrates that along with the loads of caffeine they also have sugar in the original.

A couple of years ago Coke brought out another new version – Coke Zero. This drink is aimed at men who don't want sugar and also don't want to be holding what is seen as a girl's drink – Diet Coke. Coke Zero may contain Zero Sugar, but like most things which sell themselves on a Sugar Free basis, it contains artificial sweeteners.

SUGAR FREE – SUNNY D

After the bad press Sunny Delight got when people discovered what they were selling wasn't exactly the vitamin packed fruit juice people thought it was, they decided to launch 'Sugar Free Sunny D'. In the summer of 2003 I was happily tapping away on my PC when I heard a radio advert for, 'Sugar Free Sunny D'. I am aware that BiG DRiNK will use clever wording to dupe the public, but what I heard coming out of my radio that day left me speechless. The ad went something like this:

> 'Which contains less sugar, a bowl of spinach or a glass of new sugar-free Sunny D? Yes, the answer is a glass of new sugar-free Sunny D.' They went on ... 'That's right; a bowl of spinach actually contains MORE sugar than a glass of new sugar-free Sunny D'

The statement itself is factually correct, as spinach contains good quality carbohydrates, or sugar – as the Sunny D ad liked to call it. Unlike spinach though all new 'Sugar-free Sunny D' contains artificial sweeteners, but they left that out of the ad – funny that!

H2O NO

With the bottled water market now worth over £1.5 billion a year in the UK alone, it wasn't going to be long before **BiG DRiNK** got involved. Coke brought out their own brand but it was soon taken off the market in the UK after the British press pointed out it was simply filtered tap water. This was the one rare occasion I was actually on Coke's side. They used a process called 'Reverse Osmosis'. This process turns tap water into water which is actually okay. But once the press got their teeth into it, Coke's water was dead in the water (so to speak). Outside the UK however it does great business.

It seems odd that this perfectly good water was attacked with vengeance by the media in the UK and yet the real water nasties haven't been exposed yet. I am talking here about the new breed of waters on the market. There was a time when water was just water but we have 'active water'; 'sports water'; 'Skinny Water' and so the list goes on. There is even one water which claims it's 'wetter than water' – please!

I can understand any business wanting to get involved in ever changing market trends and joining the bottled water market. I have no problem with Coke shifting to bottled water, I mean it's better than Coke after all. My objection is when **BiG DRiNK** once again turns innocent water into a not so innocent version. In front of me now I have two bottles of Volvic water with a 'touch of fruit'. When you look at the first bottle you would assume it is simply water with some lemon and lime (the two fruits pictured on the front). The label tells a different story: 5.4 per cent of this 1.5 litre (2⅔ pints) bottle is sugar. They are now adding sugar to water and putting pictures of fruit on the front. The other bottle of Volvic water with a 'touch of fruit' once again has pictures of orange and peach and a little stamp label which states 'Sugar Free'. Have Volvic realized their mistake of adding sugar and simply removed it from the original? No. Remember it's says 'Sugar Free' which means … yes – artificial sweetener. We now even have artificial sweetener added to water. If you want water with a taste of lemon and lime it's not exactly hard is it – simply squeeze a little lemon and lime juice in it. Not exactly rocket science.

Having said all of this about aspartame and other artificial sweeteners, please do not become totally obsessive. Please remember again that the body can deal with a certain amount of anything. If a person had five cigarettes a day I doubt seriously they would ever suffer any smoking related disease. It is the addictive nature of such products which cause people to have more and more and the accumulative effect contributes to the gradual breakdown of the immune system and so disease. However, if you have some 'sugar free' gum from time to time, it will not give you a brain tumour! Please use your common sense with all of this and at the same be on the look out for artificial anything. The main thing we are looking for is not so much what's on the label but the label itself.

Diet drinks of any kind do not help you to get slim, they don't genuinely quench your thirst, they don't help to reduce your intake of the wrong kinds of food – if anything they potentially do the complete opposite. If you really have to sweeten things, use Agave Nectar. It is very sweet, very natural and *doesn't* send your blood sugar sky high. It's like gold to those with an extremely sweet tooth.

DRUNK BLIND

Most people are drinking these drug-like chemical concoctions blindly: blinded by what I believe to be misleading advertising, misleading packaging and the false sense of pleasure received by the partial ending of the very mental and physical aggravations they cause. I call it the 'drunk blind' syndrome – when you are drinking something blindly, not able to see the truth. Once you can see clearly what's going on you become free not to drink them; until then you remain hooked.

All of the drug foods and drug drinks mentioned thus far play their part in knocking you down. The further down you go, the more you want a quick 'pick me up'. The irony is when you get rid of the majority of these nightmare foods and drinks from your life you won't need a 'pick-me-up' because you will already be up. The only reason why people continue with the loop is to try and get to the position they could be in if only they didn't eat or drink them.

The most common and most widely used 'pick-me-ups' of them all – and ones which are so ingrained into our culture that 98 per cent of people in the UK drink them several times daily – are our old friends coffee and tea. Now, as everyone knows, you don't have to give these up in order to get slim **BUT** if you want to calm your nervous system, calm your mind, keep your looks and tap into a level of physical and mental vibrancy you never thought possible it's time for your ...

24

COFFEE WAKE UP CALL

Yes, it's time to wake up and smell the coffee – while you think twice about actually drinking so much of it. This is one 'habit' or 'addiction' people strongly believe is difficult to break, but the reality is it can be very easy. If you don't think you need at least a mini break from coffee or tea, I can assure you your body is probably screaming for one. Luckily caffeine only takes a maximum of forty-eight hours to leave your body completely and, despite popular belief, the physical pain you have to suffer because of this will be close to zero.

The struggle people have when trying to 'give up' coffee and tea is not primarily a physical one – just like all drug foods and drinks, the struggle is mainly mental. The UK is the only place on earth where if a war breaks out people say, 'I'll put the kettle on'. These drug drinks are used as emotional crutches. This is why many people will stop putting sugar in their coffee or tea, or maybe cut down slightly on them, but get rid of them completely – not on your Nelly!

I realize that you don't need to get rid of coffee or tea in order to be slim, but by now I hope you are starting to realize this isn't simply about slimming, it's about exposing **BiG FOOD** and **BiG DRiNK** for what they are and making a decision to start making genuine choices. As I will repeat – you cannot have true freedom of choice without the freedom to also refuse. If the thought of not doing it again sends shivers of fear through you, you are hooked and as such it is no longer your genuine choice.

Clearly the odd cup of tea or coffee a day isn't going to kill anyone and if you aren't fearful and feel you do genuinely choose to have the odd cup, then continue if you want. However, I would like to put a case forward which may make you think at least 'why bother'.

Caffeine Can Be A Weighty Problem

Although it is true you may not gain weight directly because of tea or coffee (unless you are having lattes, then the milk alone would pack on the pounds) it is true that it can be a catalyst. Like all false stimulants they ultimately create the very crashes they appear to solve. This can potentially add to the overall emptiness we feel. This potentially can have us eating more to try and fill it. It is also worth pointing out caffeine causes the stomach to produce gastric acid, which *stimulates* your appetite.

Another reason you may choose to cut down or completely eliminate normal tea and coffee from your diet, is the realization there is also simply no other liquid drug drink which speeds up the ageing process quicker than caffeine. Every time you have a cup you fire your adrenal glands and put your body in an 'alert' state. The continuous revving up of your adrenal glands can potentially add many years onto you – but not in a good way!

People spend billions on *external* creams and lotions to 'fight the ageing process', 'to slow down the signs of ageing'. But why waste your money; you can't slow down the ageing process. You can, however, do a million different things to speed it up – and drinking caffeine on a regular basis is one of the best ways to do just that. Many people don't realize this because compared to most people they look okay and are ageing no faster than the majority of people around them. But the majority of people around them are eating drug foods and drinking drug drinks the same as them, all of which speed up the ageing of every single organ in the body.

YOU'RE GETTING ON MY NERVES

People often say, 'I feel like I'm living on my nerves' and the sad reality is very often they are. Every time you drink a cup of coffee or tea (or a Coke, Red Bull etc.), you jolt your nervous system. It's like being in a constant state of stress – your kidneys and liver take a battering, you overwork your adrenal glands and you rob your body and brain of water. Caffeine is a strong diuretic – meaning it makes you pee. This all helps to speed up the ageing process and literally makes your nerves stand on end. Not only that but if you keep dehydrating your body the kidneys will conserve water by making less urine. As a result of this the urine becomes highly concentrated which leads to crystals separating out. These crystals can eventually build up and produce **KiDNEY STONES**. I think I'll pass on that thank you.

The dehydration also affects the brain. Your brain is made up of mainly water and when you are in a state of caffeine withdrawal you lose some of it. Now your brain is slightly smaller than it was. Blood still has to pump through your brain in order to keep you alive. And when blood is pumping through a dehydrated brain you feel it pounding inside your skull – commonly known as a headache. On top of this you also have caffeine withdrawal which makes your nervous system feel insecure – in turn making you feel jittery. With your head pounding, your mouth as dry as the Sahara desert and your nerves in tatters what do you reach for? A nice cup of coffee!

The problem is when you drink it what happens? You do feel better, that's why you reached for it. If you didn't there would be no hook. I cannot repeat enough that what hooks people is not so much the substance itself, but what people think the substance will do for them. The drug-like foods and drinks are ultimately to blame because they have managed to delude us into believing we get some sort of genuine pleasure and relief from them. Once you have more coffee you have put more fluid into the body which helps with the pounding head and dehydration, you partially end your withdrawal from the drug itself and your nervous system actually feels calmer than it did. This all combines to make us think the opposite to what is actually happening – we are deluded into believing that the coffee helped, as opposed to contributed to, the situation.

'BUT IT'S NICE TO HAVE A COFFEE AND TEA BREAK'

Smokers think it's nice to have a cigarette break and crack-heads think it's nice to have a crack break. I realize that may come across as a rather ridiculous comparison, but the point I wish to illustrate is that it's just nice to have a break – period. When a smoker is having a 'break', they will stand outside on a fire escape in the middle of a hurricane. Do they do this for fun? To be sociable? No, they do it because they are drug addicts. Now obviously with coffee there are clear differences, and yes, I realize that on a cold winter's day a warm gingerbread latte at Costa or Starbucks is a world apart from standing outside in the freezing cold puffing on a fag. However, caffeine is a drug and if it were banned from certain places, some people would stand outside if that were the only place they were allowed to drink their drug of choice.

These drink drugs knock the nervous system so much that the person drinking them is made to believe that they won't be able to cope properly with life or even wake up without the stuff. I know many people who completely believe they simply wouldn't be able to function without a cup of tea or coffee in the morning. That's how much of a hold caffeine has over many.

Dr David Kerr of the Royal Bournemouth Hospital summed it up when he said, 'Within half an hour of drinking one or two cups, the flow of blood to the brain is reduced by 10–20 per cent. Combine that with low blood sugar and you can soon start to have palpitations, feelings of anxiety or blurred vision'. And that's just one or two cups. The average is over six, which is a nightmare for your nervous system. Please also bear in mind that when caffeine hits the central nervous system it lowers blood sugar, which increases the brain's demand for more sugar. Let me repeat that in case you skimmed by it –

When caffeine hits the central nervous system it lowers blood sugar and increases the brain's demand for sugar

This, in turn, helps to keep people rooted in the food trap. It is also worth noting that every time you drink tea and coffee our old friend insulin is released, once again helping to batter the pancreas. You have one pancreas – treat it with care.

THE NEW COFFEE ON THE BLOCK

The way we drink coffee has changed dramatically over the last few years and although we are known throughout the world as a nation of tea drinkers, we now consume more coffee than tea. This is largely due to the massive expansion of the hip and trendy coffee bars such as Starbucks and Costa Coffee. Personally I love the atmosphere in these new bars and I see why people flock there other than for just their caffeine hit. However, if you are trying to lose weight and you still want coffee, skip the lattes. Your average latte will be made from milk that came from cows fed on junk. This leads to a higher level of inflammatory omega 6s. Many don't realize the amount of milk they are consuming when having their daily lattes.

The new hip coffee places are no doubt well aware of the mental addiction people have for coffee too. In the US in particular, you see queues of caffeine junkies waiting in the cold for their first fix of the day. This is often not choice – it's a form of slavery to a drink drug. This is borne out by the fact that coffee is now the second most legally traded commodity in the world – the first is oil. The stats on this stuff are quite staggering: 70 per cent of Britons are said to visit the new 'hip' generation of coffee shops once or twice a day – that adds up to a hell of a lot of revenue, as you will discover later.

CUP OF FORMALDEHYDE ANYONE?

Now I'm not saying that everyone who goes and grabs a Starbucks is hooked on the stuff and I'm not saying that you cannot have the odd cup of tea or coffee and still be slim and healthy, because clearly you can. Places like Starbucks have a great atmosphere and as I have said many go in for other reasons than simply a coffee. If you do enter a coffee bar, most offer good alternatives which are worth trying. A Soy Thai Chi latte is gorgeous and they always have a selection of teas such as peppermint. If you are going to have your usual latte, hit the 'skinny' button. A few lattes a week won't kill anyone, but while you are in the process of change, why not have a much needed true coffee break.

Another thing to watch out for is decaf tea or coffee. Once again, the product which they market as a 'healthy' alternative really isn't. First of all, decaffeinated coffee still has some caffeine in it. Secondly, two of the chemicals used to decaffeinate coffee are turpentine and formaldehyde. Formaldehyde is used as an embalming fluid – lovely!

But remember all drug drinks and drug-like foods have no other hold over you than what you believe you get from them – once you see the truth, the belief is changed and freedom is yours for the taking. It really can be that simple. And when you do free yourself of these substances you won't believe how much calmer and more relaxed you become.

Unfortunately the truth is not always easy to see. The clever advertising, the product placements, the misinformation we have had from the experts since birth and, of course, the constant illusory 'boosts' caused by the drug-like substances all combine to keep us from seeing the truth that will set us free. And because these substances shatter and jolt the nervous system – making our lives appear a lot more stressful than they really are – this can have the knock-on effect of making us turn to yet another drug drink. The one I am talking about here makes it very difficult to see the truth. In fact it makes it very difficult to see – full stop. It is so ingrained in our society that if you don't drink it, you are questioned as to why and viewed as having a problem with it. Yet it's a drug drink which is responsible for more deaths, more violence, more suicides, more break-ups, more domestic violence, more child abuse and more heartache than crack, cocaine, LSD, ecstasy, and heroin *combined*.

It is a substance which is highly toxic, yet parents seem quite happy to give this substance to their children – often before they've reached double figures. This drug drink not only piles on the pounds, due to its toxicity, but also messes with your mind and creates overwhelming cravings for carbohydrates and sugars. It not only causes you to overeat at times but has also been known to distort the mind so much that people have been known to eat things they would never normally touch while under its influence. That was perhaps the biggest clue because, let's face facts, when it comes to food, anything looks good when you are literally ...

25

BLIND DRUNK

👹 'Okay Jason I was with you up until now. Getting shot of Coke, tea, and cheese is one thing, but if you think I am quitting my glass of wine with dinner or the odd beer when I'm out with the lads or lasses – forget it pal. This is meant to be a food freedom lifestyle and not a diet and I have no intention of going without alcohol for the rest of my life. I am not an alcoholic, I do not have a drink problem, so why should I?'

Well if that's how you are thinking you'll be relieved to hear that you do not have to quit alcohol altogether in order to have a slim, energy-driven body. However it certainly is worth looking at this highly toxic, fat-producing substance with our eyes very much wide open. This can only happen when we are sober for when we are drunk, we really do become totally blind. Blind to our feelings, blind to our emotions, blind to our behaviour, blind to what's going on around us and totally blind to what we are actually putting into our body – and I don't simply mean the insulin-robbing, fat-producing alcohol. Alcohol very rarely is seen for what it is and we all have this 'happy jolly' image and rarely take a good hard look at what it is doing to us. We need to open our eyes and realize it's not just the alcohol that piles on the pounds, batters our organs, acts as a depressant, causes lethargy, keeps us a slave and helps to once again speed up the ageing process; it's also the added rubbish we eat as a direct result of it.

Alcohol Came First Kebabs Second

I believe alcohol came first, kebabs second. Kebabs really do fit into the 'mystery food' category: big chunks of 'whatever-the-hell-it-is' meat, stuffed into a white refined pitta, the token salad (if you can ever describe it as such), topped off with blow-your-head-off chilli sauce. You see this big mound of flesh hanging up in a warm shop window for what seems like months. As you walk past during the day, neither hell nor high water could get you to put that putrefying lump of dead flesh into your mouth. Just the thought of the flies laying their eggs and defecating on it (as they do when they land on food) is normally enough to keep any rational, thinking person well away. But I did say rationally thinking person and any kind of reason or thinking goes completely out of the window when you're a couple of jars short of a coma. In fact, when you come piling out of your local pub or nightclub this lump of fly-poo-infested mystery food magically turns into the finest gourmet cuisine. And it's not only kebabs. These are also the times when the 'hot mystery food' van – which on the way into the nightclub was just a rotting old dirty van with a big fat scruffy man attempting to serve you rubbish – all of a sudden becomes heaven on wheels.

The alcohol is devastating enough for your bloodstream – the last thing it needs is a load of blood-clogging, fat-laden, sugar-infested 'food' seeping through it at the same time. But what choice do you have when you're drunk? You've lost your normal control, your sugar levels are out of sync, and your body has been stripped of essential fats, vitamins, and minerals – which all add up to an unbelievable craving for something stodgy to try and satisfy the empty feeling.

The body now has so much poison going into it that it needs to shut down in order to keep you alive. Once again it calls on eyesight, hearing and whatever consciousness is left to help it out with this red alert situation. The problem is so bad that the body just doesn't have the energy to keep you alive and awake at the same time – so it shuts down. You are now in a comatose state that even beats the Christmas dinner one. The body has such a need to repair itself that even if someone was to pick you up by the feet, swing you around the room and through the window – you still wouldn't wake up. No, the only thing governing whether you are allowed any form of consciousness is your body, and quite frankly it just has too much work to do and needs all the energy it can muster.

There is, however, one point at which the body will allow you to get up and move – when it either needs to release fluid or when it calls for fluid. If the situation is particularly bad the body may not even wake you up to release fluid – it will just do it. Sometimes, of course, it may compromise with you by allowing you to get up and move but not giving you any sense of direction – this is when you end up releasing bodily fluid either in the wrong room or in the cupboard! However, when the body wants fluid it will certainly wake you up and make you move as fast as you can to replenish lost fluid. Ah yes, the 'Sahara Desert Syndrome' as I call it. This is where you wake up in the middle of the night with what can only be described as the mother of all thirsts. The body is so dehydrated that unless it gets some water – soon – you are in a serious danger of either dying or at least causing some kind of brain damage. So the body calls to the brain **'WAKE UP AND GIVE ME SOME WATER. NOW'.** This is the point where we sit bolt upright in bed (if we ever made it there), trying to catch our breath through an extremely dry throat. Now it's sod the 'I only drink mineral water' nonsense – where's the nearest tap? Once the body can't hold any more water without bursting, it orders you back to sleep – not rest, sleep. After all, your body is hardly resting is it? So back in a coma we go. We eventually wake up to find that the Royal Philharmonic Orchestra has set up temporary residence inside our skull and our body feels like it's been run over by a truck.

So what's really going on here? Well your brain is now smaller than it was the night before – it has literally shrunk. I just want to say that again –

Your brain is smaller than it was the night before!

The water you lose because of the massive dehydrating effect of alcohol causes this. Have you ever noticed that for every beer you drink you tend to pee out three? Water is the next thing the body needs after oxygen to function efficiently. Without it you will wither and die. Every single cell and organ relies on it, including the all important head office – your brain. That little bit of water you had during the night helped a bit, but your brain (which is mainly water) is still very dehydrated – this makes it shrink in size. Every time you have a skin full it's like going into the ring with Mike Tyson. Alcohol destroys brain cells. If the brain is constantly (like a few times a week for example) deprived of water to this extent and is at the same time beaten up by the highly toxic alcohol – it can easily cause permanent shrinkage and damage to the brain. When you wake up with your brain shrunk on say a Sunday morning (the most common time) blood still has to pump through it in order to keep you alive. The pounding feeling in your head is no less than blood trying to pump through a dehydrated brain. Your head hurts like hell, your body feels weak and one more thing, your blood sugar levels – which govern hunger – are very, very low. This causes a massive empty feeling and a mother of a hunger. You see it's not just the alcohol that's the problem, or even the rubbish mystery food we eat when we are drunk, but also the rubbish we crave when we wake up with a humdinger of a hangover.

Firstly we hit the painkillers. Excellent – this is about the last thing your body needs. These tablets don't get rid of a headache; they just move the ache or cover it up. What do I mean? When you put a painkiller into your system it simply shuts off nerve endings to your brain. So you still have blood trying to pump through a dehydrated brain, only now you've taken a painkiller you can't feel it any more. However, just because you can't feel it doesn't mean it's not happening. And because you have now buggered up your body's natural action signals, you will ignore your body's calls for what it really needs – rest, nutrients, and **FLUID**.

So with the headache apparently sorted, what's next? Ah yes, the blood sugar levels which have crashed to an all-week low. When your sugar levels crash to that extent you crave an instant fix – and broccoli just isn't going to do it. You need something that's going to raise your sugar levels *fast*. You have such an empty feeling that you feel the need to load your bloodstream with sugar and fats – **ASAP**. So you crave fry-ups, white refined bread, croissants, jam, salt etc. All this drug-like food comes flooding into an already battered and very tired body. It's difficult enough for the body to try and process rubbish food like this normally, but with alcohol in the system – fat chance, literally. Alcohol is so toxic to the body that it cannot be stored anywhere; the body must get rid of it as soon as it can or it will die. This means that while the body is dealing with the alcohol it leaves anything you've eaten the night before or that morning untouched. This all adds up to the type of 'hangover' which can be with you for a long time – yes the very uncomfortable 'flesh hangover' commonly known as fat.

And we try to counteract this type of hangover by mixing some Diet Coke with the fat-producing alcohol – as if adding Diet Coke to our ten vodkas is really going to make any difference to our weight or energy levels. We not only mix aspartame with alcohol, but we also mix the new 'energy' drinks with them too – probably to try and counter the effect of the alcohol. A hip drink at the moment is vodka mixed with our old friend Red Bull. So here we have a depressant (alcohol) and a stimulant (Red Bull) in the same glass – no wonder we don't know if we're coming or going. Now if we go by one of the many myths about alcohol, you shouldn't ever get drunk on vodka and Red Bulls – after all doesn't caffeine help to sober you up? Well the answer is no it doesn't. Why people drink loads of coffee to sober up is a mystery – all you end up with is a more alert drunk. The liver can only process one unit of alcohol per hour and all the Red Bull and coffee in the world cannot speed up this process – in fact nothing can. This is because alcohol is a very highly toxic substance; in fact it is just as toxic as heroin. Let me reiterate this little known fact –

Alcohol is just as toxic as heroin

Despite this we have 'expert' doctors telling people that drinking some alcohol is better than not drinking it at all. Please bear in mind that the 'experts' once said exactly the same thing about smoking too. They will actually admit that alcohol can be dangerous, but then tell us that in small doses it can be good for people over the age of 40. Now how the hell did they come up with this? We hear this kind of nonsense all the time and yet we never really question it. Why? Because it has been put across by the 'experts' and, don't forget, part of our own addicted brain wants to believe it too. They claim that the health gains are for people over 40 who 'may' be protected against heart disease. Yet 90 per cent of people over the age of 40 do drink alcohol and heart disease is still the number one killer in the UK. If alcohol helped fight against heart disease, as is the claim, then we should be the healthiest nation in the world and our incidences of heart disease would be almost nil. But we don't and it isn't.

The reality is that alcohol kills 40,000 people a year in the UK alone, that's 100 people a day. Worldwide that figure is about 1 million people. It batters your liver, kidneys, and pancreas; it dehydrates your body; destroys brain cells and can shrink your brain. It eats away your stomach lining, speeds up the ageing process, weakens eyesight and causes impotence, diabetes, and obesity. It is a highly addictive drug that can and mostly does keep you a slave for life. It also causes unnecessary and often overwhelming cravings for carbohydrates and sugars and, despite all of this, there is still, at time of writing, no warning on the label (although this is now changing and by the time you read this warnings may well be on).

The authorities aren't about to make us more aware either – the UK government earns £10 billion a year from alcohol. We as a nation spend £25 billion on alcohol per year. To put that in perspective that's more than the annual spend on clothes, schools, and hospitals. And the conditioning experts are allowed to spend over £200 million blatantly advertising this highly dangerous, very addictive, often life- and soul-destroying drug – and just like the drug food advertisers they are certainly good at their job. The Budweiser boys are perhaps the best – with their colony of ants carrying bottles of Bud underground and partying, to their very funny Louie the frog 'bud-weis-er' ad and perhaps the most legendary and famous 'Watsssssssuuuuuup?' ad campaign.

Just like any product which is selling and promoting a false need, **BiG ALCOHOL** show images and situations over and over again to condition us into drinking their product at certain 'bell' times. They are more than aware if we do it enough and create a bell, we will feel uncomfortable and incomplete when we don't do it. For many people just the thought of going 'on the wagon' creates feelings of fear and apprehension.

Like any drug the need for alcohol is created by alcohol. Before we started drinking it we didn't need it. I don't know about you but I can't remember coming home from a bad day at school and saying, 'I've had a pig of a day mum, I could murder a pint'. We all have our apparent reasons for drinking alcohol, but rarely if ever do we question those reasons. For example, we often say we drink because we love the taste of alcohol, but do you remember your first alcoholic drink? For most it was horrible. All that happens is we persevere due to wanting to look 'grown up' and eventually we acquire a taste for it.

We often also say that alcohol helps us to relax, yet when you see someone having a fight in a pub, do you think 'Quick, give them more alcohol, they are clearly not relaxed enough'? Surely we only feel relaxed when drinking alcohol in already relaxing situations. If you are in a bath and have a glass of wine, you should feel relaxed, but not because of the wine, because you are soaking away the stress of the day. When you are in a pub after a day's work, the main level of relaxation you feel is the fact work is over and you are with friends. The question shouldn't be do we feel more relaxed with a drink, but do we feel unrelaxed without a drink. If so, how has that happened and what caused it? Clearly the alcohol itself.

We often say it helps to give us courage, yet when we see someone of three foot nothing ready to take on Arnold Schwarzenegger after a few beers, we know that's not genuine courage – it's stupidity. Alcohol removes fear and as such prevents us from ever overcoming our genuine fears or apprehensions in certain situations. In order to be courageous we must overcome fear, in order to grow as a person we must overcome fear: if alcohol has taken away your fear there is none to overcome – this means you are not being courageous. By taking away our ability to overcome fear on our own, we prevent our courage muscle from ever growing and ultimately our courage is diminished with alcohol.

We often say alcohol makes us happy, yet it is common knowledge that alcohol is a depressant and we have all experienced this effect at times. If you are feeling down, you can drink all the alcohol in the world, but you will still feel down. And look at all the trouble and violence on Friday and Saturday nights – the people causing it look happy don't they? Have you ever been unhappy despite the fact you are drinking? If so, and if alcohol as a substance transported people into the world of happiness, why can that situation ever occur?

We often say alcohol helps us to socialize, yet when we see someone who is drunk during the day the last thing we want to do is socialize with them. It also makes you slur your words, makes you repeat the same point constantly and eventually makes you pass out – hardly sociable. It is sociable to meet people and go out, but if one person is drinking a non-alcoholic drink and the other an alcoholic one, does it mean they aren't being social? If I was at dinner and I had a different meal to someone else, it doesn't mean I am being boring or unsociable.

The Happy Illusion

Everyone has this 'party', 'good time' image of alcohol – not only because that is the side which is constantly advertised, but also due to the fact that most of the situations where we drink alcohol are 'good', 'fun', and often 'party' occasions: Christmas, birthdays, meals out with friends, the weekend, watching the game, New Year's eve, on holiday etc. But aren't these all good times anyway? Didn't we enjoy these times before we started drinking without the need for alcohol? The problem is now we have alcohol 'bells'. We have such a link with alcohol and these situations that we believe these situations wouldn't be the same without it.

It's time to realize that alcohol doesn't make a party – it just happens to be drunk at all parties because we have been conditioned to do it. I have been to plenty of parties where the alcohol was flowing and it was a good night, but I have also been to many parties where the alcohol was flowing, yet it was still a lousy party. Why? Because alcohol itself doesn't make a party, it's the company, the banter, the interaction and the music which all determine whether the party is a success or not. The truth is that alcohol may not have made any parties, but it has certainly ruined many. It's funny how **BiG ALCOHOL** don't ever appear to advertise the reality of their product. I can see why they don't as I somehow think it wouldn't be as appealing. Imagine if we revamped the famous Budweiser **TRUE** commercial with the 'What's Up Just Chillin" theme.

'Watsssssuuuup?'

'Just chillin', in fact i'm bloody freezing standing here half-cut waiting for a cab at 3 a.m., all because i can't bring my car when consuming this drug drink — true'

'Watsssssuuuup?'

'Just chillin' here with a beer-gut the size of the Napa valley, watching the game — true'

'Watsssssuuuup?'

'Just chillin', destroying brain-cells, shrinking my brain, not making head nor tail of the game — true'

'Watsssssuuuup?'

'Just chillin', passed out, missing the game — true'

'Watsssssuuuup?'

'Just chillin', watching the game on a hospital bed waiting for a liver transplant — true'

And it's obviously not just the Bud boys; the whole industry is at it.

Does all this mean you can't have a glass of wine with a meal or a pint with your mates? **NO, NO, NO** and in case you missed it **NO!** You can do whatever you like – the idea, remember, is to feel free and the odd glass of wine or pint is really not going to prevent you from getting slim and healthy. At the same time though I also want you to feel free *not* to drink. We are under such pressure from other people who drink that we often simply feel pressured into 'joining them'. Alcohol is the only drug on earth you have to constantly justify not taking. By the time you finish this book I want you to feel free to go out and experience a non-drink night and love the experience for the sake of it – you never know you just might get hooked.

'i had a great night last night — i must have, i can't remember a thing'

In case you are wondering, I personally stopped drinking many years ago and I really have no desire to start again. Yes the extremely odd glass of Champagne has crossed my lips at certain events, but me having Champagne is almost as rare as finding WMDs in Iraq. I even wrote an entire book on the subject (*Stop Drinking for Life … Easily*). You might be wondering why I choose not to drink? Well it's not because I can't drink, because I obviously can whenever I want to. It's also not because I'm a couple of haloes short of a sainthood either, and it's not because I'm what society would describe as an alcoholic. It's because I can't see any reason on earth to get drunk any more. I go out more now than ever before, I don't have to worry about driving my car or how I will feel for work the next day. I socialize more because I have the freedom *not* to drink alcohol – a freedom most do not have. I can stay out later and I wake up earlier. I see much more of life and I have my Sundays back. I also never, ever get a hangover. So why would I want to drink the stuff, what would it do for me? About as much as it would do for a child – nothing. It wouldn't make me happier (as it's a depressant) and it wouldn't help me to socialize (as it makes me slur my words and stupefies me – then it makes me pass out). It wouldn't help me to relax (as it overworks the organs and shatters the central nervous system). It certainly wouldn't improve my watching of 'the game' (the game doesn't change because you've got a beer in your hand). It wouldn't give me energy (as it takes tremendous nerve energy to deal with it) and even though it's a liquid, it wouldn't quench my thirst, only cause dehydration. It would also drain fluid from my brain, destroy brain cells, beat up every organ in my body and it would rob my accounts of insulin and calcium. Plus – which was always a biggy for me – it would cause fat to be stored in my body. So yes I can drink alcohol whenever I want to, it's just call me fuddy-duddy – I just don't want to spend my one and only life exercising constant control, week in week out, over a drug drink which gives no genuine benefits whatsoever.

The only time I have any kind of alcoholic drink is for ritual purposes and nothing else. If someone's cracking open a bottle of bubbly to celebrate a special occasion, even though I may not agree with the conditioning around Champagne, I'll take a glass, say cheers, clink my glass with others, take a swig and go back to my normal drink. The hook would only occur if I thought that a particular occasion wouldn't be the same without actually drinking a certain amount of alcohol.

Clearly there are people who can and do have the 'odd' drink and it is their genuine choice, but the reality is that it is rare. For most people the thought of having any kind of social gathering and not drinking would create tremendous fear within them and fear of that kind = **HOOKED!**

UNDER THE INFLUENCE

Clearly it's your choice and you may well not be hooked and be perfectly happy to just have a couple of glasses of wine with your restaurant meal, but be aware. What we think is our genuine choice is far from it.

Our actual decision to take this drug drink is due to being under the influence. Most people think they are 'under the influence' when they actually imbibe alcohol. The truth is that the only reason why people even want to drink this stuff is because they are already under the influence. Under the influence of advertising, under the influence of misinformation, under the influence of others, under the influence of social pressure, and under the influence of the illusion created by the drug itself – which all adds up to the 'drunk blind' syndrome.

And as you can now see we have not only been eating all kinds of drug foods blindly, but drinking all kinds of diet, soft, energy, and alcoholic drinks blindly too. You should also now see that there is a tremendous potential price to pay on the health front for what is essentially a very short-term illusory set of pleasures. Not only do we pay heavily on the health front, but these empty foods cost a fortune too. It does seem odd that we even pay for the privilege of being mentally and physically abused by all this rubbish. It's not just your body's bank accounts of enzymes, insulin, and calcium that get robbed, what about your financial bank account? **BiG FOOD** is making a mint from our addictions and now you know that, just like **BiG TOBACCO**, they often add chemicals to deliberately make their foods and drinks 'habit forming', you may think twice about handing them your hard earned money. **BiG FOOD** and **BiG DRiNK** can certainly help you lose pounds, but only it seems from your bank balance. Not only does **BiG FOOD – BiG PEOPLE** but **BiG FOOD** also equals …

26

VERY BIG FAT PROFITS

BiG FOOD equals **FAT PROFiTS**, the kind of profits that are hard to get your head around. The profit margin on highly sugared syrup drinks and foods is tremendously high, even as much as thousands of per cent. This kind of food is very cheap to produce and even when sold what appears cheap, the profits are very high. As most are habit forming and addictive, they get to repeat the high profit over and over again.

GROWING VERY FAT ON THEIR PROFITS

As a nation the UK spends over £7 million a day on drug-like fast foods from places like McDonald's, Burger King, etc. – that's seven million pounds a day. That doesn't include what we spend on all the crisps, cakes, chocolates, biscuits, 'energy' bars, sugared sweets, and the like. We now spend, wait for it, over £4 million on crisps per day. That's a least 12 million bags a day in a nation of 60 million. That's just crisps. A product which costs pennies to produce and yet can sell for over a pound. When I was growing up crisps appeared cheap, but now we have 'designer crisps' and I have seen bags for over two pound each – that's £2 for a bag of crisps.

The Coca-Cola company made $5 billion worth of sales in just one quarter. Cadbury made annual pre tax profits of nearly £100 million. The amount of money we spend on **BiG FOOD** and **BiG DRiNK** doesn't really compute. Here are a few examples of what these things cost over a lifetime. The average chocolate lover will spend an average of £8,000 in a lifetime on chocolate, and that's only with a very conservative spending of £3 per week. I used to grab some kind of choc bar on my way to work every morning and one on the way back. That's easily more than £3 per week, especially if I add the extra choc bought on 'special' occasions – birthdays, parties, mood swings, friends coming round, the weekend etc., etc. This would be okay if it genuinely boosted us, but when you think it's simply an empty drug-food with very clever and mind manipulating advertising, it's a massive waste of money.

Then, of course, we have the tremendous amount of money spent on **BiG DRiNKS**. And what a fortune we spend too. Alcohol alone will set the average person back over £100,000 in their lifetime. That is how much the average drinker will spend; for many the figure is a lot higher. That's **ONE HUNDRED THOUSAND POUNDS** to put yourself in a state where we often fail to remember a large part of our lives. One hundred thousand pounds to suffer all of those hangovers, and so it goes on.

Then you have the 'soft' and 'diet' drinks. In the UK alone we consume ten billion cans of fizzy drug drinks every year – five billion of which contain that lovely stuff aspartame or another artificial sweetener. The cost of this works out to be in the region of £3–4 billion a year. Then there's coffee and tea. These two are very nice little earners for people like Starbucks, Costa Coffee, the PG Tips boys and, of course, the McDonald's gang. Yes, not content with just selling their own coffee in their 'restaurants', McDonald's have decided to give Starbucks and the like a run for their money with the launch of McCafes. They want a piece of the coffee bean pie and who can blame them. Your average latte in Starbucks will set you back over £2. If you have two a day, seven days a week, you will spend nearly £80,000 in your lifetime on lattes. They aren't called Star*bucks* and *Costa* Coffee for nothing. If my Uncle George were alive today he wouldn't believe what has happened to the world. We not only pay for bottled water, which would freak him out, but it has become normal for a single cup of coffee to set us back £2.50.

SUGAR RICH

The section of **BiG FOOD** that pretty much has silent shares in *all* **BiG FOOD** is **BiG SUGAR**. I have mentioned that white refined sugar is the Cocaine Of The Food World and like cocaine, it brings **BiG PROFiTS**. Unlike cocaine, **BiG SUGAR** isn't underground and can be very open about its business. Sugar used to be eaten only by the very wealthy and if you were overweight it was a sign of wealth. In our twenty-first century world it tends to be the poorer we are the more sugar we consume. The more sugar we consume, the fatter we become and the richer **BiG SUGAR** become.

According to official figures, we consume over **ONE HUNDRED** lbs (45 kg) of the stuff per person each year. I believe it's more than that, especially when you take into account that just one can of Coke contains seven teaspoons of the stuff, ketchup is 27 per cent sugar and it is in pretty much all packaged processed foods. Our slavery to this stuff keeps Messrs Tate & Lyle laughing all the way to the bank and leaves us, not only financially worse off, but physically poor too. **BiG SUGAR** have a great deal of influence in this world and just like **BiG TOBACCO** they will do anything to defend their product (as you read earlier). Sugar is highly addictive and causes premature death – but it will be many, many years and a few court appearances before **BiG SUGAR** come close to admitting their substance can possibly cause harm. Unlike tobacco, sugar is a food and so the arguments are much harder. However, even if the arguments are harder, it doesn't alter the facts.

ADDED COSTS

The financial costs of consuming **BiG FOOD** doesn't simply end with the cost of the substances themselves, you also have to take into account the indirect costs of these drug foods and drinks. We could talk about the average alcohol drinker spending £18,000 on taxis in a lifetime alone or that they spend a huge amount on cover-up drugs to try to counteract their hangovers, but far more important is the cost to your health.

The National Health Service may be free, but I think it's fair to say that it's at breaking point and more and more people are now going private. Even those who cannot afford to go private soon find the money when their life is at stake. I mean, how much is your liver worth? How much for your kidneys? Your heart? These are times when people really wake up and realize that money means jack when it's a matter of life or death. The idea is to wake up *now*, do something *now* – not when you reach that stage. It's much, much easier to prevent than it is to cure. Having seen four family members pass away due to cancer I am more than aware of this fact.

Another added cost to perhaps think about is the reality of the effect the wrong foods have on our appearance. So if you don't make the change after you've read this book, make sure you keep plenty of money aside for the tummy tuck, the liposuction, the face-lift, and the expensive anti-ageing creams. And while we are talking about the money spent treating the symptoms, let's not forget that $32 billion was spent on different diets, 'nutritious' shakes, slimming pills, and other weight 'cures' in the US in the year 2000 alone. On top of that, $23 billion was spent on work time lost due to drug and junk food related problems.

Isn't it mad? We spend an absolute fortune on drug foods and drinks that make us feel and look sluggish, fat, old, make our lives hell and cause depression – and we then spend another fortune treating the symptoms they cause. It wouldn't be so bad if we were spending all this money on stuff that made us happier, but it doesn't – in fact it does the opposite, that's why you are reading this book.

**'You can fool some of the people some of the time
but not all of the people all of the time'**

I don't know who said that but it appears they were wrong. **BiG FOOD** and **BiG DRiNK** have been fooling virtually all of us for years. We have been seemingly happy to part with our hard-earned cash because we have been blinded by the advertising and blinded by the illusory 'pleasure' of injecting a shot of this stuff into our bloodstream to end the low it caused. But we have also been blind to people's greed to make money out of us – no matter what the cost to our health. Until the blinkers are off we remain mentally trapped.

Breaking free of this trap doesn't take 'positive thinking' or willpower as we have also been totally conditioned to believe, it just takes a full understanding of the nature of the trap you are in and a simple route out. The following chapter should go some way to getting that full understanding; I will then give you the simple way of thinking which will set you totally free. Firstly, to help you see this particular trap in a very bright light, I would like to show you …

27

THE MOUSE TRAP

A mouse is put in a cage and given natural food, water, and a funnel containing pellets of a drug (which look like food). There is a button to the side of the funnel which dispenses the drug pellets. In order for the mouse to get the drug it must hit this button with its nose. The natural food and water have always been in the cage, but the funnel containing the drug pellets is new. So out of curiosity the mouse hits the button and receives its first dose of the drug. The pellets have also been sweetened to cover up the foul taste of the drug, which the mouse would naturally be repelled by.

The drug pellets are designed to shatter the mouse's nervous system and at the same time create a *false* hunger and a *false* need. They are designed to play havoc with the natural, finely tuned chemical balance of the body by rapidly raising the blood sugar levels of the mouse and then making its blood sugar fall rapidly. It's the instant rise and excessive fall which they are hoping will trick the mouse into choosing the pellet drugs over natural food – just like any other drug addict. To add to the fun the pellets are also designed to cause dehydration. In other words the pellets are ultimately designed to create a void and a false need.

The scientist now removes the natural food and the mouse is left with just the pellets and the water. However, to make matters worse, the scientist replaces the water with a liquid drug. Once again, just like the pellets, this liquid drug has been heavily sweetened to trick the mouse into believing it is something good. This liquid drug is designed to do exactly the same things as the food pellets, except that it dehydrates the mouse even faster than the pellets.

Having no choice the mouse then hits the button, eats the drug pellets and drinks the liquid drug. Because of the nature of these substances, the mouse very soon starts to feel the effects of low blood sugar and dehydration (let's call this the withdrawal period). As soon as the mouse begins to feel these effects, what does it do? It hits the button for a pellet and drinks the liquid. Does the mouse now feel better and calmer than it did? Does ending this aggravation create a feeling of pleasure? The answers are yes and when this happens **BOOM** – it's hooked. Physically, of course, there is no hold and if the mouse just stopped hitting the button it would return to normal. But it won't stop because it's now *mentally* hooked on a false belief. I cannot repeat enough that it's the delusion which is the real hook, not the physical element of the drug. The mouse has no way of knowing what is really going on as the empty, insecure, void feelings are just the same as normal hunger and normal thirst and the minute he eats and drinks the substances those feelings subside – for a short while at least.

After the mouse has hit the button for a few days, the scientist puts the natural food and water back into the cage alongside the drug pellets and liquid drug. When the mouse feels hungry it recognizes the old natural food and takes some. But in no time at all it goes straight for the button again. After a while the mouse ignores the food and water altogether and chooses the pellets and liquid drugs. Why? Because the natural food and water will not instantly satisfy the mouse any more. The natural food will only satisfy a genuine hunger; it cannot *instantly* feed the false one. The false one needs to be starved out, in a similar way to withdrawal from a drug. The natural food was not designed to send sugar levels sky high in an instant, because sugar levels are not meant to fluctuate at this tremendous rate – it causes an imbalance in the body and mind.

The blood sugar levels would need time to level out for the body's natural balance to be restored. The mouse has no way of knowing this; it just feels an insecure, hungry feeling and so is not about to wait for the feeling to go away naturally. As far as the mouse is concerned it won't just go away naturally, it's hunger and if you ignore it you die. It is programmed, like all animals on earth, to feed a hunger if possible. This hunger needs to be satisfied, and the natural food just isn't instantly doing the job. All animals are designed not to ignore hunger, it is the single biggest driving force of our lives and our existence depends on ending it. When we feel hungry, we feel insecure and restless, it affects the way we think and our concentration. This is the body saying, 'forget everything you think is important – it's time to survive'. So when the mouse feels the crashing effect of such low levels of blood sugar it has an insecure feeling and it knows that feeling as hunger. If the drug food was taken away from the mouse when it felt these feelings, it would panic. Even though there might be plenty of natural food around, it won't give the mouse that instant 'hit' it's looking for. If it starts to feel apprehensive about this or starts to panic, what will happen? More empty, insecure feelings occur, identical to that of very low blood sugar or hunger. So the *overall* empty, insecure feeling is now huge and if the mouse still cannot find any instant 'hit' food or drink, even greater panic will set in and an even greater insecure feeling will occur – the majority of which is caused by mental panic.

So you can see that even though the mouse might be left with plenty of natural good food – which would help to rectify the fine chemical balance of its body and ultimately solve its problem – it would still go into a frenzy looking for some food that provided an instant hit (very similar to humans on a diet don't you think?). Can you also see that if the cage was the only place for the mouse to get the instant drug food you could leave it wide open and the mouse still wouldn't escape? If you think about it, it can't escape for it's no longer the cage that's keeping it there – it's the lack of truth. The mouse is mentally trapped by a simple physical confidence trick.

The truth is it would be too scared to leave the cage because just the thought of not being able to find more drug pellets would send it into a panic. Don't forget the mouse actually believes it cannot survive without the pellets – that is how much these things have affected its nervous system and way of thinking. Can you also see that even if the mouse gained weight, became tired and lethargic, or became diseased and knew that it was indeed the drug pellets causing those particular problems, it still would not stop hitting the button? Why? Because it's still *mentally* trapped. The same insecure feelings would occur, the same panic and the same low blood sugar. And in that moment, when the sugar levels crash and the empty, insecure feelings begin, the mouse would feel insecure and the mental desire to end the insecurities ASAP would be greater than a desire to be slim and healthy. The second the insecure feelings go away, the mouse can think straight once again – but by then it's too late.

This is the food trap and we are the mice. And white refined sugar, additives, chemicals, and white carbs are the pellets.

In the actual experiment with the mouse, the drug affected the mouse so badly that it physically shook when it was in withdrawal. When it hit the button the shakes stopped. But in no time at all its nervous system began to be affected again. The shakes started again and what did the mouse do? Hit the button. Did the mouse feel better? Yes! But only better than it did a moment before and nowhere near as good as it felt before it pushed the button for the first time. Did it feel a sense of pleasure? Yes! But only the pleasure you would feel by putting down some heavy shopping – it's just the ending of the aggravation. The poor mouse has no idea that its central nervous system is slowly being destroyed by the drug; the drug is fooling the mouse into thinking that it is helping and there is a genuine pleasure in getting the instant hit. In other words the mouse is hitting the button blindly. The more the mouse shakes the more it hits the button, the more it hits the button the more it shakes. The mouse builds up such an immunity and tolerance to the drug that it still shakes even while it hits the button and is under the influence of the drug; just slightly less than a moment before. After a while the mouse just continues to hit the button, hit the button, hit the button – until it dies.

Believe it or not the scenario above is not something I made up – experiments like this are routinely carried out in drug tests (though I have changed certain parts to illustrate the point I want to make). I do not agree with this type of experiment, but it perfectly illustrates the principle of the food and diet trap.

This is why there are hundreds of thousands of highly intelligent people who are constantly struggling not to eat certain foods. And this is despite the fact that they know these foods are bad for them and cause weight gain, lethargy, misery and all kinds of disease. The saying goes, 'what you don't know can't harm you' but it's not true in this case. What you don't know could eventually kill you.

If you look at the experiment it is exactly what I was doing when I was hooked on drug foods and drinks, and it is precisely what you and millions like you have been doing probably ever since you were first weaned. Once you hit the button a couple of times you really do become the mouse. The difference is that we had our first dose of refined sugar before we were old enough to think for ourselves. We are all meant to have a sweet tooth as fruit and nuts are our natural foods, so we were easily fooled on the taste front. And on top of that we have the advertisers actually encouraging us to hit their button and become their mouse. The more they get us to hit the button, the more money they make. And the fatter and more tired we become, the more we think we need this stuff to keep us going. See the loop?

FREE BLIND MICE

Just like the mouse, we cannot see things for what they are while we are pushing the button – especially if we are surrounded by millions of people all doing the same thing. Drug foods and drinks appear to have the opposite effect to what they are really doing, so until someone points it out how the hell is anyone meant to see? These so-called foods were suppressing my nervous system so much that I believed in the end that I could not enjoy myself or live properly without them. Knowing what I know now, I wonder how I lived properly *with* them.

The insecurities and strong apprehensions I felt at just the thought of getting rid of this rubbish was all caused by the drug foods and drinks themselves. Just like the fears the mouse had were ultimately caused by the button. Now I am out of the cage it is easy to see. The reality is that there is nothing to fear or feel apprehensive about by escaping from the trap and everything to fear by staying in it.

This book is about stepping outside of yourself so that you can see what is really going on. If the mouse had the opportunity to see what it was actually doing, do you think that it would continue to hit the button? Do you think it would continue even if the drug pellets tasted sweet? Do you think it would continue if it knew that the insecure feelings would just go if only it stopped hitting the button? Would it continue if it knew that the button was the cause and not the cure? Do you honestly think for one second it would stick around if it were armed with the facts?

FREEDOM OF GENUINE CHOICE

The mouse never had a genuine choice, it was never its choice to hit the button, it was simply lured into a very clever trap, and ended up believing it was choosing to hit it. Exactly the same thing happened to me and exactly the same thing is happening to you and millions like you. No wonder we hate ourselves for eating this rubbish. We know it's bad for us, we know it's making us fat, and we often hate ourselves for doing it, but we've missed the main point – we never really understood why we *were* doing it. Everyone is so busy focusing on why we should-n't eat rubbish (as if we don't know) they have failed to look at the simple chemical reactions created by the drug foods themselves; chem-ical reactions that cause false hungers and delude us all into believing we can't quit because we love these 'foods' too much.

Starve the false hungers from the body; get rid of the brainwashing from the mind; change your diet to one of the No Label variety and you are free – no more food problem ever. Having been routed in the food and diet trap myself it is almost hard to describe how good it feels to have a Food Freedom mentality. To know that you will *never* be over-weight again is an amazing feeling, one I now take for granted. It is a feeling of total freedom. To feel light and have the raw energy to liter-ally suck the juice from life is just the best feeling in the world. To wear what you want when you want to is amazing. To feel energetic, confi-dent, slim, and actually like the way you look and feel is like a new world. The best feeling of them all though is just not having to control what you eat: to be free from the constant battle with food. No more weighing food, no more weighing myself, no more feeling bloated, no more drug food hangovers – bliss. I have been fat and I have been slim, the difference is like the Earth and the Moon – two completely different worlds.

The irony is that the only things keeping people in the food trap are their own thoughts and beliefs. The actual physical 'withdrawal' from these drug foods and drinks is hardly even noticeable. Our thoughts and beliefs about certain foods and drinks have been influenced by years of brainwashing, conditioning, and total bullshit from **BiG FOOD** and their clever advertising friends. The excellent news is that the door to freedom is wide open and always has been; we have, in fact, been our own jailers – trapped by what we believe we get from these foods and drinks. The only reason people struggle when they go on a diet or try to change what they eat is because they strongly believe they are giving up a genuine pleasure that they think they can't be without. The fear is in the thought of missing out, the belief we are making a huge sacrifice and that our lives will never be the same again. Change the belief, see the truth and you realize there is nothing to fear. Once that happens you can break free, easily.

Up until now I have given quite a comprehensive outline of all the disadvantages of eating drug-like junkie foods. I would like to balance the argument and I have dedicated the next two chapters to firstly the advantages of eating junk foods and secondly the sacrifices you will be making when you make the change. You need to know what you are up against.

28

THE ADVANTAGES OF EATING JUNK

29

THE SACRIFICES YOU WILL BE MAKING

... that's right — NONE!

30

DIET MENTALITY

The Twelve Steps To Failure

The only reason why people find it difficult to change their diet permanently is simply because they go about it the wrong way. Here are the usual steps most people go through whenever they attempt a change of diet – see if you can spot any flaws:

1 Believe you are making a huge sacrifice and that your life will not be worth living.

2 Work yourself into a mental tantrum, like a child being told they can't have a toy.

3 Get extremely irritable and obnoxious with everyone around you (if you do this for long enough the people who told you to go on the diet will probably tell you to eat and leave them in peace).

4 Allow all of your waking moments to be dominated by thoughts about the foods and drinks you feel you have 'given up'.

5 Feel sorry for yourself at all times.

6 Stay in and feel constantly deprived. On no account go out and have fun until you are slim.

7   Drive yourself mad waiting for the desire for these foods and drinks to go away (unless you change how you think about these foods and drinks please expect this step to last for the rest of your life or until your diet ends).

8   Hate and envy all your friends who are 'allowed' to eat and drink what you feel you are being forced not to.

9   Weigh yourself every day to really feed the depression.

10 Binge when no one is looking, and when they, are eat some salad.

11 Spend all the time you are on the diet moping around for something which you hope you'll be able to resist.

12 Starve your body so that you are also physically fighting against the most powerful instinct known to mankind – survival.

Spot any flaws?

If you followed all the steps that people usually follow when trying to get slim, do you think for one second you would feel happy about making the change? Do you think there's a chance in hell you could do this for the rest of your life? Can you see why 95 per cent of diets fail? I believe that the figure is 100 per cent, for how do you gauge success? By how much weight is lost? By how long they have kept it off for? By how much energy someone has? If someone is still using these 'steps' to stay slim or to stay healthy then they have only been successful in using tremendous amounts of discipline and self-control and continue to do so. If you are still mentally craving certain foods and constantly using your discipline and self-control not to have them, you are not a success, you are still using 'diet mentality' and you are still rooted in the trap.

I know not everyone reading this book is doing so to lose weight, but I have yet to find anyone who doesn't want more energy, better health and a strong immune system to help prevent the now 'normal' degenerative diseases. Those people who are already slim and are trying to change what they eat still use the same mentality as those trying to lose weight; in other words they are still using the diet steps and are stuck in the food and diet trap.

I personally used these steps many, many times as they seemed a logical way to go about it. Simply build up all the reasons in my head why I shouldn't eat the rubbish, hang on in there and hope for the best. Logically it should work, but as I have repeated throughout this book, addiction and logic have no place together. I always believed that the reason I could never stick to a diet was simply down to the fact I was just weak-willed when it came to certain foods. I now realize willpower had nothing to do with it; I just had no idea what was happening in my bloodstream and that I was chemically and therefore emotionally addicted to drug-like foods.

The term 'drug food' has never been used so how is anyone meant to know it's the food that is the problem and not them. How are we meant to know that the very foods which we are using to try and feed an emotion are in fact part of the very cause of that particular emotion?

The *Stronger* Willed You Are The *Less* Chance You Have Of Succeeding On A Diet

The reality is: it's not about how much willpower, discipline, and self-control you have; in fact you know you are free when you no longer have to use huge amounts of willpower to control your intake of certain foods and drinks. For those of you who are convinced that changing your diet must require willpower and self-control and I am mental for suggesting anything to the contrary, let me illustrate this point clearly.

Imagine two people in a room, one strong-willed and the other weak-willed, each with a chocolate bar in their hand ready to eat it. If you were to remove the chocolate from them and tell them they are not allowed to have it, who do you think would kick up more of a fuss and tantrum? Clearly the *strong*-willed one. Now imagine the same two people in a room with chocolate bars near them, but neither had any desire for the chocolate at all. What would happen if you were to come in and remove the chocolate in this situation? Which one of the two will kick up more fuss? The answer of course is neither of them. Why? Because they don't *want* it, they have no desire for it, and they don't believe their lives would be enhanced by it. If you have no desire for something it becomes completely irrelevant whether you are weak-willed or strong-willed. However, if you still believe certain foods retain a genuine benefit and you use the diet steps to try and do without them, then the *stronger* willed you are the *more* of a fuss and tantrum you will make and the harder it will be.

The problem is every time we repeat these diet steps, all we are doing is reinforcing over and over again that life with the junkie foods is a hell of a lot better than life without. Every single time you are on a diet and using the steps, you build these foods up in your mind to be something which they are clearly not. You believe they can enhance your life and mood in some way, therefore you feel deprived whenever you think about them. The more deprived you feel the more precious those foods become, the more precious they become, the more deprived you feel. It doesn't take long before you say, **'SOD iT'** and crack. Now try to imagine going through this mental tug-of-war while starving your cells at the same time. No need to imagine, if you have been on any one of the common diets you have already experienced it. On most diets we are not just putting ourselves through a mental trauma, but also a physical one. Most diets involve nutrient and food deprivation – this is called starvation. When the body senses it is starving it starts storing fat. While you are starving, your body begins to eat your muscle tissue, leaving the fat till last for energy. You are now starving your body of food and nutrients to an even greater degree than normal and it's not even getting enough bulk to sustain a reasonable quality of life. Your sugar levels remain at a lower level than is comfortable, thus creating a knock-on effect in the mind which is now screaming to feel satisfied. No wonder you get ratty, irritable, want to beat people up and say 'sod it'.

The fundamental point I wish to make and repeatedly hammer home is: are we happy once we have finally given in to our own mental tantrum? Well, initially the answer is yes. We feel better because we've just been through mental torture and, depending on the particular diet, we have also been physically starving ourselves at the same time. It is no wonder that we feel an immediate sense of total relief when we stop the mental tantrum and feed the body something other than cabbage soup.

On top of that, when we are using the ridiculous diet steps we avoid going out where possible, and if we do brave the outside world we're constantly looking at all the food other people are 'allowed' to eat – so either way it's hell. We constantly feel deprived, so we strongly believe we are making huge sacrifices. When on a diet we can go through this mental tug-of-war for hours, days, weeks, or if you are some kind of truly amazing human (or masochist), months or even years. So when we say 'Oh sod this for a game of soldiers' and decide to bring the madness to an end –we are bound to feel better than we did. However, this is only because we have put ourselves through mental hell in the first place: once again the satisfaction and pleasure we feel is in the ending of a massive low. This simply compounds the false belief that changing your diet is hell and eating crap is great fun.

The problem is, when we finally decide to 'give in' on a diet, we don't realize that the relief and pleasure we then get from eating the foods we were craving is just the ending of a massive mental and physical aggravation which *we* have caused in the first place by the way we are thinking and the self imposed tantrum we put ourselves through. The pleasure this gives simply confirms in your mind that you are a miserable, boring, unsociable, and ratty individual *without* those types of food and much happier with them. This only adds to the ingrained belief that these foods are very precious and pleasurable, and help your mood. We deduce from all of this that we are indeed happier because *of* these drug foods and drinks. Yet the truth is we are happier because we have stopped a mental tantrum, which we and only we were causing.

Treating The Symptom With The Cause

It wouldn't be so bad if the battle came to an end when we did eventually decide to give in, but we need to ask ourselves what caused the mental battle in the first place? This mental battle is of course caused by the very 'foods' and 'drinks' we think will end the battle. Effectively we are using the foods which caused the battle to begin with as a tool to try and end it. This is why the battle doesn't come to an end by simply going back to the same old ways. By having these foods again we may be happier than we were on the diet, but only for a *very* short time. It's usually only halfway through the piece of drug food we eat, because we soon realize what we have done and start to feel like a weak-willed failure once more and delude ourselves that this 'one off' won't hurt and all will be okay. But too late – the drug food parasites have reared their ugly heads and you have just seemingly had confirmation that you were missing out. The dripping tap has well and truly started and now you are using each mental diet step but now magnified 1,000 per cent. The battle has not come to any kind of an end with that 'sod it' moment – it's just become a whole lot tougher.

You then spend the next couple of days or weeks deluding yourself that you are still on 'it' and yet are seemingly blind to all the secret eating you are now doing. After all, it's one thing for you to know you have failed, it's another to tell the world. So it's salad in front of your friends and pig-out when you're by yourself! After you have had enough of hiding the fact that you are now eating this rubbish again, you then let everyone know by blaming the diet itself or your genes (always a good one). You say you have been on 'the diet' for much, much longer than you actually were, and as the people around you only actually saw you eating salad, they believe you. You then start to eat the same way as you did before you went on the diet, only now you binge slightly more, subconsciously trying to make up for all that lost time. After a couple of months of 'living' like this, with all the physical side-effects that go along with the intake of drug-like foods, you realize you really can't live like this and so try and solve the problem once more by doing what? Yes, the latest diet. But nothing has changed; no matter which 'diet' you now choose, you are still going to have a battle because the problem is *mental* not physical. So we end up going nuts spending our lives on a semi-permanent diet, constantly trying to control our intake of foods and drinks which are controlling us, while still keeping all the physical symptoms of being a drug-food addict and overeater.

The 'diet steps' only remove the food and drink causing the physical problem – in fact many diets don't even do that – but you are still left with the brainwashing, conditioning, and false belief these junkie type foods can be used as an emotional crutch. The food problem is in reality *95 per cent* mental and only *5 per cent* physical – the complete opposite to popular belief. If you only remove the physical element you are still left with a very, very big problem. You are still left with the very strong belief that you are missing out. You are still left with the belief that you cannot enjoy or cope with your life in the same way without these foods and drinks. In other words you still have the problem and you are still hooked. The 'hook' is a mental one that creates an emotional pull, very similar to a bad relationship.

Any Type Of Food Addiction Is 95 per cent Mental and Only 5 per cent Physical

There are many people who have stopped eating certain foods, but still have a problem with them. If they've quit but six months down the line are still craving all those drug and junk foods, using their control not to have them, then these people still have a food problem – even though they don't actually eat these foods. Even if these people do get slim, they still have a food problem and because of this the chances of them staying that way are not good.

This is why many 'Fat Camps' and health breaks rarely work. People pay huge sums of money to be locked in some building in the desperate hope that when they are 'released' they will be slim. But the cause of the problem isn't tackled at all – only the symptoms. They are still using the diet steps when they're in these places, which means as soon as they're 'released' they will immediately reward themselves for being 'good'. And what do they reward themselves with?

The Win-Win Situation

According to conventional wisdom then, the choice seems to be one of two options. Either eat the drug-like foods and suffer the daily mental and physical consequences or try to stop consuming them using the 'diet steps' and suffer the daily consequences of that nightmare. Either way you still suffer and you still have a food problem.

There is of course one other option that no one seems to have thought of – see the junkie mind-controlling, body-destroying substances that they really are and jump for joy to be finally free not to have to eat them.

There are many 'food gurus' who have made millions out of helping people who are overweight, but are far from ecstatic about being free themselves as many aren't in fact free. Many might be slim but they still believe they are making many sacrifices when it comes to certain foods and drinks; they just believe that the sacrifices are worth it. But as the previous chapter illustrated, all the sacrifices are made when you are having to eat this rubbish day-in day-out, not when you finally stop the madness. All the sacrifices are made when you suffer the mental and physical problems these so-called foods create. These people should be elated to be free from the fat, the lethargy, the restrictions on what they can wear and the slavery to these types of food. But many of them are still mental slaves to these foods, even though they might be physically trim now.

As far as Rosemary Conley, the big weight loss clubs and virtually all the 'food' gurus are concerned it's all about exercising control. Sarah Ferguson, the Duchess of York and one of the 'faces' of Weight Watchers, said of the overweight people featured on a TV programme on obesity, 'It will be a lifelong battle for all of them'. And the sad thing is it *will be* unless they see the truth – if they see the truth they can be free. Do you want to exercise control for the rest of your life or do you want to be free? I met Sarah Ferguson when I was on the Steve Wright in the Afternoon show on Radio 2. I said I had mentioned her in my book and that it would be nice if people realized there could be another way and stopped portraying as fact that it will always be a battle. Just because nearly everyone finds it a battle, doesn't mean it has to be – it simply illustrates what happens when the vast majority of people go about something that can be incredibly easy, in a very difficult way.

Cutting Down Isn't Always A Stepping Stone To Success

Instead of achieving mental and physical freedom from these drug-like foods and drinks most of us simply 'cut down' on the amount of the *same* food we were eating in the first place – smaller portions and weighing scales. The calorie counting madness that has been the heart of the diet industry for decades is all about counting and cutting down. But when you 'cut down' on these foods, not only can you rarely achieve your goal of total mental and physical freedom, but you once again make these foods and drinks appear more precious than before – making the 'hook' even stronger. After all, the longer you hear a baby crying the more pleasure you feel when it finally stops!

There are people out there that can tell you exactly how many calories are in virtually every food – and I mean to the exact number. During the obsessive counting calorie days, which to be fair are far from over, some people even worked out that a cheese sandwich had exactly the same amount of calories as semen! Then you have slimming clubs not only doing their completely pointless counting the points stuff, but also the food diary nonsense. But how is writing down everything which passes your lips meant to help you get slim and healthy? Any dieter knows that if you eat anything while you are standing, or from someone else's plate, or you just take little bites of something every now and then, you won't put it in your diary because in any of these situations IT DOESN'T COUNT! And anyway, who the hell has got the time to actually list everything they eat and drink? More importantly why on earth should we want to?

It seems slightly mad, that as intelligent human beings we think that if we do somehow manage to cut down on the junk, keep a food diary, weigh our portions of food correctly, check what time we are allowed some more food, see how many 'points' or 'sins' we've got left for the day etc., etc. that it proves we are in full control of our food and sorting out our problem. But if you think about it, the opposite is true. If you have to do any of this it proves you are far from in control, in fact it proves you are being controlled by the very things you believe you are in control of. Remember –

if you are having to exercise control over anything, then that something must be controlling you

The idea is to stop trying to control and just free yourself both mentally and physically – then you become truly in control. In reality people like Rosemary Conley, and most people on a diet, are constantly moping around for certain drug-like foods and drinks which they hope they won't have. Can you imagine doing that? Once again, there's no need to imagine it as we have all been guilty of making the whole process of changing what we eat very hard for ourselves by doing precisely that. And this is the real madness of it all, the fact we

Constantly mope around for certain foods and drinks which we hope we won't have

Isn't that just a touch insane? Isn't it bonkers to spend your life moping around for certain things which you hope you won't have? And this is the main reason why we all seem to think it's difficult to change one's diet and get rid of certain foods and drinks from our lives. Yet if we just stopped the moping and the self-imposed feelings of deprivation – and actually felt good about the fact we now have a genuine choice and are totally free not to consume the crap any more and free to say up yours to **BiG FOOD** – we just might find the whole process not only easy but extremely enjoyable.

We have had it back to front for so many years that many find it hard to accept that the process of changing your diet is one of the easiest and enjoyable things you could ever do. We are so conditioned to believe losing weight is hard that many can't even get their head around the fact it's stupidly easy if you go about it the right way. We are effectively our own jailer and the key lies with us. The key is simply to stop the whinging, tantrums and moping around for foods and drinks which we hope we will not have anyway. Seriously think how absurd it is to get angry or upset because you can't have something, which you hope you won't have anyway!

I CAN'T

On that note, this is another stupid thing we say to ourselves over and over again which simply confirms the false belief that changing your diet is hard – 'I Can't'. We constantly tell ourselves we can't have this food or that food when in reality we can do what the hell we like. I used to have chocolate most days, but there would be times when I just didn't have any for many days. Did it bother me? No. Was I using willpower in the time I had no desire for it? Again no. Did I suffer any withdrawal or tantrum? No. And many of you reading this book will have had many occasions where you have gone for days without having certain foods and drinks and yet it hasn't bothered you in the slightest. But the very second you tell yourself you **CAN'T** have these things any more, boom! – you experience the 'forbidden fruit' syndrome. When this happens the 'forbidden' foods and drinks become a thousand times more precious than they were before you told yourself you couldn't have them. The result? You immediately feel miserable and deprived, even if you would normally find it easy to abstain for a few days.

Kicking the vast majority of junkie food from your life is ridiculously easy; the *only* reason why people struggle is because after they kick them they continue to mope for something which they hope they won't have. If you ever get caught up in this mental tug-of-war for whatever reason I have one simple yet highly effective approach to stop it:

Either Have The Food Or Drink and Shut Up or Don't Have it and Shut Up ... but whatever you do ... SHUT UP!

It's only the mental tantrum that causes the problem. So either have 'it' and shut up or don't have and shut up, but **SHUT UP!** Be aware though if you do have it, you will find it very hard to shut up. Drug-like foods trigger the 'need' for more and you will have a much larger mental battle than before you had the first dose. Even if you are one of those people who believe it must require willpower because that's just how it is, please realize that any degree of willpower goes up by a 1,000 per cent once you have 'just the one'. **BIG FOOD** even tells us this but we don't seem to believe them. Didn't Pringles warm us that 'Once You Pop You Just Can't Stop' and weren't we also warned by another member of **BIG FOOD** that 'One Nibble And You're Nobbled'?

Get It very clear in your mind that when you get rid of the drug-like foods and drinks from your life, you **CAN** consume them whenever you wish, just as I can whenever I wish. I just don't wish. You **CAN**, after all, take heroin whenever you wish; nobody in the world is stopping you, so why don't you? Because you don't wish to. I am not your teacher or parent, you **CAN** do whatever you want after you finish this book – the choice is yours. But please remember you will no longer have a choice if you *do* consume all these drug-like foods and drinks. Drug addiction of any kind takes away the freedom of genuine choice. It must be crystal clear that we are not talking about a habit or a genuine pleasure or even genuine food – it is drug-food addiction, nothing more and nothing less.

Bear in mind though that the addiction is virtually all psychological. If you tell yourself that you can't then you will feel deprived and miserable. What we should be saying is, 'I can have these foods and drinks, but what on earth would be the point, what would they do for me?' The answer to that question is crystal clear – **NOTHING**. There is just no point in eating or drinking these nightmare substances, other than in emergency situations and when you are genuinely hungry and there really isn't another choice. Remember, although we are talking about drug-like foods, they have no actual lasting hold over you at all, it's all about your perception.

Just saying the word 'can't' or actually believing that you can't would be the only thing that could make it remotely difficult for you to quit the drug foods. I have a couple of great acronyms for the word can't –

Constant And Never-ending Torture
and
Constant And Never-ending Tantrum

That is exactly what we put ourselves through when we keep telling ourselves we can't – constant and never-ending torture. Look at Rosemary Conley: judging by an article I read she is, at certain times, suffering from the **CAN'T** syndrome. She wrote the incredibly successful *Hip and Thigh Diet* years ago, which would strongly suggest she is doing the 'never-ending torture' bit quite successfully. But why put yourself through a completely unnecessary mental torture?

Once you are out of the cage you can go back in whenever you want. You can suffer the daily nightmare of being dependent on drug-like foods that are essentially doing nothing for you. You can remain fat, lethargic, and hooked, but if you now understand what is going on, why on earth would you ever want to? The point is that you *can have* whatever you want whenever you want – not that you *can't*. What you say to yourself determines how you feel about any situation. By understanding at any time that you always can but that there is no point to it, you instantly remove the T, which is where the torture lies. All we need to do is shift from the diet mentality, which is –

'i want but i *can't* have'

to the correct way of thinking –

'i *can*, but i don't want to have'

Or more accurately:

'i can, but i don't *need* to, or *want* to — i'm elated to be free'

When I first made the change myself many of my friends and family would say, 'Oh I forgot you can't have that can you' or 'Let's look on the menu to see what you can have'. What they fail to realize is that I can have whatever I like – often they are the ones being controlled by their eating habits, not me. I am now completely free around all food and it's like night and day compared to how I used to live.

We have all at some point in our lives suffered from the 'can't' syndrome. It's the syndrome everyone experiences when they're quitting smoking or alcohol or are on a diet. The mad thing is it's self-inflicted and so easily remedied.

Would You Adam & Eve It? – It Can Be So, So, Easy

Personally I am not overly religious, but one story can help to illustrate my point. The story of Adam and Eve perfectly outlines the power of 'can't'. After all, being told 'you can't' didn't stop Adam from picking an apple from the tree. Even being told he would die if he did, didn't make a difference. Why? Because …

C.A.N'T. overrides death

And there are many people who, at this very moment, are being told either to diet or die. I have already given two examples in this book of two 15-year-old girls. One from the UK, Georgia Davis weighing in at 33 stone (209 kg) and one from the US, Terriny Woods, weighing in at 41 stone 12 lb (over 260 kg). Georgia Davis has been told she needs to 'diet or die' on several occasions, but that hasn't helped her any more than it helps a smoker to state the obvious or someone heavily addicted to alcohol. I sincerely hope Georgia doesn't die because of the insidious nature of this trap and **BiG FOOD**'s insatiable appetite for **BiG PROFITS.** I hope by the time you read this she has got the genuine help she needs. I for one, at the time of writing this book, will be contacting her and asking if she wants to be a guest at my health retreat. That way we can deal with the mental as much as the physical aspects of this trap. Whatever happens I hope she gets the correct help she so desperately needs.

Many, unfortunately, will die: not because they are weak-willed or have some genetic disposition which cannot be overturned, but because they are caught in a very clever trap and are under the illusion that they will not be able to enjoy or cope with their lives without what they perceive to be their friend, crutch or pleasure. A documentary entitled *Half Ton Mum* fully illustrated the desperation and ultimate tragedy of what being caught in this trap can cause. Renee Williams weighed over 70 stone (445 kg). In her desperation she had gastric bypass surgery, which carries its own risks. She was the largest person in history to have this operation. Although the operation went well, she died soon after. And for what? What did she ever genuinely gain from her addiction to **BiG FOOD** and **BiG DRiNK** apart from tremendous amounts of weight? The sad truth is absolutely nothing. It seems odd that it's okay to say **BiG TOBACCO** has plenty of blood on their hands but I don't think we have quite reached the stage where we can say the same about **BiG FOOD** and **BiG DRiNK** – but they have and I am saying it first, and more blood in my opinion than **BiG TOBACCO**.

Remember the words of Eric Schlosser from his wonderful book *Fast Food Nation*:

> **'it is the ultimate consumer technology, designed to manufacture not a tangible product, but something much more elusive: a brief sense of hope. That is what Las Vegas really sells, the most brilliant illusion of them all, a loss that feels like you're winning'**

As I mentioned earlier, Eric was talking about gambling, but again I need to remind you that is what **BiG DRUG FOOD** and **BiG DRUG DRiNK** are also selling – the most brilliant illusion of them all, a loss that feels like you're winning. When Half Ton Mum Renee Williams gave herself a 'lift' from drug-like foods she no doubt felt, in that moment, she had won. Clearly there was no winning taking place at all, simply degrees of losing. The only way you win is to see this sinister trap for what it is and jump for joy to break free.

Mind Your Language

The language you use when you change your diet is extremely important to finding it easy or difficult – in fact it's all in the words. In particular, and to hammer this home, never underestimate the power of **CAN'T**. It appears on the surface to be just a word, but we should never underplay the power of words. Words, after all, are the only things preventing people from changing their diet – it's simply a case of what they are saying to themselves. As soon as Adam told himself he couldn't have that apple, he was doomed. Adam simply fell victim to the 'can't syndrome'. Tell yourself you can't and you will want whatever it is you think you can't have a thousand times more. Understand you *can* – that nothing is preventing you but that there is just no point in having it, that you don't actually want to – and you won't struggle – at all. It isn't hard and for the first time ever you can genuinely feel free.

It is also extremely important never to use the expression 'given up'. When you use the expression it implies immediately that you have made some kind of sacrifice, but all of the sacrifices are made when you are eating rubbish, not when you finally stop. You are sacrificing your health, your money, your peace of mind, your self-respect, your courage, your confidence, your money, and your freedom. You are 'giving up' being able to wear the clothes you want, to be the person you want to be. You are 'giving up' the opportunity to move your body the way you would love to. 'Giving up' the real pleasure of ending a genuine hunger and being free around all food. You are possibly even 'giving up' an amazing intimate love life and above all you are 'giving up' being who you truly are. **ALL** of the sacrifices are made by *not* making the change and above all you need to fully understand there is absolutely nothing to 'give up' by making the change, so mind your language and never use the expression 'I have given up' when there was nothing to 'give up' in the first place.

It is Not Your Genetic Make Up Or Your Addictive Personality

I cannot emphasize enough that the reason why people find it difficult to quit the kinds of foods and drinks that are causing them so many problems have got nothing to do with their genetic make-up, character, or personality: it is simply down to a feeling of mental deprivation – a mental moping caused by the belief that they are missing out on some kind of genuine pleasure. They feel mentally upset because society's attitude has perpetuated the belief that if you don't eat and drink these drug-like substances, *you* are the one making the sacrifices (and, of course, this is reinforced by the illusory effects of the drug foods themselves). You believe that these substances are affecting *your* life, but most people can seemingly eat and drink this stuff without the same problems. This is simply not true – the need itself, the actual desire to consume these drug foods and drinks is the problem. Putting these substances into your body is the problem. The need to try and exercise constant control is the problem. And that's without the physical side effects of fat, tiredness and lethargy.

PITY DON'T ENVY

Get it clear, everyone who feels the need to consume this rubbish on a regular basis and struggles to stop eating this way is in the cage and has the problem. Whether they actually admit it or not is irrelevant as we need to bear in mind that all drug addicts lie – including drug food addicts. The last thing we should be doing is envying the people who still remain in the food and diet trap; instead we should feel genuinely sorry for them. If you take the Mouse Trap analogy and you saw your best friend in the cage hitting the button over and over again would you envy them? Would you feel as though you were missing out? Or would you attempt as best you could to explain exactly what they are doing so they too could be free? The point is simple – don't envy these people, why not change what you have always done and actually start to pity them instead and feel euphoric about the fact that at least you are free? Start to realize they will be envying you.

No wonder we all believe it's hard to lose weight, gain health and have physical and mental vibrancy – we have all been going about it back to front. People start their attempt to get a slim, energy-driven body believing that it will be very difficult or nigh on impossible. They dread it and who can really blame them? They strongly believe they will be making huge sacrifices and that their lives are about to change for the worse. They believe that in order to get to their goal of landing in Slim Land, they will not be able to have certain foods any more; that they are going to feel constantly deprived and miserable; that they are going to envy everyone they see; and, if they do manage to reach their ideal health and weight, in order to stay that way they will have to use 'control' and 'willpower' for the rest of their lives. It sounds like living hell and no doubt if you have tried to change what you eat in the wrong way you'll have realized it is exactly that.

But as I can personally testify, if you do it right, then you can approach the change feeling not just positive but excited and elated. We have been so brainwashed into believing that a problem with food is a lifetime battle – that it is strange not to consume chemical concoctions masquerading as food – that we all begin our attempt to quit this muck by feeling sorry for ourselves, as if we have just made a massive sacrifice. This is instead of feeling liberated and elated at the knowledge that we have just freed ourselves from one of the worst forms of addictive slavery from which we will ever suffer; that we have just stopped what is a progressive disease in its tracks. When you get rid of these foods from your life and step outside the cage, mentally and physically, it is the end of a disease and should be a wonderful feeling. But people using the 'diet steps' never get that wonderful feeling of freedom.

When Can We Feel Free?

When people are on a diet they wind themselves up into a mental tantrum. The theory is that if you can suffer the tantrum for long enough the cravings for certain foods will eventually go and you will reach the stage where you can tell the world, 'Have you heard the news? I don't need to eat that rubbish any more – I'm free'. Let me ask you a question: at what stage did Nelson Mandela realize that he was free from his captors? At what point was he free never to return ever again? Was it a year after he was released? A month? A week? A day? Or was it the very second he was released? Do you ever think he gets a craving to go back in? Of course not – he's over the moon to be free.

But at what point can the ex-drug food and drink addict say, 'Have you heard the news? I've done it. I'm **FREE**: I'm free not to consume this rubbish any more. Isn't it wonderful?' At what point in their lives can they become elated that they are free? At what point will the 'craving' go? At what point can they be over the moon to be free? The answer is never, not while they believe that they are still missing out.

The problem is that the attitude of society, the brainwashing and the years upon years of advertising all combine to give you the impression that if you are *not* eating fat-causing, life-destroying foods that you have indeed made a genuine sacrifice; that you will be the one who is missing out, that you will become boring and unsociable. So when people quit these nightmare foods and drinks they don't start by celebrating the fact they are free from substances that have been mentally and physically abusing them, but rather with a feeling of complete despondency wondering when, not if, they will fail.

The big trauma that the 'dieter' goes through when they stop eating certain foods and drinks is *not* caused by the withdrawal of the drug-like foods leaving their body, or by anything in their genes, but simply by a feeling of **MENTAL DEPRIVATION**. I cannot hammer this point home enough, remove the tantrum and the problem is over – it's that simple. People only continue to feel deprived because they don't know the full nature of the subtle and sinister food trap. You, on the other hand, now do. Which would make it even more ridiculous for you to continue pining for this rubbish after you break free from it. It would be the same as Nelson Mandela pining for prison or John McCarthy getting upset because he is no longer in Lebanon!

You now know all the lies and rubbish we have been subjected to since birth about certain foods and drinks and some of the tricks of **BiG FOOD** and **BiG DRiNK**, which means you have the unique opportunity to free yourself from drug foods and be happy about it. And now that you do have an understanding of drug foods, drug drinks, the hoodwink advertising and the misleading labels you are finally in a position to deal successfully with the physical symptoms of being a mental victim of the food and diet trap. Years of nutrient deficiency and increased toxicity will have left its toll. In all likelihood you will probably have been left with excess fat; battered organs; elevated sugar levels; an acidic system; a clogged colon; and probably some kind of definite medical condition will have been diagnosed, such as arthritis, asthma, or diabetes. You have probably clogged your system so much over the years that there is a good chance that your colon has a build up of waste matter which has gradually hardened and stuck to its walls, reducing what is normally a 6 cm (2⅓ in.) wide tunnel to one as small as just a few millimetres. This has led to the UK getting the unenviable title of –

The Most Constipated Nation In The World

There are now well over 20,000 new cases of bowel cancer every year – that's just bowel cancer. There are so many people dying from all kinds of diseases as a *direct* result of what they are eating and drinking that it's frightening. I also don't simply mean people who actually die; I am also talking about people like Renee Williams, whose life was effectively over many, many years before she actually died. It's not just how long you may or may not survive, it's the quality of your life while you are here that is equally, if not more, important.

BIG FOOD = BIG MEDICINE

The way we tend to treat the physical symptoms of years of **BiG FOOD** and **BiG DRiNK** consumption is with **BiG MEDiCiNE.** The problem with **BiG MEDiCiNE** is that they think 'a pill for every ill' is the solution to our health problems, or at least the solution to **BiG MEDiCiNE'S** next holiday home! (Have you seen the size of GlaxoSmithKline's building as you enter London from the M4?) I mentioned in the 'Pharmageddon' chapter the kind of money that is involved in **BiG DRUGS**. Drugs are not the solution to the obesity epidemic nor are they the logical approach for the treatment and prevention of most disease. However, as you cannot patent nature's healing and nourishing foods, **BiG DRUGS** will always bring out their latest block buster all-dancing and all-singing 'medical breakthrough' for whatever ailments you may have. When it comes to twenty-first century medicine the **BiG DRUG** to get under your pharmaceutical company belt is of course an FDA approved **FAT PiLL**. These approved pills are worth billions and yet do as much for obesity as George W Bush did for peace in Iraq.

It seems mad that **BiG PHARMACEUTiCALS** are all trying to find the super pill answer to weight loss without any harmful side-effects and yet it is right under their noses. No doubt after they read the next chapter they will be rushing out to the part of our planet where this natural **FAT PiLL** grows so freely. Not only is it effective in the treatment of obesity, but all aspects of disease. **BiG MEDiCiNE** are looking for it, most humans are hunting for it and many organizations and individuals would pay tremendous amounts of money for what I can quite confidentially describe as …

31

THE FAT CURE

Imagine receiving a call from your doctor about news of an amazing breakthrough in health and obesity science. It is the biggest breakthrough the medical profession have ever had. Nothing whatsoever has ever come close to the health promoting, disease preventing and in particular weight loss powers of this set of pills. They are so effective in the area of weight loss that they are being hailed as 'The Fat Cure'.

The 'The Fat Cure' has no adverse side effects and doctors have no vested interest in the pill at all. The doctors' only interest is genuinely to help as they know this amazing breakthrough in weight loss and health technology will help every single aspect of your health.

Unlike conventional pills, these are designed to be eaten. The thought of eating a pill may not appeal, but each one is designed to taste delicious and feed the body with genuine nutrients. Some of the pills come with a tough outer layer which you simply take off and eat what's underneath, while others come with a thin protective layer and you can just eat the whole thing. These pills have been specially designed to feed and nurture every single cell in your body. Unlike any fat pill before it, the manufacturers have made sure that the combination of pills they recommend, contain *every single* vitamin, mineral, and nutrient required by the body to function.

The design of 'The Fat Cure' is even more remarkable as each one contains over 80 per cent organic water. The incredibly high water content helps to transport the nutrients directly where the body needs it and helps to flush out the waste. The pills require little or no digestion as they also contain their very own digestive enzymes and have more or less been pre-digested. As no digestion is needed for breakdown and disposal of the pills, energy can be freed to be used for repairing damaged tissues and organs, and for the removal of excess fat. The pills have been designed to satisfy a genuine hunger, leaving you feeling satisfied for longer and, due to the incredible amount of water they contain, they also are designed to meet the body's requirement for fluid. They are also specially formulated to help build an incredibly strong immune system in order to help to protect against all disease. The Fat Cure range of pills also help to strengthen bones and teeth, and improve breathing. They are designed to feed the body and the mind. They also improve concentration and mental agility, and have the amazing ability to enable you to sleep like a baby.

Having heard this from your doctor you may well think The Fat Cure sounds too good to be true. Well, before you get too excited, as with any pill you must be prepared for the inevitable side effects.

The Fat Cure Side Effects

There have been many independent studies in the group of pills, and continued and regular use of the pills has, as you would have imagined, brought with it many side effects. The side effects include:

- Increased energy levels
- Shiny hair
- Strong teeth
- Hard nails
- Strong bones

- ❦ Beautiful glowing skin
- ❦ Increased libido
- ❦ Improved breathing
- ❦ Increased confidence and self-respect
- ❦ New clothes
- ❦ Improved mental agility
- ❦ Slim body
- ❦ Slim body
- ❦ Slim body!

Overall the message on the label is crystal clear:

WARNiNG:
These pills will seriously improve every single area of your life

The Fat Cure set of pills also come in hundreds of mouth-watering flavours, some with an unbelievably sweet taste. Here are just a few of the amazing flavours they come in: peach, pineapple, banana, mango, paw paw, orange, apricot, avocado, tomato, blackberry, strawberry, blueberry, melon, nectarine, kiwi, apple, tangerine, cherry, grapefruit, lemon, lime, grape, cucumber, sweet pepper, and hundreds more.

You don't need a prescription for these life-changing pills, because there are no adverse side effects whatsoever. The pills are suitable for all ages, and can even be taken by pregnant women. You can also purchase them virtually anywhere you go. Not only that but they are also relatively inexpensive. Given the money you save on drug-like foods, these hunger satisfying, health pills can save you a small fortune. Luckily for us the ingenious scientist who invented this amazing set of pills did so not in order to make money, but simply for the genuine wellbeing of others (what a concept). If you have your own garden you can even grow the pills yourself for free and often when you do this they are even more effective.

Having weighed up the pros and cons and listened to what your doctor has to say, would you be interested in trying The Fat Cure set of pills? Not only would you be interested but you would no doubt want them **NOW.** Would you be happy and excited to take them? **YES.** How much willpower would you need in order to start taking them? **NONE.** Not only would you not find it a penance but you would be itching to start taking them immediately.

As you've undoubtedly guessed, as simple as it sounds, fresh ripe sweet delicious fruit is 'The Fat Cure' range of 'pills'. But then you hardly need to be Inspector Clouseau to work it out once it's been explained properly do you? Yet for some reason it has never been advertised for what it is and what it does, although I read that is all to change – thank God. Finally schools will be giving fresh fruit to pupils. In addition, an advertising scheme is to be tested that will encourage children to choose fruit for themselves by making it 'hip and trendy'. I said advertising works and how's this for evidence? Children were shown videos featuring fruit- and vegetable-loving 'dudes'. They were told if they too eat these foods, they can join the struggle to defeat the evil General Junk and his Junk Punks. The results were mind-blowing. Among children who watched the video, which contained snappy phrases and catchy songs, the consumption of fruit and veg increased **FOUR-FOLD**. That's simply amazing and in terms of the next generation's health it's a good start.

Fruit is the very food which we are, without doubt, biologically adapted to eat over any other food. No other food even comes close to the health-giving and cleansing properties of fresh ripe fruit. Scientists and food 'experts' can bang on as much as they like about what we should or should not be eating, and continue trying to create pills for health and weight loss, but no one can dispute that humans have the digestive tract of a primarily fruit-eating primate and the Fat Cure pill has already been invented. It tastes delicious, satisfies a *genuine* hunger and enables weight to melt away. When I say fruit, I am also talking of 'vegetable fruits' – anything with a seed is a fruit, so that includes avocados and cucumber and the like.

'AN APPLE A DAY KEEPS THE DOCTOR AWAY —
AND THE LiPO SURGEON TOO'
(with a few apricots, oranges, bananas, avocados, cucumbers, and nuts thrown in)

Hippocrates, the so-called 'father of medicine', knew only too well the power of fruit and veg. 'Let food be thy medicine' was his catchphrase and he was certainly right. If you are fat, you are ill; if you are tired all the time, you are ill; if you have arthritis, you are ill. If you feel like crap all of the time, you are ill. Mounds of fat are your body's way of telling you it is at dis-ease with itself: in other words, it has a disease and you are ill. And the only thing physically keeping all that fat there is a lack of nutrients and available energy. The body spends so much time trying to digest the rubbish we put in it that it simply doesn't have the time or energy to shift the excess fat, repair damaged organs, or to give us some mental or physical energy when we need it. If we just learn how to 'free up' energy in the body and provide it with a high-powered nutrient workforce, then the actual physical side of getting a slim, energy-driven body is very, very easy. The body just needs some help – and fast, nutrient-packed food is what it's crying out for.

I will repeat this point once more as I want you to really get this – the human body was specifically designed with fast food in mind, and once again I don't mean burgers and fries. I mean foods that are fast to digest, fast for the body to assimilate and fast for the body to eliminate. I mean real, genuine fast food: foods that will quickly inject nutrients into every cell in your body, giving it a brand new workforce that is specifically designed to clear out excess fat and wastes; foods that contain antioxidants which help to build a defence against cancer and other diseases; foods that contain massive amounts of what our body thrives on and cannot do without – water. This amazing group of foods not only taste incredible, but also help to replenish your already depleted enzyme and life bank accounts.

And they don't leave you feeling bloated and guilty, but instead lift your spirits and keep you looking and feeling fantastic.

FRUIT AND VEG – THE DYNAMIC DUO

Even when I say it, it sounds too simple. But, yes, fruit and water-rich, easily-digestible vegetables are nature's ultimate fast foods and the benefits of eating these incredible foods every day last a lifetime. I know we hear all the time we must get our five a day, but I fear it goes in one ear and out of the other. Also, and as sad as this is, many people don't even know what is classed as a vegetable. In a study in the US they asked a group of schoolchildren what their favourite vegetable was. Eighty-seven per cent answered: French fries!

Fruit and vegetables are about the only genuine foods that you could stick the following label on and in no way would it be misleading the public:

- No artificial colouring
- No preservatives
- No additives
- No added sugar
- No added salt
- No E numbers
- 99.9 per cent fat free
- Non dairy
- Water rich
- Calcium enriched
- Vitamin and mineral enriched
- Suitable for old, young and can even be taken when pregnant
- Totally natural
- Pure goodness

And because they are natural, in the genuine sense of the word, they don't even need a label. It is super-fast, super-rich, super-charged nutrition. Fruit takes little or no digestion and so leaves the stomach very quickly, usually after about half an hour. It then goes straight to the intestines where the nutrients can be absorbed. It requires no washing up, tastes wonderful, looks amazing, satisfies a genuine hunger, is cheap compared to most other things, and the high water content helps to transport the life-giving nutrients to every cell in the body and flush the system of waste matter. Yet often, humans get hold of this amazing food, stick it in a pan, heat it to death, cover it with loads of drug-like sugar, sprinkle on some drug-infested cocoa, give it some pretentious French name and call themselves 'Master' chefs. We are the only creatures on the planet that turn something highly nutritious into something detrimental to our health and then brag about being 'masterful' because we have managed to do such a thing.

However, there is one thing that humans have done with fruit and veg which can only be described as truly masterful. Using the enzymes and live nutrients found in all fruit and vegetables, they have managed to produce something, which is even more powerful and effective for fast fat removal.

What I am talking about here is the ultimate in fast food and nutrient technology. It is the single most powerful fat-blasting, colon-cleansing, nutrient-packed weapon known to mankind.

No false hunger can possibly survive when you are *mentally* equipped with knowledge of the food and diet trap and *physically* armed with …

32

PURE JUICE POWER

Before I get into the truly unbelievable health and weight loss powers of freshly extracted juice, I want to make clear – you do not need to juice to get Slim For Life. I am only mentioning juicing as it is a great tool and wonderful catalyst to the land of the slim in super fast time. However, if you feel juicing is not for you for whatever reason, as long as you follow the Slim For Life principles (page 337) you will arrive safe and sound in Slim Land before you can say smoothie.

Having said that, I sincerely hope that after reading this small chapter, you will at least introduce juicing into some part of your life. Personally, and as corny as it may sound, juicing saved my life and I know of hundreds of thousands of people who have testified to juicing saving theirs. I feel it would have been an injustice not to mention juicing, especially when I know how incredibly effective it is.

Since this book was first published I have written a few books on juicing and have received thousands of emails from people all over the world thanking me for introducing juicing to them and their families.

For many people reading this book, your health and body will be in an emergency situation. I never underestimate the situation people find themselves in after years of eating the wrong foods and unless we get some 'live' nutrition in the system fast, things could get worse. This is where pure juice power comes in.

Freshly extracted fruit and vegetable juices are without question the single most powerful and fastest way to get live nutrients through your clogged system and into every cell in your body. It's almost like employing a super-fast nutrient courier bike to weave in and out of all the built-up rubbish to deliver the liquid life-force directly to where it's needed. There is no chemically-manufactured pill, 'nutritious' shake, processed food, canned fruit, bottled or carton juice that comes anywhere near the nutrient power service supplied by freshly extracted fruit and vegetable juices.

Why Juice – Surely Eating It Is better?

Not in our twenty-first century world it isn't. It is thought that due to certain farming practices the fruit and vegetables of today are far inferior to that of yesteryear. For example, a twenty-first century apple has around a third of the nutrients it had in the 1950s. This means you would need to eat three apples today to get the same nutrient value as one back then. Where it is hard for most people to eat three apples at once, everyone can easily juice three apples and drink it. If you feel some of the nutrients have been wasted we need to understand that we are one big juice extractor anyway. When we eat any fruit or vegetable all the body effectively does is extract the juice from the fibre – fibre cannot feed the body, it's the juice contained within the fibre that feeds the body. We need fibre of course, but you will get this from all the other food you will eat. Remember, juicing is a tool and I am not suggesting we use this tool so much we turn 'juiceorexic' (if there is such a thing). What I am suggesting is that due to the fact most people who read a book of this nature have excess weight and health problems, you use juicing as a food and as a medicine to rectify the situation.

All you are doing when you use a juicing machine is you are giving your body a much needed rest. The juicer simply does the work that your body normally has to do. It extracts the nutrients from the fruit and vegetables and disposes of the waste in what's called a 'pulp jug'. In nature the waste would have come out in other areas!

Fruit and vegetables are easy for the body to digest, use and dispose of anyway but what makes juicing them so wonderful for an already tired and abused system, is that it takes even *less* work and time for the body to get what it needs from juice. When we eat vegetables and fruits the body uses energy trying to squeeze the liquid it needs from the fibre. When you put fruit and vegetables through a juicing machine – you've effectively done the body's work for it. By drinking the freshly extracted juice you have skipped the digestive process and efficiently furnished your cells with a wonderful supply of live nutrients. What many people don't realize is that although vegetables like carrots, broccoli, beetroot, swede, etc. contain tremendous life-giving nutrients that are of huge benefit to our cells and immune system, they are not always easy to get at. The body can have a tough time trying to break down hard vegetables like carrots and broccoli in their raw state, especially when it is already tired and weak. This is why we tend to steam or cook them to make them easier to digest. The problem with this, as you will recall, is that when you apply any kind of heat you kill a large percentage of the live nutrients and at the same time increase the waste that needs to be disposed of. Juicing is a completely different ball game. The juicing machine breaks down the hard vegetables for you, it then sucks out the live nutrition and puts it in a liquid form that is extremely easy for the body to use and assimilate.

Fresh fruit is a lot easier for the body to break down than hard vegetables. Whole fruits only take thirty minutes to leave the stomach which, compared to any concentrated food, is extremely fast. Juice, however, is even faster. Freshly extracted juice is on the fifteen-minute express service, making it by far the fastest food on earth.

Live nutrients begin to flow through your bloodstream within minutes. Not only that, but only a tiny percentage of these powerful nutrients needs to be used by the body for digestion and disposal. This leaves a surplus of raw energy in the body (something it probably won't have had for years). This surplus energy is used for the breakdown and disposal of excess waste (Fat).

LIQUID GOLD

In terms of 'life' for the body and mind, let me make it quite clear – a daily intake of freshly extracted juice is like the largest ever lottery win. The biggest difference with this lottery is that all you have to do is simply buy your juicing ticket every day and you are guaranteed to win. In terms of true wealth, all the money in the world becomes totally meaningless if your body's 'enzyme' bank account is overdrawn. This type of overdraft can manifest itself in many, many ways: headaches, lethargy, rapid ageing, a clogged system, stored fat, a lack of energy, heart disease, cancer, diabetes, arthritis, and asthma – to name but a few. This affects the way you look, think, breath, work, and play. In other words, it affects every single thing you do. In terms of sheer quality of life we need to replenish our enzyme account every day.

As Dr A. Rosenberger puts it:

> 'You lose enzymes through **stress, alcohol,** and **processed foods.** You can't get them back from **Diet Coke, hot dogs** or **coffee.** You can **only** replace them with **raw, wholefoods** – including **juices.**'

Freshly extracted juice is quite simply liquid gold for your body and mind. Every time you drink a glass of freshly extracted fruit or vegetable juice you can literally feel the goodness pouring through your system within seconds. It's like injecting a brand new workforce into your body whose mission it is to lift out excess fat and breed a new life into you; blast out the fat and gunk, promote supreme health and give you a new lease of life. The taste of the juice you make yourself is also in a different league from the nutritionally-dead versions you see on supermarket shelves masquerading as the real, 'pure' thing. Even vegetable juice, when made in the right way, tastes incredible. Of all people I can't believe I'm saying that. Me, Mr – I would rather stick hot pokers in my eyes all night than eat broccoli – Vale, is now enthusing about how wonderful vegetable juice tastes.

Most people have never tasted freshly extracted vegetable juice and it's the idea more than anything that's off-putting. Plus, of course, most people don't know the right way to make vegetable juices – some of the versions I have tried tasted just a few rats short of sewer water. But I can assure you that when you taste just how smooth, sweet, and creamy they can be you will be converted for life. As far as I'm concerned even if they tasted disgusting, given the amazing change in my weight, health, and thinking, I would just hold my nose and pour the stuff down. Fortunately they do taste incredible and even the ones I found a bit strange at first, I now love.

THE FUTURE'S BRIGHT, THE FUTURE'S ORANGE (AND GREEN)

We all know that vegetables contain incredible amounts of antioxidants which help us build a strong immune system. The dark green ones like broccoli, spinach, and kale contain something called chlorophyll (nice name). This stuff is simply sunshine for your cells. Chlorophyll traps the energy of sunlight and when the plant is broken down the energy is released – this is the best form of carbohydrate known to mankind. The antioxidants and chlorophyll found in vegetables all drastically help to decrease our chances of getting cancer, heart disease and God knows how many other diseases. This is all excellent. However, for most of us, the idea of sitting down to a plate full of raw broccoli, kale, spinach, celery, and carrots doesn't exactly make us want to do somersaults in the snow. In fact, the average person's daily intake of raw live nutrition in the form of fruit and veg is somewhere between 0 and 5 per cent – that pretty much equals suicide! So here's where juicing once again comes into its own.

IF YOU CAN'T EAT THE STUFF – DRINK IT

There is just no way on this planet with my busy schedule that I could get an adequate amount of easy-to-digest nutrients circulating in my system if I didn't juice vegetables every day. I am not a great raw broccoli, kale, celery or beetroot lover and for me juicing them is a very neat way of getting the amazing goodness into my body without having to eat them raw. We are, remember, primarily fruit-eating primates and root vegetables are hard for our bodies to break down and use. But if we drink them instead we are doing our bodies a massive favour and helping to 'free up' even more raw energy. At the same time we have, for once, used our incredible know-how to gain access to the live nutrients in hard vegetables without putting a burden on our digestive system.

> 'i know that if i do not drink a sufficient quantity of fresh raw vegetable juices every day then, as likely as not, my full quota of nourishment enzymes is missing from my body.'

Dr Norman Walker

Dr Walker died peacefully in his sleep, disease free, at the age of 113. Another US doctor whose diet also consisted of large quantities of fruit and vegetable juice died at the age of 96 but, to be fair, he didn't die of natural causes like Dr Walker. He was killed by a freak wave while surfing. Yes surfing at 96 years of age – that's my kind of guy.

GREEN, GREEN, GREEN

Jay Kordich, the juice man in the US, is well known for his statement: 'All life on earth emanates from the green of the plant.' The late Dr Bircher-Benner, who founded the famous Bircher-Benner clinic said, 'There is nothing more therapeutic on earth than green juice'. If there was ever a time to go green now is it. Good quality organic where possible fruit juices are incredible, make no mistake, but it's the green ones that will really supply pure sunshine to every living cell in your body in the fastest way possible, and make a truly unbelievable impact on your health, looks, and energy levels – which really can make others green with envy.

What do Goldie Hawn, Gwyneth Paltrow, John F Kennedy, Sean Connery, Madonna, Donna Karan, Nastassja Kinski, Jordan, Jennifer Anniston, Sarah Jessica Parker and Ross Mansergh have in common? Yes you guessed it – fresh juice, usually of the veggie kind. Ross Mansergh has perhaps the most remarkable story when it comes to juice. Ross who? Yes not many people have heard of this remarkable man. He is (as the headline read) …

The miracle man who beat cancer with carrots

Well carrot *juice* to be more specific, with a few apples, leeks, and red cabbages thrown in for good measure. He went through 75 lbs (34 kg) of carrots a week, 60 apples, six red cabbages, and 25 lbs (11 kg) of leeks. In his own words, 'The best way to beat cancer is not to poison the body further, but by feeding it the right nutrients'.

He now feels fitter and healthier than he has in years. He no longer needs 75 lbs of carrots a week but still gets through at least 15–20 lbs (7–9 kg). Why? Because the best way to prevent cancer and heart disease (the two biggest killers by far) is to feed the body the right nutrients on a regular basis. If you don't, the live cells which rely on nutrients and oxygen will be slowly starving to death. The huge amount of fruit and veg Ross juiced every week also illustrates how meaningless the 'calorie counting' business is. When he was on his anti-cancer juice regime he was drinking 5,000 calories a day for two years. Yet he never ended up the size of the Napa Valley; in fact he lost some weight and it made him fitter.

You may not be surprised to hear that the 'expert' doctors questioned about this case were not convinced. Dr Ian Smith, consultant at the Royal Marsden Hospital in London, called the treatment 'scientifically unproven'. **UNPROVEN?** The man's alive and spankingly well. What more proof do you need? Science is 'that which works' and this clearly worked. There is at least one doctor I know of who cannot say enough about the power of juice – Dr Charles Innes. He is 100 per cent convinced that carrot juice saved his life by fighting a brain tumour he had and is even more certain that it stopped him going blind. But the majority of doctors are dismissive of the idea that juicing can have this kind of impact. I have had many 'experts' tell me that some of my theories are 'scientifically unproven', but I am living proof that what I do works and there are many thousands more out there who can testify to the remarkable effects of freeing yourself of the need and trap to eat crap, and the physical raw energy gained by getting juiced every day.

Broccoli Juice Is Helping Me Beat Cancer

Above was another newspaper headline in reference to the effectiveness of freshly extracted juices. Cancer patient Ray Wiseman was told he wasn't expected to survive, but five years on he is alive and well and puts it all down to his daily tumbler of broccoli, carrot, and apple juice. The scans show his cancer has stopped spreading and he is feeling fit and well. Cancer Research UK even asked for the recipe to further study the vegetable's benefits. My question is simple – haven't Cancer Research thought about studying vegetable juice before now? We are in the twenty-first century and in such a 'BIG MEDICINE is best' train of thought that we seemingly can't see the wood for the trees. Isn't it ridiculously obvious that all fruits and vegetables help in the prevention of all disease? Isn't it also obvious that if our digestive systems are battered and we cannot extract all of the nutrients from these super foods that extracting the juice with a juicer and drinking the liquid fuel will benefit in areas way beyond any medical science.

Juicing isn't some kind of new fad either, it's been around for a while. Using raw vegetable juice for healing goes back to the nineteenth century. At that time of course they didn't have electronic juicing machines. No, back then if you wanted a juice you had to squeeze crushed or chopped vegetables through muslin – a process which took an eternity. Do you think that anyone would have gone through that amount of grief and hassle to make juice if it did no more for a person than the whole vegetable? Never in a million years. Vegetable juice is very nutritious and has an extremely powerful effect on disease of any kind. Max Gerson MD found that when he put his fifty cancer patients on a juice therapy regime all recovered through his natural 'gentle' treatment of cancer (for further details see his book *A Cancer Therapy: Results of Fifty Cases*).

This isn't a book on juicing so I have little time to fully get across just how powerful freshly extracted juice can be. If you do nothing else in your life the finest investment you will ever make in terms of your health is to buy a juicer. Not only to buy one, but to use it! Luckily, we have progressed considerably since the days of the muslin cloth and we have now entered twenty-first century broadband juicing. Juicers these days have wide funnels where you can put three whole apples in at once. They are also easy to clean and making a juice takes minutes. (See page 381 for a list of the best juicers). If you don't get a juicer and follow the Slim For Life principles you will clearly still get slim. The reason why I am such an advocate of juicing is that you get certain raw foods into your system which you would otherwise never consume. I hate celery with a passion; raw beetroot makes me gip and eating a raw broccoli stem doesn't exactly make me jump with excitement. However, when juiced and combined with the gorgeous sweet flavour and creamy texture of freshly extracted apple juice, it tastes wonderful. Pure raw goodness, feeding every cell in my body and helping to shift the fat while protecting against disease. Why wouldn't anyone juice? This book isn't a recipe book nor a set plan, but as juicing may be new to you I have included a few juice recipes to get you started (page 361). If you want more get hold of *The Juice Master Keeping It Simple*.

The spark of mental and physical energy you will feel once you are mentally free and physically juiced has a wonderful knock-on effect that helps to change literally every aspect of your life. It not only helps you free yourself of the disease of being fat, tired, and lethargic, but also helps you to free yourself of another disease which is sweeping our nation. Nearly every person who walks into my seminars suffers from it in one form or another and it is spreading fast. It is a disease which affects every muscle, cell, and organ in your body. It affects your circulation, your breathing, your energy levels, the way you look and the way you feel. It is an insidious disease which affects the shape, tone, and muscle structure of your body. It is, of course ...

33

FURNITURE DISEASE

'What disease?' Furniture disease – the disease you get from sitting or laying around on various bits of furniture for too long. And we do more of it now than at any other time in history.

It seems odd that a great deal of our time is spent sitting on various bits of furniture, usually staring at the television. The average person in the UK now watches between four to six hours of television a day. That's about thirty-five hours a week. At that rate if they live till they're 80 they would have spent at least **TEN YEARS** of their one and only life sitting on furniture watching furniture. I'm not saying don't watch TV (I couldn't live without *Friends* or *My Name Is Earl*), just that we often don't realize just how little we move our bodies and just how much modern technology has contributed to our lack of oxygen. The average child in the US now spends twenty-one hours a week watching TV – that's one and half months of TV a year (and what happens there soon happens in the UK). And while they're watching the box they'll be subjected to thousands of TV commercials – of which the majority will be for food.

Personally I love the new 'techno toys', it means we can now do things a hell of a lot faster than ever before – but it has also brought with it an unbelievable increase in lethargy. We have become so 'advanced' that from the time we wake up to the time we go to sleep we can run our lives from the comfort of our armchairs. Even the shopping can now be done by sitting on furniture tapping your fingers on more furniture. We can order everything from the Internet if we wish and have it delivered to our door. Our bills can be paid without us having to leave our chair with the help of telephone banking and the Internet. All of this is just great, but it also means that our bodies are slowly being starved of a good supply of oxygen. Drug-like foods clog the system, as you now realize, but at least we used to have to actually get up and walk to get the stuff. Now we don't even need to get out of our car to reach for a Big Mac or BK Flamer – we can just 'drive through'. In fact for many brands of drug food we haven't even got to leave the house. When I was fat and lethargic and well and truly mentally stuck in the food trap, pizza seemed like a godsend. All I had to do was pick up the phone, oh, and go to the door to pay – which at the time seemed like a lot of effort!

PLAYSTATION GENERATION

When it came to furniture disease, I was no amateur. I mean I had it down to a tee. Play football, are you mad? I can of course play it on Sega! Go skiing? Don't be silly, not when you can pretend on screen. I used to sit up all night some weekends puffing on fags, drinking beer, eating drug foods, and playing computer games till daylight with my friends. I am not exaggerating – that is precisely what my life was like, day in day out. I knew exactly what all the characters in the soap operas were doing, but what was I doing? Many hours of my day was spent watching fictitious characters leading fictitious lives on television while chucking dose after dose of drug food down my throat.

So am I saying never use telephone banking, the Internet, delivery services, computer games or watch television? **NO**, of course not. I use all of these and where would I be without my weekly fix of *Frasier*? I am just saying that if you want a level of health that so many people simply wish they could have, you need to turn off the TV and move your body.

A report in the medical journal *Pediatrics* showed that children who watch TV burned the equivalent of 211 calories fewer per day than if they did absolutely nothing at all. Yes, you read correctly – TV hypnotizes us so much that our metabolic rate slows down and we burn less calories than if we sat on the sofa doing nothing! So turning off the TV and getting moving will do you more good than perhaps you thought.

The human body is an incredible vehicle, but even the finest fuel in the world will only do so much. As we are all too aware, this fine vehicle of ours was designed to be driven. That is exactly what this book is all about – how to mentally and physically get a light, slim, and **ENERGY-DRiVEN** body. There is no question that quitting drug foods, eating some fruit and veg and drinking the rich juice contained within, will go a long, long way to getting you the body you crave. However, physical movement is the best weapon of them all.

You can go weeks without food, days without water, but only minutes without oxygen

An abundance of oxygen is vital for the life of our cells, and I am not talking here about just the shallow incorrect breathing we do every day or the amount we get from just walking up a flight of stairs. That amount of oxygen keeps us going – just. Athletes are something like nine times less likely to get cancer than 'normal' people. What do they do a lot more of than most people? That's right – **MOVE**. And when they move they breathe in a certain manner which feeds tons more life-giving, fat-blasting, blood-circulating, energy-producing oxygen to the cells. By doing this on a regular basis they also automatically keep their lymphatic system free from the build up of billions of cells that are dying every second in the body.

BECOME A LYMPHOMANIAC

What exactly is your lymphatic system? It's a network of vessels that carry lymph – or tissue-cleansing fluid – into the circulatory system. In layman's terms, lymph transports nutrients to the cells and carries away waste products such as dead cells. The system relies on a good supply and flow of oxygen to pump lymph around the body. We have four times more lymph fluid in our body than blood. The blood has its own pump (our heart), but to keep the lymph fluid cleansed it is essential we keep it flowing with the power of deep breath. A good supply of oxygen created by breathing in a certain way cleans the lymph system out.

it's amazing what happens when you breathe properly: Breathing Restores Energy And Total Health

This doesn't happen for most of us because we are the only creatures in the world that suffer from furniture disease. If we just moved a bit (well a lot), the lymphatic system could just get on with its job and we would feel good. The fact is the human body was designed to **MOVE** and unless we drive our magnificent vehicle we are slowly starving our body and mind every day of the single most vital ingredient of them all – **OXYGEN**.

Often when we feel tired and hungry it is as a direct result of not moving enough. The system becomes clogged and the cells begin to be starved of what they need most – a good blast of oxygen. Have you ever felt tired and hungry at the end of the working day, but made the decision to go for a blast down the gym instead of just sitting down and eating? (Okay it might have been some time ago now). Have you noticed that when you've finished your workout you are *less* hungry and certainly nowhere near as tired as you were before you started? This is because you have given your body what it thrives on and what it was being deprived of more than anything else – oxygen. I must point out that I am not talking here about walking for ten minutes on a treadmill while thinking about the extra 'points' you are earning. That obviously only adds to a false mental desire and false physical hunger. I am talking about when you move your body until you sweat.

EXERCISE (Now there's a sod of a word if ever I heard one)

Exercise, a lot of people simply hate the word and it's another favourite of 'The State The Bloody Obvious Brigade' who regularly inform overweight people, 'You know you really should do more exercise, it would help you lose weight'. As if they hadn't figured this one out for themselves. I used to get this all the time when I was overweight. But here was the problem: I was tired, I looked awful and I felt lousy most of the time. Just the idea of running for an hour on a treadmill made me reach for a cream bun! The thought of joining a gym with all those slim people was very daunting – I mean, come on, I was fat. And besides all that, **i HATED iT.** I'd tried 'exercising' many times and it just wasn't for me – or so I thought.

Just as I could never imagine drinking vegetable juice, eating salad and not eating chocolate, so I would never have thought in a million years that I would feel so juiced that I would want to move my body every day. But then that was before I discovered the single most effective and most enjoyable exercise programme in the world. Now you can't stop me doing it – I love it. And as unbelievable as this may sound to you at the moment, you will too.

I actually discovered this exercise programme many years ago but only started to do it again after I got juiced, so to speak. It is one that you may even have done in the past yourself but at the time you simply didn't realize that what you were doing was ...

34

THE BEST EXERCISE PROGRAMME IN THE WORLD

So what exactly is it? Quite simply – **THE ONE YOU ENJOY DOING.**
It's no good some fitness expert telling me that the best form of exercise for me is to go on the rowing machine for half an hour, because I hate it. So I won't do it. You can have the finest exercise machine in the world but if it bores the pants off you you're not going to use it. It is therefore not a good exercise programme *for you*.

'Can young Johnny come out to burn some calories please?'

You won't hear that – ever. Children 'exercise' all the time (well they used to before the new techno toys came along – although Wi consoles are changing that slightly) but they don't call it exercise, they say can we go and play. They don't give two hoots whether they are playing aerobically or anaerobically, they just enjoy playing. They don't know if they are 'fat burning' or 'sugar burning' they are just moving. The mental energy you gain from feeling free from the food and diet trap and the physical energy you gain from putting the right nutrients into your body, will give you that spark again to go and play.

I went to a very big seminar some years ago in the States. On sale was a machine that was being hailed as, you guessed it, 'the best exercise programme in the world'. This machine gave 'the ultimate workout' in just four minutes. The price of this incredible machine?

TEN THOUSAND DOLLARS!

I had a go – and had about as much fun as I would plucking my nasal hairs with a fish fork! For me the machine was about as effective as a cat-flap in a hippo's house. It's bad enough when you watch the dust settling on the running, rowing or home exercise bike which cost a few hundred quid, but can you imagine owning a $10,000 machine that you only ever use for a few days every new year?

The best exercise programme in the world is one that's enjoyable and fun – for you. If someone got on that $10,000 machine and loved it, had fun on it, had the money, then magic – they have found something that works for them. Luckily for me I found something which costs an average of £10. It's called a football. All I need is a ball, a park and I'm as happy as pie. And if there's a goal with a net still up in it then I'm quite simply in heaven. I also love tennis, squash, rounders, aerobics, surfing, cycling, table tennis, swimming, water polo, basketball, running, water pistol fighting, and rebounding.

The way you move your body changes the way you feel, the way you feel often determines what you put into your body, what you put into your body changes how you feel

The reason why I didn't 'exercise' in the past wasn't because I was lazy. It was because I wasn't physically or mentally juiced. I didn't like 'exercise' so I wasn't mentally inspired, but I did like having fun. My only problem was that I was simply out of practice on the physical, fun side of things.

You can get rid of all the drug foods and drinks and feed your body with tons of super-fast nutrition, but unless you are mentally inspired to move your body, you will still suffer from a lack of oxygen to the cells – otherwise known as furniture disease.

There is no such thing as laziness, just an uninspired mind

You tell any lazy, so-called couch potato that they've just won £12 million on the lottery – see how they move then. So what am I saying? That we need a lottery win every day to make us move our bodies? **NO** (although it would be nice). I am saying that we just need to find something that will mentally inspire us to move our body. Look at children – the minute they see snowfall they're running, leaping, throwing snowballs, making sledges from baking trays and having lots of **FUN**. When it snows it stimulates a 'lottery-win' chemical reaction in the mind of the child (or adult). They smile more, laugh more, feed oxygen to their brain and cells, and get all the exercise they need without ever calling it exercise. They build up an incredible appetite, so enjoy their food more and, afterwards, they sleep like a baby. Not only that, they also interact with others, make more friends and expand their lives. Somehow running on a treadmill in your house doesn't quite hit all the same notes, but finding the best exercise programme in the world for you, gives you all those things and more every single day.

We often put our reluctance to play down to our age, or a lack of time (always a good one), but that doctor I mentioned earlier was still surfing when he was 96 years old. He died doing 'The Best Exercise Programme In The World' – for him. There is no question that surfing gave that man much, much more than just physical exercise. And there is no question that when you start to move your body in a way that stimulates your mind and body, it will give you so much more than just a slim body. Physical movement improves your daily quality of life in so many different ways. Not only does it feed your body and mind with the life-giving, fat-blasting, energy-increasing oxygen it so desperately craves, it makes you feel lighter, happier, and more relaxed. You sleep better, think clearer, have more energy and get such incredible pleasure from ending a genuine hunger that even your meal times are a complete joy. That's not all, when you play – instead of 'exercise' – your body produces anti-cancer chemicals. I kid you not, there is a man in the US who managed, with the help of laughter, to beat his cancer. This illustrates why walking on a treadmill, stressed out of your head is not really the best way of getting yourself moving – although it's better than a clip around the ear with a wet kipper. **FUN**, that's the key. If you enjoy the feeling you get from a good blast on the treadmill – then do it.

Children love to play and if truth be known so do we. In reality we are all kids who happen to play at being an adult most of the time. Kids come back from school and they just want to play. I'm now back in the position where I am so mentally and physically juiced that when I've finished work I too want to go and play. I am now disappointed if for some reason I can't go to the park or the gym – and that's some-what of a turnaround I can tell you.

I have more mental and physical energy now than I can ever remember having in my adult life and more importantly I have more FUN in my life now. I often don't even wait until after work to go and play – as soon as I wake up I put my favourite music on and jump up and down on my mini trampoline. Am I mad? Probably, but I love it, and it's much better than waking up uninspired, tired, lethargic, groggy, and reaching for a coffee to give me a false kick-start.

Do you remember bouncing on the bed when you were a kid? Wasn't it fun? Do you remember dancing in your room to your favourite tune just for the fun of it? Do you remember playing football, hockey, squash, netball, rounders, badminton, or tennis? Do you remember how much fun roller skates were? What about games in the pool as a kid or games in the street which required just physical movement and pure unadul-terated imagination? Four things all of them had in common – they all required physical exercise, they were all fun, they all made you totally oblivious to any problems you thought you had and perhaps the most important thing – they all made you feel good. When you move your body to the point where you sweat it just makes you feel so good.

And isn't that what we are all working so hard to achieve – just to feel good? Maybe it's not a lottery win we need, or a promotion, but simply some team games, some physical movement, a bit of stimulating music, and some fun. In fact, if you think about it, some of the best nights in or out seem to involve some kind of physical movement until we sweat (I was actually talking about dancing!).

Does this mean that a nice long walk in the country is no good for you, that you have to be bouncing around every two minutes in order to get some benefit? No. Any kind of physical movement (especially if it's outdoors) is fantastic. There aren't many things as nice or as therapeutic as a long walk in the woods or along a beach. But in order to really supply your already starved body with some dynamic fuel at the same time as having fun, you really do need to find the best exercise programme in the world – and do it till you sweat.

Many Tools In Your Physical Armoury

We are not talking here about just one thing either, the beauty of the best exercise programme in the world is that it could be many different things to you depending on the day, the weather, the people you are with etc. All these factors will play a part in determining exactly which physical movement I am going to do on any particular day. If it's a sunny morning, I will head for the park with my football or go outside and jump on my mini trampoline. If it's raining, I'll do a high-powered aerobics class at the gym. Yes me, Mr – I'd rather stamp idiot on my forehead than do aerobics – Vale, doing aerobics at 7 a.m. and loving it. If I am in Cornwall I get my body board and off to the beach I go. Even if you feel you hate all physical movement and nothing you do will seem like playing, you can easily train yourself to like exercise. I know many people who hated running, but after a few weeks they are almost addicted. Running is wonderful. You just need a pair of trainers and off you go. Running is also a wonderful escape from the world when you just need to cut off.

IF MUSIC BE THE FOOD OF OXYGEN – PLAY ON

Have you ever been out for dinner with a group of friends and felt too tired to go dancing afterwards? In the end you go because everyone else is bugging you to. But then what happens? One of your favourite tunes comes on and **BOOM** – you're shaking your tail feather. The more you move your body the more alive you become – why? Because you are feeding oxygen to your cells, getting an adrenaline surge and having fun. People just come alive when they are doing something which is fun for them. You've done God knows how much 'physical exercise' but because it was fun, you never called it exercise and it never felt like exercise. I also believe that music has something to do with it. The best music in the world is an unbelievable stimulus for getting you moving. What is the best music in the world? The one you love, the one that gets you going, the one that inspires you. My iPod is just as important to my daily health as my juicer and mini trampoline. I change my playlist every week and add tunes that inspire me. Jumping up and down on my mini trampoline is fun, but add some funky music and it just increases the pleasure ten fold. I now love running, but without music it's nowhere near the same. The iPod (or MP3 player) is one of the finest inventions of the twenty-first century. You can change your playlist in seconds and the order the songs are played in – couldn't exactly do that with the old personal tape players.

JUST DO IT

Whatever you choose on any given day to be the best exercise programme in the world for you, make sure you go beyond just knowing what it is – do it. After all, by simply 'joining' a gym you get nothing. You will find that even if you hate the idea of a gym and can never envisage liking anything it has to offer, just like 'changing your diet', it will soon be such an integral part of your life you couldn't imagine not going. I now actually like running on a treadmill to music – it gives me time to think and de-stress after a hard day, and I feel so good afterwards. So even if at first you don't particularly like 'exercising' at the gym, you will soon be hooked. Thirty per cent of people who join a gym stop going in the first month and that figure goes up to a whopping 80 per cent after just three months. Some people continue paying every month for years, yet never go. My gym has over 2,000 members, yet you see the same twenty people every night. There are two main reasons why people who find what they enjoy, then fail to actually do it. One is that their body can sometimes be so tired from a lifetime of abuse that they physically cannot participate. In this case a few weeks free from the food trap and the help of some super-charged juice will make them feel lighter and give them a better opportunity to at least slowly join in the fun. The second reason why people fail to do the physical acts that they would love to do is by far the most common. It is caused by an awful phobia that seems to be on the increase. Virtually everyone I meet on my retreats has suffered from it at various times and there is no question it prevented them participating. It is so insidious that it can stop people swimming, playing rounders, beach volleyball, doing aerobics, dancing, and even having sex!

You will have no problem whatsoever enjoying the best exercise programme in the world to the fullest once you are free not just from the food and diet trap and physically nourished, but also totally free from …

35

PEOPLE PHOBIA

People phobia, a truly life- and soul-destroying phobia that can, and so often does, prevent people from expanding their world. More importantly it is the very thing that can prevent you from doing the best exercise programme in the world. Not everyone suffers from this to a large degree, but I do believe we all allow people phobia to control our lives at times. Once you get this one licked, your quality of life will explode and you will feel freer than you've felt in years.

WHAT IS PEOPLE PHOBIA?

People phobia is when you are so worried about what other people may think of you that it stops you from truly living and expanding your world. I used to suffer from this phobia to a large extent. It was hardly surprising when you consider that I was fat, had bigger breasts than your average supermodel and was covered from head to toe in a horrific skin disorder called psoriasis. I used to cover myself with two towels before jumping into a swimming pool; I would keep my top on, on a hot summer's day, even if I was sweating heavily. If I ever did go to the gym I would come home to shower and change, despite the fact they had showers, steam-rooms, and saunas at the gym; and I always kept the lights very low or off at 'bed' time (if you catch my drift). But I realize now that I did all of those things, not because I was fat or my skin was bad, but because I was suffering from 'people phobia'. After all, would I have kept my top on if I was by myself and there wasn't a soul in sight? Would I have wrapped two towels around my body if it were my own private pool? Would I have gone home in my sweaty clothes after a session in the gym if it was my gym and I was alone? **NO!** I would have felt free to be me. And that's what I am talking about here, being truly mentally free.

How on earth can we ever be truly free to do what we want if we are constantly worrying about what other people may or may not think of us? The bottom line is we can't. Unless we nip this in the bud now people phobia can stop you from sucking the juice from life and living a truly free and playful life. Life is just too short ever to have to suffer from what is a pretty egotistical way to think anyway – yes you heard me correctly – egotistical. When I was overweight, lethargic, and suffering from a skin disorder I certainly never considered myself in any way egotistical – after all what on earth did I have to be egotistical about? However, when you really analyse it, if we don't do the things we would love to do for fear of what others may think of us, then we must have not just egos, but super egos. What makes us think we are so special that everyone's going to look and talk about us? And what makes us think that even if they are making a comment about us that it is in some way negative? And quite frankly who cares anyway? If they are the kind of people who are that critical and judgemental you don't want to be associated with them anyway. The truth is that most people just aren't looking at you and couldn't care less what you are doing or how you look. How often have you looked at someone that was a bit different? Do you continue staring at and talking about them twenty-four hours a day? No. You look, think about it for a millisecond and just get on with your life. So why do we think that just because we happen to a bit fatter, thinner, older, younger, or out of step, that everyone is going to be talking about us? Get it clear – **THEY'RE NOT**. Yes they may look, but then don't we all tend to look at someone new? In fact don't we just tend to look – period. It's what we do; it's why hidden cameras and fly-on-the-wall documentaries are so popular – people like watching people. The problem only lies in the way we are thinking about ourselves. If you believe you're too fat, too old, or too whatever, you are always going to believe that everyone else is also thinking about you in the same way, but it's time to realize **THEY DON'T CARE.** When I was overweight and had an unsightly skin disease I was so paranoid I believed 'they' were judging me, yet I now know that most people in a gym actually admire anyone who comes and has a go, *especially* if they are overweight. They tend to look in admiration, and anyone who looked at my skin problem was looking out of concern – not revulsion. I am free from the stupid egotistical belief that the world is looking at me and talking about me. We need to realize the problem is not what other people are thinking, but what we believe they are thinking and the fact we allow this to alter our behaviour. It is *our* thinking that is the problem – not theirs. If we change the way we think, the problem simply cannot exist.

Whose Problem Is It?

When I was covered in a skin disease people would say I had a skin problem, and I did. There was no question that I made my skin much more of a problem than it ever needed to be. I always thought I was being judged, stared at, and talked about. It affected just about every area of my life and dominated my thoughts. The point I wish to make is that it needn't have. Every now and then I get a mini flare up of my skin and when I do sometimes people will comment and say, 'I didn't now you had a skin problem', to which I reply, 'I don't'. If anyone has a problem with my skin, then surely it's now their skin problem. If I don't allow it to be a problem to me and yet it bothers someone else, surely it's their problem.

This same principle applies to a weight problem. When I was overweight I allowed the excess weight to be much more of a problem than it needed to be. When I changed my diet I knew it would take a little while actually to get rid of the excess fat – but because I was so elated to see the food and diet trap for what it is and so excited about the change, I removed my weight problem the very day I made the change. Others around you may have a problem with your weight, even though you are changing your diet and will soon be slim. If they do, please realize **iT'S NOW THEiR WEiGHT PROBLEM!**

'Poor is the man whose pleasure depends on the permission of another' – Madonna

People phobia can prevent you from doing just about anything: dancing the way that expresses who you are, joining a gym, doing aerobics, sunbathing, wearing certain clothes, going swimming – and yes, if you are paranoid about your weight, your age, your skin etc. It can even stop you having intimate relationships.

I don't want anything to get in the way of your success and part of that success comes from giving yourself permission to go out and play again – it's the very essence of the best exercise programme in the world and in a way the very essence of life. Many people would love to join a gym but don't do it because they think everyone will look at them. They're worried about not being able to keep up or do the right steps and movements in an aerobics class. They're concerned what people will think of them if they don't have the right clothes. They're worried about the shape of their body or whether they're going to fit in. How do I know? Because that's exactly how I felt for years – right up until the point where I realized that it just didn't matter. I remember stepping into my local gym in about 2000 to do my first ever aerobics class with Mad Theo from L.A. Gym in Peckham (now closed down – real shame). Not only had I never done aerobics, but I was fat, I was new and I was a man. In fact, apart from the instructor, I was the only man in there. But I just didn't care any more. I'd heard from a friend that this class was fun (key word) and I actually felt mentally free to just do it. What I didn't realize was that I had walked in to perhaps the highest impact class ever devised. I did all the wrong moves, stood out a mile and had to stop quite a few times as I wasn't the fittest cookie in the biscuit barrel. But the music was good, I was having fun and it felt good. Then I had the added advantage of everyone in the class liking me – why? Because I made everyone look fantastic! I was the most out-of-step, out-of-shape person in there and they loved having me there.

A woman in her seventies sent me a beautiful letter a couple of months after attending one of my seminars. She explained how her life had completely changed since she'd not only freed herself from the food and diet trap, but of her people phobia. She had started line dancing in her mid-seventies, had met loads of wonderful people and made many new friends – and she feels younger, fitter, and freer than she has felt in years. In her words, 'I feel like a child again and I love it'.

It is such a cliché to say it but it is so true – we get one life and we cannot afford not to live it to the full because of pointless worrying about what people (most of whom we have never met) may think of what we are doing. Who cares what they think? Young children don't care either. Just by watching them we can learn so much. Children tend to live by two very simple rules and if you follow them, **BOOM** – no more phobia. Children tend to:

Move like they can't be seen and sing like they can't be heard

Whenever you hit a situation where you would have previously worried about people looking at you or judging you, simply walk, talk, breathe, and move like you are the only person there – and quietly smile to yourself. (People in their cars at traffic lights who pick their noses seem to have this off to a tee). What I am talking about is a frame of mind where you simply do things freely, where you are free to be you and free to play: a frame of mind that allows you to walk around the pool without the towels wrapped around you, one that allows you to dance and act a bit silly when you want and one which allows you to join that class and not give two hoots if you're a little bit out of step. If you do happen to do an aerobics class, stand at the front and just feel how liberating it is. Wear the brightest colours if you want to – if you are going to stand out at least do it in style.

NO NEED TO RETREAT ANY MORE

On my retreats, we make sure that People Phobia is dealt with on day one. We get people of all ages and all shapes and sizes. Most people travel alone, some for the first time in years, and many have health issues other than their weight. On one particular retreat we hire a beautiful place in southern Turkey. It is cut off from the rest of the world and even has its own island. On the first day of the retreat I have everyone get into their swimming costumes and get in the sea. This is after a full day's travel and is often on the evening of arrival. Many of the people there haven't been in a costume for years, one lady even mentioned to me it had been over twenty-five years since she had been in public in her swimming gear. Most are extremely apprehensive at first, but after the first mini talk on People Phobia, everyone gets in. It is one of the most liberating feelings and it expands their world for the rest of the week. By 'pulling the thorn' (as I call it) and just doing it, it means they are free to do it every day of their holiday. If they had plucked up the courage to go in on day four or five, they would have seen there was nothing to worry about, enjoyed how liberating it felt but they would have missed out on the full enjoyment of their retreat.

There was one particular lady who will always stay with me. She suffered from severe alopecia and wore a wig. To look at her you would never know. She was incredibly athletic, but clearly her hair was causing her a great deal of problems. On day three of the retreat the group saw a lady they didn't recognize swimming in the sea (we are cut off from everywhere so we are the only ones there). She plucked up the courage to remove her wig and swim in front of everyone. It was extremely liberating and moving and proved once again that if she didn't have a problem with her hair, she didn't have a hair problem. If others do, what was her problem becomes theirs.

So if you want to join a gym – go do it. If you want to jump on a pair of roller-blades regardless of your age or weight – go do it. If you want to pick up a hairbrush and sing to Elvis and wiggle your hips in the mirror – go do it. If you want to jump on a mini-trampoline to some funky music

– go do it. If you haven't been to a club for years and you're in the mood to have a boogie – just go do it. If you want to go hiking in the Lake District – go do it. In fact, whatever you want to do – **GO DO IT.** And do it **TODAY.**

If you feel free from the start you are free from the start

And that is what this whole book is about – your freedom. It's about freedom to move in a way you haven't done in years; freedom to eat and drink what you choose, not what **BiG FOOD** and **BiG DRiNK** wants you to eat and drink. It's about freedom from the need to consume drug foods; freedom to wear what you want when you want. Freedom to be with other people eating drug foods and not envy what they are doing but, for the first time ever, genuinely pity them for the poor drug food addicts they are. Total freedom to be yourself every day no matter who is there or what you may look like; freedom to enjoy the process of becoming slim and energy-driven; freedom to do the best exercise programme in the world whenever you want; freedom from the diet industry for the rest of your life; freedom from 'people phobia' and freedom from the life-destroying **FOOD** and **DiET TRAP** forever. I am talking about being and feeling totally free. That is exactly how I feel – **FREE.**

This kind of freedom is yours for the taking and the only thing that can possibly prevent you from getting there is fear. The fear that you won't be able to cope or enjoy your life without certain foods or drinks. But remember this fear is just yet another symptom of being a drug food addict. Think of the mouse in the cage. The drug had slowly shattered its central nervous system so much that in the end it was fearful of not being able to hit the button. Any outsider could clearly see the mouse should have been fearful about continuing to hit it, not stopping. And this is exactly what drug foods and drinks do to people. The key to freedom is not to feel deprived because you are no longer hitting the button, but be totally relieved and euphoric that you have finally stepped out of the cage, set yourself free and are in a position where you no longer have to hit the button ever again.

The reason people feel so gloomy when they're on a diet is because they believe they are 'giving up' something worth having. They go through what amounts to a mental grieving process, as if they have lost some kind of friend. But what kind of friend is it that physically and mentally abuses you every day? What kind of friend shatters your nervous system? What kind of friend undermines your confidence and keeps you their slave? What kind of friend beats you up and then pretends to help you out? What kind of friend demands you feed them at the cost of starving yourself? **FRiEND?** Who needs enemies? Drug foods and drinks are not your friends, they are your enemy. These so-called pick-me-up friends have been undermining your confidence; taking away your self-respect; keeping you a slave; keeping you an addict; keeping you fat, tired and lethargic; stealing your money; and, behind your back, they have been planning your death. So I wouldn't have any qualms or feel nervous about kicking them out of your life. Drug foods are designed to shatter the central nervous system and create a degree of false insecurities and fear – so if you are in any way nervous about the change I would simply feel the false fear and rejoice in starving it to death.

There is nothing to fear from making the change but everything to fear from not making it

It is only fear that keeps people hooked on drug foods and drinks. It is only fear that keeps them looking for ways to try and control these nightmare substances instead of just letting go of them completely. It is only fear that prevents them from gaining the quality of life they ultimately crave. Don't allow this false fear to keep you hooked for the rest of your life. That is exactly what these fears are – FALSE. Just like the false pleasure, the false comfort and the false hungers these nightmare substances cause, the fear they create is also very false. I once heard a great acronym for fear:

False Evidence which Appears Real

One which is more apt in this case would be False Eating which Appears Real. The fear people have of changing their eating habits appears real because of the illusionary effects of the drug foods and drinks. The illusions are giving false evidence which appears real to you. Using the mouse in the cage as an example – the fear of just running out of the cage and being free appeared real to the mouse, but it was false. The drug was causing the feelings of insecurities and dissatisfaction, yet the false evidence indicated the opposite to the mouse. This caused it to fear life without the drug and this is why even though the cage was open it was still trapped – by a false feeling of insecurity and fear. And it's exactly this false fear that keeps people rooted in the food and diet trap. But when you open your mind and see behind the brainwashing and through the fear, what is there to fear by making the change? What is there to be scared of? In fact it's all good; there is no down side whatsoever to breaking free and changing your diet, but quite a bit to fear by not making the change.

Fear can hold you prisoner ... the truth will set you free

There is no question that if you have understood what I have said so far then true freedom around all food is yours for the taking. All you need to do now is make a very simple choice based on your newfound understanding of the food and diet trap. You can either carry on as you are for the rest of your one and only short life on this planet, sinking further and further into the trap – getting more lethargic, more overweight, more insecure, more enslaved, more people phobic, or you can lift yourself free. To put it another way, the choice you have is quite simply this: it is time to either ...

36

GET BUSY LIVING OR GET BUSY DYING

I want to make this point very clear: the food and diet trap is like quicksand and unless you get out it will suck you further and further down. You cannot simply sit on the fence when it comes to this decision because there is no fence, it's one or the other – either get busy living or you get busy dying.

THERE IS NO IN-BETWEEN

All drug addiction is a form of disease and slavery, including drug food addiction. And like any disease it doesn't just get better one day and it doesn't just disappear if you ignore it – **IT WILL CONTINUE TO GET WORSE.** Each day you will become just a little more tired, a little more lethargic, a little more diseased, a little more starved, a little more insecure, a little more hooked, a little more stressed, a little more unhealthy and just a little more overweight. Each day adds to the next and that 'little' soon becomes a hell of a lot. People think they just wake up one day with heart disease, cancer, irritable bowel syndrome, gallstones etc. One day they were fine, the next – **BOOM!** They then look for what could have caused 'it'. Of course it can't have been their crap diet, after all they have been eating and drinking the same stuff for years, seemingly with no major life-threatening problem – so naturally it must be genetic. And how do we tend to treat this – toxic drugs!

ONE FAST FOOD BURGER HAS NEVER KILLED ANYONE BUT THEN NEITHER HAS ONE CIGARETTE

It's the *thousands* that go along with it that are the problem. Drug food and drink addiction is a chain reaction for many people, each one creating the false mental and physical need for the next. Each one causes an imbalance in the body chemistry, thus creating additional empty feelings which only seem to be filled with more of the same. The more empty drug foods and drinks you consume the larger the void, the larger the void the more you consume – it's a trap. That is why simply trying to cut down by going a restrictive diet doesn't work, in fact it makes it worse. All you do is exercise more control over the very things which are in reality controlling you. Unless you step outside the cage and see for yourself exactly what's happening and break the chain completely it will continue for the rest of your life and you will never be free. If you choose not to open your mind to what's really going on, if you choose not to starve out the false fear and the little drug food parasites and leap to freedom, you will spend the rest of your life a slave to drug foods and drinks – being mentally and physically beaten by them daily.

YOUR FUTURE IN THEIR HANDS

Most people think you only have two choices: either eat these foods, feel guilty, get unhealthy and fat and wish you hadn't; or exercise willpower and control not to eat them and feel miserable, deprived and envy the people who are eating them. Either way you have a problem. With the foods or without them, you'll be miserable. Imagine having to spend the rest of your life doing this – what a living nightmare. But there is another option and it makes the whole process of getting a slim and energy-driven body so easy. Simply see these so-called foods for what they really are, see behind the advertising and glossy packaging, make a decision to dump them from your life and jump for joy that you are finally free *not* to eat them. What a concept – a happy non-drug-food eater. No more doom and gloom, only total elation at solving your food problem for life.

This is where everyone gets it wrong. It seems the whole world believes that if you don't have these nightmare substances flooding your body – making you ill and fat, and controlling your life – *you're* missing out on something. But there is nothing to miss, it is all one huge confidence trick, one massive illusion. There is nothing to give up, there is no struggle, and freedom from the food and diet trap is easy. It is, after all, very difficult to get depressed or feel deprived when nothing has been taken from you. If you've understood what I have said so far it should by now be crystal clear that it's not you who will be missing out or giving up – it's them. It's the poor drug food addict that's missing out on just about everything and they are the ones who are constantly giving up. They're giving up their health, their money, their energy, their life force, and their freedom. And all for what? What do they get in return?

NOTHiNG

I want to make it very clear that all the sacrifices are made when you are eating and drinking these kinds of foods, not when you quit. All the sacrifices are made if you don't have liquid energy flowing through your bloodstream feeding your cells every day. If you are a tired, lethargic, overweight drug food junkie then you make sacrifices in every area of your life – from your physical and mental vibrancy, your health and energy levels to your relationships and the amount you can get out of your life.

iF YOUR LiFE iSN'T EXPANDiNG — iT'S SHRiNKiNG AND iF YOU'RE NOT LiViNG — YOU'RE DYiNG

I know that no matter what state of health you are in at this time, or how badly addicted you think you are or not, you can easily turn everything around. I was a chain-smoking, dope-smoking, heavy-drinking, drug food, and drug drink addict who was fat, badly asthmatic, covered from head to toe in psoriasis. I come from a one-parent family, I left school at 15 and used to live on a council estate in one of the worst parts of south east London – North Peckham Estate. I was mugged over ten times growing up, had knives at my throat and my mother had her fair share of absolute nut cases that we both had to deal with. The kind of nut cases who would threaten her with violence, put knives up to an 11-year-old boy's throat and bring out a hand gun on the street.

My point is this. It doesn't matter where you are at this moment, what you have tried, what you have been through, or what your story is (believe me, we all have a story), it really doesn't have to be hard work or a struggle to make the change. It's simply down to the correct frame of mind. *Not* making the change is hard work. It's *not* doing anything about it that creates tremendous pain. Your present state of health is a direct result of the decisions you've made in the past, but let me make the next point very clear:

The past does not equal the future

If you are driving your car and you want to go forward do you stare in your rear view mirror? Of course not. Remember the past does not equal the future, it's what you do today that counts. So many people carry unwanted failures with them through life, fearing they can't succeed because of what happened yesterday, or last week, or last month, or ten years ago – **RUBBISH.** You will succeed and it's easy. It doesn't matter how long you've been eating your particular diet, how much you used to eat or how many times you have tried in the past – anybody can find it easy and enjoyable to change their brand of food and get moving for life. All you have to do is:

UNDERSTAND THE NATURE OF THE TRAP
AND FOLLOW THE INSTRUCTIONS

You must get it clear in your mind that all the knowledge in the world is nothing without the final ingredient – **ACTION**. So many people know what they need to do and sometimes they even know how they can do it, but they actually fail to do it. It's not what you know that counts; it's what you do with what you know. What sets apart the successes from the failures is the ability to take action; the ability to go beyond simply talking about a good life and great health; the ability to go that one stage further than just thinking about the change; **the ability to truly decide.**

A TRUE DECISION = CERTAINTY
HOPE = UNCERTAINTY

The key to lifelong change is just that – to truly decide. Not to hope but to *know for certain*. If you hope you are going on holiday, it doesn't mean you are actually going anywhere, but if you know for certain – then you will go for certain. Once you book your place you are as good as there. It's the same with the food trap: it may take a while to shift the physical symptoms left over from being a victim of the food and diet trap for so many years, but the second you make a concrete decision to make the change – a concrete decision to starve the false hungers – then you are as good as there. Once you make a true decision you cut off any other possibility. That is what decision in its Latin form means: 'to cut off from', 'to terminate'. You remove any other possibility so that whatever happens in your future life, good days or bad, reaching for drug-like food to help with an emotion of any kind is simply not an option. It's the equivalent of turning to heroin in such times; it is something that you simply wouldn't consider because you know it won't actually make the situation better. You have moved on and you are free. Happiness, after all, is not a tub called Ben And Jerry's!

When you make a true decision you give your brain an air of certainty which it thrives on; when you hope things will turn out okay you give your brain an air of uncertainty which creates doubts, insecurities, and fears – and this wears you down. So it's time to stop talking supreme health and a slim body – it's time to **DECIDE** to have it. The minute you decide, really decide and have the correct mental and physical recipe to follow – it's yours.

WHATEVER YOUR DECISION IT WILL DETERMINE YOUR FUTURE LIFE

Let's make something very clear, the decision actually to change your diet, to get busy living, to choose health over disease, to choose slim over fat – is without doubt the single most important decision you will ever make in your life. Nothing even comes close to just how important this decision is. You cannot buy your way to the land of the healthy and slim – you can only do it. All the money in the world is meaningless if you are tired, lethargic, fat, miserable, and constantly battling with drug foods and drinks and your weight. All the money in the world is of no use if you are in the cage. It's no good being a wealthy prisoner is it? The good news is it's easy to escape – the door has always been open. You are your own jailer, so make the decision to walk to freedom – it's a decision that will totally change the quality, and very likely the length, of your future life.

Some people say to me, 'Yes but you can get run over by a bus next week' and yes of course you can, but would you take heroin just because you could get run over by a bus next week? **OF COURSE YOU WOULDN'T.** There is a bus coming along for all of us – it's the daily quality of our lives that counts. It is how we feel **TODAY**. It's making sure that we are in control of our lives before the bus comes along that ultimately counts – making certain that we live and not simply survive before our bus arrives.

So remember, the past does not equal the future – it's what you do today that counts. The decision to act or not act on the information in this book will determine your future life – sink even further or jump to freedom? I cannot stress enough just how easy it is to change what you eat and how enjoyable it is to get moving again – it's simply down to how you think. And when you look at it, when you really simplify it, it really only comes down to just a couple of things: decide to kick the rubbish foods from your life and don't pine, mope or feel down about your decision – rejoice and jump for joy from the start.

That's it. It really can be that simple. It is only the indecision, the pining, the moping, the counting days, and feeling miserable about it that makes it difficult. But what the hell is there to feel down or miserable about? **NOTHING**. You're not going on a diet, you're not going to be avoiding certain situations, you're not going to be starving yourself, you're not putting a stop to dinner parties or going out, in fact you're going to be free to eat, free to move and free to live. Remember:

This is not a diet and this is not a rigid, boring exercise programme. it's total freedom

You can now look forward to a future where you can eat freely, move freely, and live freely. So instead of the usual doom and gloom feeling people start diet and exercise with and wonder why they fail: get excited, you are about to get busy living – really living. You are about to go on a journey that will literally shape your entire destiny and clearly your body. You will sleep better, think clearer, feel lighter, feel sexier and freer than you have in years. Every part of your life will be affected, from your work to your everyday relationships. And you'll find your confidence will explode. It really is hard to put into words how I was and how I am now – the difference really is like night and day. Your food problem is being solved for life and you are off to the land of the slim and healthy and for you it will be easy.

At this stage I cannot blame you for being like a dog on a leash, straining to get on with it, dying to just get started. But wait –**YES PLEASE WAIT**. Before you start your journey you need to be *fully* prepared. There is an old saying:

if You Fail To Prepare You Prepare To Fail

As cheesy as that saying is, it's bang on the button. You may well have struggled in this area for years and it's not going to take long to read just a few more short snappy chapters. They could mean the difference between 'Slim and Healthy For A Week' and 'Slim and Healthy For Life'. You need to know exactly what to expect on the journey so that nothing throws you. To make absolutely certain of your success before I give you the principles there are a few of things you need to watch out for. First up it's …

37

THE FOOD POLICE

Yes – the food police. This is the squad that goes around watching everything you eat and drink. These are the people who, knowing you have changed your eating habits or knowing you have read this book, will pick up on anything you eat that's not fresh fruit or vegetables. This is the force that believes you have somehow committed a crime by breaking free from the constant need to eat crap; that you are a do-gooder and it's their job to pick up on any 'normal' foods you do eat and ram it down your throat (figuratively speaking that is). Yes the food police are out there in full force, and on your journey to the land of the slim and healthy, they are all too ready to pounce – so be very alert.

You would think that people would be pleased for you if you were out of the cage and no longer hitting the button, especially those closest to you. You would think they would be happy that you have changed what you eat and are on the road to being slim and healthy wouldn't you? Well yes you would think so, but in order to have a pleasant journey there is one thing you must realize when making the change –

Nobody minds you changing what you eat and drink, nobody minds you going to the gym, nobody minds you declining a dessert … **providing of course you are miserable about it!**

It's sad, but true. If you are moping around, getting uptight, depressed, and moaning that you 'can't' have what you want, then they are fine – in fact they secretly quite like it. But if you are happy about quitting the rubbish – if you are enjoying eating and drinking fresh produce, and loving the journey to the land of the slim and healthy – they hate it.

Why?

Because you are a constant reminder of what they feel they should and, in reality, would love to be doing. Every time they see you eating fresh produce and having no desire for drug foods and drinks it makes them feel even worse than they normally feel after consuming rubbish. This leads them to try and justify their reasons for eating and drinking this stuff, and to cries of 'health freak' and even feelings of resentment. This is why they join the food police. They just can't wait for you to commit a 'food crime' so they can slap you with a humiliation fine. They can't wait for you to fail and will often do anything in their power to bully you into changing back, or use their persuasive powers to lure you back.

No drug addict likes to be the only one taking it – including drug food addicts

If I was offering apples to all my friends and they declined I would have no problem eating one. I wouldn't feel ashamed, I wouldn't call them names or claim they have flaws in their personality because they choose not to have one – would you? Yet with drug foods it's different. If you say no to a dessert, the drug food addicts can't just leave it there. They say things like 'Come on you boring bastard', 'Live a little', 'Stop being so unsociable', 'I remember when you were fun', 'It's only a bit of choco-late, it's hardly going to kill you', 'What's the matter with you?', 'Life's too short', 'You could get run over by a bus tomorrow'. But how on earth does not having a piece of sugar loaded refined fat laced cake make you boring, unsociable, unfunny or mean you're not living any more? If someone doesn't want a grape they don't get this crap do they? They don't have to justify why they don't want one. Why? Because grapes are a natural food and we don't feel instinctively stupid eating them. But with drug foods we do. This is why if you do say no to them, the drug food addict will do everything in their power to make sure you 'join them'. If someone else is doing it they feel better – in exactly the same way as a smoker will feel much better smoking in the company of at least one other smoker.

'YOU HEALTH FREAK'

Yes you'll definitely hear this one; time and time again. It's without question the favourite of the food police: 'You health freak'. You will hear it when you first make the change and to some degree for the rest of your life – and I'm not kidding either. Yes, when all else fails they will try to make themselves feel better about what they are doing by calling you a freak. But I wonder how they'd feel if you responded by calling them a 'Disease Freak'? How on earth does eating well and doing a bit of exercise suddenly turn you into a freak? In reality there should be no such thing as a health freak: it shouldn't be seen as 'freaky' to be healthy – it should be totally normal. The fact that it is seen as freaky shows just how far most people are sinking in the food and diet trap and just how strong the hold **BiG FOOD** and **BiG DRiNK** have. We are the only creatures on the planet that consider it odd or freakish if one of our own kind is not poisoning themselves on a regular basis, and we're the most intelligent – apparently.

It's ironic that **BiG FOOD** spends literally billions of pounds every year advertising its wares, yet the biggest sales force they have actually pays them. It's the drug food addicts themselves – the very people who are hooked are the ones who do the biggest advertising for these organizations. The next time you are at a restaurant just listen to how the person who wants a dessert describes it; how they 'advertise' these drug foods to their friends. The words they use and their facial expressions and the ums and rrrr's would be worthy of any Saatchi & Saatchi advertising campaign. You see all they need is just one person to join them and they are happy, it means they can then 'indulge'. But if everyone says no, nine times out of ten they will also decide to skip dessert themselves.

Why? For the simple reason already stated but worth repeating – when you are doing something which you instinctively know is pretty stupid you will feel less stupid if someone else is doing it with you. If they do get someone to join them with a dessert just listen to how they talk about it when it arrives. They constantly try to make you jealous, making all kinds of noises as they eat it, but what the hell is there to be jealous about? The image the menu gave and the words the drug food eater used to describe this 'delight' is always a far cry from the frozen lump of sugar and cow glue covered in theobromine-laced cocoa that has arrived at the table – oh with the squirt of 'cream in a can' on the side of course. And how do they feel after they have eaten it – not so happy then are they? Virtually every time they'll say 'Oh I wish I hadn't had that'. And even if they don't actually voice it, they will be thinking it. How do I know this for sure? Because not only have I treated thousands of people who all testify to this type of thinking, but more importantly because I've been there myself.

So watch those around you, unless you are aware of why they are saying the things they are saying they can pull you back

When people are *on a diet*, others around them don't mind as the person on the diet is almost doomed to misery and failure before they start. On top of that the dieter is constantly feeling deprived and voices how much they would love what the others are having. This simply confirms the false belief that people not on a diet are getting something special and the dieter who pines for, but declines, is the one missing out on some kind of benefit. This makes the non-dieters feel okay, in fact it makes them feel sorry for the dieter. However, because you are not going to be *on a diet*, not moping and will actually be pitying them for the poor drug food addicts they are, a part of their brain will resent you. Your change is affecting them because they would ideally love to be in your position but feel as though it's out of their reach. So if they can't get to where you are the next best thing is to try and tear you down.

So when you hear members of the food police banging on about what you eat or don't eat, please remember it's only because they feel, on some level, insignificant around you. This leads them to justify their actions very loudly at the same time as bringing you down – it's simply a need to feel significant. You will get exactly the same reaction from 'The Gym Police' when you are regularly participating in the best exercise programme in the world – so be prepared.

HOW LONG HAS IT BEEN? HOW LONG HAVE YOU GOT LEFT?

You will also get the 'how long has it been' and 'how long have you got left' gang. These people will say things like 'Well how long has it been? I wouldn't speak too soon it is, after all, early days yet'. These are the people who gauge your success by length of time and by your past 'attempts' to change. But what they won't know is you are not 'attempting' to do this and you are not *on a diet*. You have made a true decision, you have changed your diet and therefore have already done it. And what the hell has time got to do with it? Does it really matter how long you've been free as long as you are free? What these people don't realize is that you are free from your old eating habits for LiFE. And that freedom started from day one. The last thing you'll be doing is counting the days. That is what dieting is all about: sitting indoors counting the days, waiting for the day you might actually be happy with your decision, waiting for the day you can say to the world, 'I've done it. I don't need to eat that rubbish any more. I'm going to start living. I'm free'. But the point I want to hammer home is why wait? The truth is you can say it from day one. If you do not say it on day one then when are you going to say it?

You are free from the start so rejoice from the start

Did Nelson Mandela get this nonsense when he was released from prison? Did people say, 'I wouldn't celebrate yet Nelson, it's only been a week'? Length of time means nothing. It only means something while you are waiting for your release date, but once released – it's over at that moment. Nelson Mandela only counted the days he was in prison. Once you are free you are free. But you need to realize that the food police don't understand the concept of having changed your diet as opposed to being on a diet and it often freaks them out. The truth is they don't want you to be eating healthily, moving your body regularly and being cheerful at the same time.

Remember they don't mind you changing – providing you're miserable.

So just watch out and be aware of exactly why people do what they do. And don't forget that the same thing that got us all lured into the food trap in the first place is still out there – the advertising, brainwashing, and conditioning. Yet remember the biggest advertising is actually done by the very people who are slap-bang in the food and diet trap themselves.

Am I saying that everyone will do this kind of thing? No. I am just pointing out that some people will behave in this way and that it will happen most during the first few weeks. This is why it is essential for you to know exactly why they are doing it. It is also essential for you to recognize certain physical and mental triggers, which, unless fully understood, could lead to a jump back to diet mentality. These triggers happen automatically, sending certain thoughts to your mind during the adjustment period. These can be caused by the 'bells' (cinema equals popcorn for example) or by the false physical hungers (drug food and drink hangovers). Such triggers are nothing to worry about, but you do need to know why they are happening so that you don't start to panic.

As I have repeatedly said, it's easy to make the change but your brain needs a little time to adjust to any new situation. So please – and this is one of the most important instructions I will be giving you – during the first couple of weeks it is essential to …

38

GIVE YOUR BRAIN A BREAK

Your brain is the most ingenious computer in the world and it will adjust to any new situation, but please understand that as magnificent as your brain may be, it will take a little time to adjust fully to your new lifestyle.

ADJUSTING TO THE SWITCH

It's a bit like when you change your car. Sod's law the indicator switch seems to always be on the other side. What happens when you want to indicate on the first day of driving the new car? You put your windscreen wipers on. Why? Is it because you secretly wanted to wipe the windscreen? Is it a sign from the universe that you want your old car back? Is it your brain's way of telling you that you don't deserve a new car? Of course it isn't – it's just your brain adjusting to the new situation. The first day you drive the new car, every time you take a corner you put the windscreen wipers on by mistake. Not sometimes – *every single time*. Do you get stressed, get massive insecurity attacks and say things to yourself like, 'Oh my God I'm never going to adjust to this, I need my old car back'? Clearly not. All you do is switch the indicators on and get on with driving in the direction you want to go. Even though you put the wipers on every single time that you want to indicate on the first day, you never think for one second that you won't adjust to it. This is because you are not *hoping* you are going to adjust – you *know for certain* that you will. This is why you don't go to bed the first night worrying about whether the same thing will happen the next day or every day for the rest of your life. All you think about is how wonderful it feels to be driving your new car. The second day you drive the car, the amount of times you wipe instead of indicate is literally halved. The next day, it's halved again, then halved again and again and within no time at all you have fully adjusted to the new car. And exactly the same thing will happen with what you are doing.

MENTAL WINDSCREEN WIPERS

You may find that certain situations and feelings will make you automatically think about certain drug foods and drinks – for example when you enter a cinema and think of popcorn and cola or nachos. But just because you think of them it doesn't mean you still want them or have a genuine desire for them – it's just your mental windscreen wipers and it's essential you fully understand this. Whenever you are in any situation where out of the blue you find certain drug foods and drinks pop into your head, all it means is that something, either a false mental hunger (a bell or trigger situation) or a false physical hunger (drug food and drink withdrawal), automatically made you think about them. But again, this doesn't mean that something has gone wrong with the way you are thinking – it's simply part of the adjustment. It would actually be abnormal for these thoughts not to pop into your head every now and then.

It's like if you go on the same route to work every day for months or years. You become so 'conditioned' to the route that you can find yourself heading there even on your day off when you planned to go to a completely different place. The point I am making again is once you realize that you have headed in the wrong direction, do you go to work anyway simply because you're already halfway there? **NO WAY.** You realize what's happening and do a sharp U-turn. And you will find yourself doing exactly the same thing in various situations when it comes to certain foods and drinks.

OFF YOUR TROLLEY

Another good example of this is the 'supermarket shopping route'. Anybody who regularly shops in the same supermarket will have one of these – a set route planned in your mind before you even enter the store. This is why supermarkets are forever changing things around; they know we have a set route that we stick to and they know we will automatically go to where things used to be not just once, but several times until we get used to their new position. The point is because you have been travelling on the same 'food' route for years it is perfectly normal, especially during the first three weeks, for your mind and body to automatically start heading in the direction of your old brand of food and drinks. If you find yourself doing this at times, just like the route to work analogy, don't panic – **DO A SHARP U-TURN AND FEEL RELIEVED THAT YOU NO LONGER HAVE TO GO THERE.**

There are many situations that can create automatic thoughts with regard to certain foods and drinks. Remember these are only thoughts. All kinds of things can trigger a thought, but a thought is just a thought. A thought holds no power over you other than the power you give it. We think of all kinds of things, but do we act on all our thoughts? **NO** – if we did we'd be arrested! Thinking about drug-like foods and drinks is not the problem – it's what you think *about it* that matters. John McCarthy was locked up for seven years in Lebanon: did he think about Lebanon when he was first released? Of course he did. In fact, he probably thought about it more during the first few weeks than at any other time. The point is yes he did think about Lebanon and yes he had to experience a period of adjustment after his release, but I can guarantee he loved the adjustment – no matter how strange it felt at first. And I can be certain that when Lebanon was in his mind he never thought,

'Oh I'd love to go back there for a treat'! His overriding thought was, 'Thank god I'm free'. That's exactly what I thought when I was first released from the food trap and it's precisely what I think now – 'Thank God I'm free' 'Thank God I'm Not Part Of That Trap'.

DON'T TRY NOT TO THINK OF CHOCOLATE

Another mistake we tend to make when trying to kick certain foods and drinks is to try not to think about them. We even try to keep ourselves busy so that our minds are occupied with other thoughts. But does this work? **NO**. Once again this is diet step stuff and it has completely the opposite effect. You cannot try to not think about something – it's impossible. If I said to you please try not to think about Michael Jackson, what are you immediately thinking about? Michael Jackson. And exactly the same happens if you try not to think about something like chocolate. If you try not to think about anything you are bound to think about the very thing you are trying not to think about. The idea is not to avoid the thought, or try to think of something else, or worry that you are thinking it: the answer is to acknowledge it for what it is and jump for joy you don't have to act on it any more – that you are free. Remember, thinking about the drug foods and drinks that you have dumped from your life doesn't matter a jot – it's what you think about it that counts. In fact, in order to have food freedom for life, I want you to make a point of thinking about them. The people who forget about what these so-called foods really are tend to be the ones who get sucked back in again.

STARVING THE PARASITES

It's worth reminding ourselves that some of the 'mental windscreen wipers' (automatic thoughts) are directly caused by the physical drug-like food and drink parasites calling for their fix. Remember, what makes the food and diet trap so ingenious is the way the industry has managed to create a false need for their consumers. Drug foods and drinks actually create *additional* feelings of emptiness (hunger) that seemingly are only instantly filled with more of the same. The more people consume, the bigger the emptiness they feel, the bigger the void, the more they try and fill it – this is the essence of the food trap and should be crystal clear by now. People stay mentally locked in the food trap because drug food and drinks appear to fill the very emptiness they helped to create.

Under normal circumstances it is quite natural to feel insecure, get stressed, and panic if you are hungry and believe you can't end it for whatever reason. We were specifically designed to feel insecure and fearful. Hunger is, after all, nature's way of saying **GO AND EAT.** A slight physical hunger can blow into full-blown mental panic if you think you will be deprived of food. However, all you need to remember is that as long as you are getting a good supply of natural 'no label' food and feeding every cell in your body, there is nothing to panic about. If you do feel any hunger between your meal times, you can be assured these are simply the *false hungers* and they will soon be gone for good. They cannot be fed with natural food and they cannot go away with drug foods, for they are the cause. These empty feelings only appear to go away with drugs foods – that's the food trick if you recall. The only way to get rid of these false hungers is to recognize them for what they are and rejoice and love the feeling of starving them to death.

DRUG FOOD TERRORIST

If you do ever get a thought that makes you believe that it is **YOU** that wants these nightmare foods during the adjustment period, remember why you are reading this book, why you are making the change, why you have made the decision to get busy living. It's not *you* who wants them, you want to be free – it's what I describe as your 'drug food terrorist' demanding to be fed. So change the thought from 'I want' to '**iT** wants'. 'It' being the drug food terrorist daring to rear its ugly head in a desperate attempt to survive. It is common knowledge that you should never negotiate with terrorists as they will only demand more. Don't negotiate with them here, realize it's them asking and not a genuine need you have.

In fact if you get any thought at all, whether it is a drug food terrorist demanding that you feed it, an empty insecure feeling or a mental trigger or 'bell' during the first couple of weeks do yourself a favour – blame it all on the terrorists and experience how wonderful it feels to say, **'STUFF YOU, I'M FREE.'** Experience how brilliant it feels to know that each time you don't feed the blighters, each time you let them starve, you are one step closer to ultimate freedom and one day closer to the land of the slim and healthy for life.

Am I saying that you are going to be pestered with the parasites calling all the time? No. On the contrary, with the help of the fastest food in the west and the good wholesome solid foods that you will be eating, most of the time you won't be aware of anything at all. Of course the proof of the pudding is in the eating, but the majority of people are so nourished and so euphoric they don't notice a thing.

NATURAL ENERGY

Depending on the amount of false stimulants (or drug-like foods and drinks) you were consuming, you may or may not experience a dip in energy over the first 24–72 hours. For some it can extend for a few more days, but this is very rare. If you do feel like you want to sleep all the time you must go with it and under no circumstances have any false stimulants like coffee to try to 'lift you'. This is the trap remember. The body is so used to relying on false stimulants that it needs a couple of days to learn to fire on its own natural energy stores. Even if you feel like death over the first few days, you will find you will hit a 'health high' at some point during the first week – a high that money can't buy. You feel light, you feel your system flowing with natural energy (not nervous false energy) and you feel great that you starved the little parasites to death and have come out the other side. You may also get genuine physical symptoms from the withdrawal of certain drug-like foods and drinks such as coffee, Diet Coke, and refined sugars and carbohydrates.

This usually manifests itself as an unusual tiredness and a headache. The headache for some can be quite big. If you do get one, get plenty of water, eat some fruit and go for a lie down if you can. During the first few days if you are a member of a gym and can use a sauna and steam room to help with the withdrawal process please do so.

Please remember that whatever withdrawal symptoms you are experiencing, (tiredness, empty insecure feelings, slight anxiety, headaches etc.) it not because you have stopped consuming certain foods and drinks, but because you started in the first place. If you stopped eating bananas, apples, cashew nuts, grapes, avocados, fish or any other 'no label' food you wouldn't suffer any withdrawal symptoms. This once again proves just how harmful drug-like foods and drinks are, they cause withdrawal symptoms just like any other drug – natural foods do not. This means that if you are constantly eating drug-like foods you are *always*, to some degree, suffering from a level of withdrawal. This withdrawal feels like hunger and so no one ever knows it's addiction like any other. Unlike nicotine though, clearly these drug-like foods *do* supply the body with some nutrients in order to sustain, but they simply keep you ticking over, while withdrawing from your health bank account and battering your organs. They keep you in a constant state of withdrawal and keep you on an emotional rollercoaster, whether the person realizes or not.

Remember then, above all over the first few days any feelings/ thoughts/headaches you may be having are there not because you have *stopped* consuming drug-like foods and drinks, but because you *did*. The sooner you allow these feelings to die, the sooner you come out the other side and the sooner you feel totally free.

Any feelings you do have, especially the false hungers and calls for certain foods and drinks, you can use as a positive tool to help you. Every time you get the feeling, instead of saying, 'I *can't* have this or that' you will now simply think, 'I *can* have it, but what's the point, what will it actually do for me?' You will find when you do get these feelings of adjustment over the first few days/weeks you will smile as you now can see them for what they are and you know any feelings of withdrawal go away quickly when you brush them off. If you give them power, then and only then do they spiral. I know many people who love the process as for the first time in years they feel in full control of something that was controlling them. They get a kick out of the 'drug-food terrorist' rearing its ugly head asking to be fed and simply seeing it for what it is and letting it starve to death.

I mentioned at the start of this book that if you fully understand the nature of the food and diet trap and follow the simple instructions not only can the change be easy but also enjoyable and for some who are deep in the trap, even euphoric.

WELL DONE – YOU'VE PASSED

Understanding this book is a bit like passing your driving test. When you first pass your test the liberating feeling is amazing. I remember waving my pink slip at people at bus stops on the way back from the test centre with the biggest grin in the world on my face and yelling, 'Yes, Yes, Yes!'. I wasn't simply happy when I passed my driving test – **I WAS EUPHORIC.** But just like every single person in the world who passes their driving test – I couldn't actually drive when I passed. Now you may think that my examiner made a mistake by passing me, but the truth is nobody can drive when they first pass their test – they learn to drive in the few weeks after they pass. The first week you're still thinking about clutch control, looking in your mirrors etc. If someone talks to you while you are driving you tell them to shut up because you need to concentrate. But in no time at all you're talking, changing the radio station and driving at the same time without even thinking about any of the mechanics – it becomes automatic. Each and every day you become a better driver. Your brain soon adjusts and something you once thought difficult becomes automatic. And exactly the same goes for the change you are making here. In no time at all your new regime of juicing, eating, breathing, and doing the best exercise programme in the world becomes as automatic as brushing your teeth. The exciting news is that if you have already made the decision it means that you've already passed and you are already mentally free, even if you aren't fully aware of it yet.

TOTAL FOOD FREEDOM

One final aspect of food freedom mentally is to make sure you do have *total* food freedom. This means having the freedom of genuine choice and not becoming evangelical about food or becoming the health food police. We are in a twenty-first century world of dinner parties and real life and in order to have lifelong success we must above all …

39

BE FLEXIBLE
And Let Common Sense Prevail

In order for you to have food freedom for life you must be flexible. Do not become evangelical about food and do not label yourself, as it puts too many unnecessary restrictions on you in times of genuine need. I am not a 'vegetarian' nor am I a 'vegan' or a 'fruitarian', and I'm certainly not a 'breatharian'. I am a human being who eats wonderful food when I'm feeling hungry. Although I am not a big meat eater, if there wasn't anything else available, it was good quality and I was really hungry, I would eat it. A few pieces of organic grass fed chicken are much better, health-wise, than a plate full of white refined pasta. Some people will choose to quit meat on other grounds; if so fine. But if you're considering quitting it on the grounds of health, remember that white meat is often a good option.

I did once label myself 'vegan' for over two years. I found myself not eating at times when I was genuinely hungry and felt deprived because of it. I felt deprived because I was, at times, being deprived – I should have eaten. If you are in an airport, it's often tricky to get something you want. The salads are often a waste of time (mainly iceberg lettuce and nothing else), the fruit looks like it's been there a month and everything else smells good. Remember, there will be times like these when you deviate from your change of diet, the key is not to lose sleep over it or start saying stupid things like, 'Oh no I've blown it all now'. The key is to be free to do this – that's the point. Just eat the best choice available and enjoy ending a *genuine* hunger – you can always clean-up at the first possible opportunity. Once you understand it, it becomes almost impossible to 'blow it'.

Whenever I went up to see my Auntie Hilda in Halifax she would have been highly offended if I didn't have some of her homemade cake and quite rightly. My body, and yours, can easily deal with a bit of cake to be polite. I don't particularly want the cake, but when I have it, I enjoy it, I don't feel guilty and all is well.

For some people, certain foods and drinks are like nicotine: they can trigger an almost instant reversal of dietary behaviour. When someone has been without cigarettes for weeks, months or even years, just a single puff can trigger the old pattern of behaviour, and they are back on a packet a day before they know it. The same principle can apply to food, or to be accurate, drug-like food and drinks. Even a slight indiscretion can lead some people back to all their old eating habits. If you are aware that you are one of these people then be very careful if you ever have a dietary indiscretion. For some just breaking the seal can lead to the road to Fatsville once again. For most though, there is no need for it to spiral out of control as long as you are aware of what's happening and you 'clean up' the next day.

Use your common sense, choose the best option available wherever you are and be flexible at other times – it's vital for your sanity and freedom for life. There will be times we find ourselves in Starbucks, at a dinner party, in a situation where although there may be a better choice health wise, we simply just fancy something else. If so, and as long as it is the exception rather than the rule, be free to consume what you like.

WHEN IN ROME

Being completely flexible also allows for the 'when in Rome' way of living. It means that if you go to Jamaica and want to know what Jerk Chicken tastes like – you are free to do so. If you are in Tunisia and are curious about curried goat – you are free to tuck in. If you are in France and want some snails – go for it. If you're in China and you want some dog – well maybe not! You haven't always got to apply the 'when in Rome' principle and when it comes to places like China I don't blame you for not doing so, but it means if you do want to try the food of a particular country – **YOU ARE TOTALLY FREE TO DO SO**. This is why I don't label myself veggie or vegan and this is why I advise you don't either.

As long as you're not evangelical about food, you take action and change your diet, free yourself from things like 'people phobia' and really start to live as opposed to survive, then you will have what few do – total freedom from the food and diet trap and a daily quality of life many simply dream of. The real key is to keep to the Seven 'Simple Steps To Be Slim For Life' (coming up soon …), that way you can be as flexible as you like. I don't know what your story is or just how deep you've sunk into the food trap, but one thing's for sure – as from now it all begins to change.

Don't forget to enjoy the journey as much as arriving there and don't forget when you wake up each morning you have a choice: you can either get busy living or you get busy dying – as always it's up to you. Remember, there is no in-between – you are either sucking the juice from life or it's sucking the juice from you. With that in mind it's worth reminding yourself as you go to bed each night that you are finally on your way to the land of the slim and healthy for life. When you open your eyes each morning, get excited because in case no one has told you up until now, or in case you have forgotten …

40

YOU'VE GOT A TICKET TO THE BIG GAME

Have you noticed how children can't sleep on Christmas Eve and how they are up at 4 a.m. asking if it's time to open the presents yet? Ever noticed how excited they are, how alive they are, the look of joyous anticipation that lights up their face? It's a very different story though when they have to get up for school. If you *have to* get up to do something which doesn't inspire you it's tricky lifting your head off the pillow. Yet if you're going on a once-in-a-lifetime holiday you're up like a shot! Well it's time to start getting up like a shot because you have a unique ticket to the big game. The only question is – what are you going to do with it?

I see it like this. Life is a holiday lasting roughly a hundred or so years if we are very lucky, for many it will about eighty or ninety. Now even on holiday you have good and bad days. The problem is many people believe they've got a lousy deal from their holiday firm and have been landed with the holiday from hell. What they fail to realize is that …

WE ARE OUR OWN TOUR OPERATORS

This means it's up to us, not 'them' to design the holiday of our dreams. We get the unique chance each and every day to write the script and play in the big game. You can be sure of one thing, if we don't write our own script, if we don't take charge of our own game, there are millions of people who are paid massive amounts of money to write the script and play the game for us. You have seen this with the food companies and the way they use advertising and chemicals to write your script for you and use your big ticket for their financial gain. The idea is to take charge of your life each and every day, because we only get one ticket and each day really is a once in a lifetime day.

> **'Life is what happens while you're busy making other plans'**
>
> John Lennon

We get about 85–100 Christmases, and that's if we look after our incredible machine. We get the same amount of birthdays, and the same amount of **TODAY**s. Once it's gone – **iT'S GONE**. You can't just 'do it later', because in terms of today, there is no later – today only happens once. It's a one shot deal. This is why feeling physically and mentally vibrant is so important – it gives us a chance to play the game. And there is no question that you play a much better game when you feel light, clear-headed, and alive. Each day is unique, each day is part of the game and as long as the clock's ticking (your heart) – you're still in it.

We are all so busy working for tomorrow that we so often fail to appreciate or capture today, this moment, this second of our lives. As John Lennon wrote, 'Life is what happens while you're busy making other plans' – so don't miss it while you are busy making plans.

CARPE DIEM (SEIZE THE DAY)

Many people play the 'I'll be happy when …' game. And it's one you never win. I'll be happy when I earn this amount of money. I'll be happy when I get this new car. I'll be happy when I reach the top etc. This amounts always to living in the future, thus missing today – right now. I still play the 'I'll be happy when …' game, but I've changed the rules slightly. Now I'll be happy when … ever I feel like it! So don't say, I'll be happy when the weight comes off or I'll be happy when I'm healthy. If you do that you've missed the point and all you'll be really saying is, 'I'll be miserable *until* I've lost the weight' – but why? There's no need, that's the 'Diet Steps' remember? The whole point, the whole message of this book is to make you see the process is easy when you're not sitting around waiting for something to happen and it's the process that's the good part. It's about enjoying the journey, not just getting there so:

Don't be a weight watcher

If you are overweight and you follow the simple instructions then the excess weight will come off – but not tomorrow. You don't need to be Sherlock Holmes to figure out that it takes time to lose weight. So don't sit there staring at it each day to see if there's a difference and don't jump on the scales every day or week to see if you've dropped a few pounds. In fact – **THROW YOUR SCALES AWAY** and really set yourself free. It is not normal to weigh yourself, it only appears normal because so many people do it. If you watch a kettle it seems to take forever to boil and if you watch your weight the fat never seems to budge – so get on with living your life and delegate the process of fat removal to your body, it will do it for you. Just give it time.

THE FINEST DRUG TO BOOST YOUR GAME

One of the biggest joys of no longer using drug foods or drinks to try and change my emotional state, was the realization that we already own and have twenty-four-hour access to the finest drug in the world in its purest form and **IT'S FREE OF CHARGE.** It's also the only drug that genuinely boosts every area of your game: pure adrenalin – life force. It's the buzz and excitement of being and feeling alive: growing each and every day, actually facing and meeting new challenges instead of first turning to, or trying to hide behind, food or drugs; the confidence to go out and truly live, regardless of what people may or may not think; the courage to just do it, whatever it is in that moment.

Drug foods and drinks are not only dead nutritionally, they also kill your life force. They slowly make you die inside. The problem is, because it happens so slowly, so gradually, most people don't notice it happening. People who are stuck in the food trap, hooked on drug-like foods and drinks, have no idea just how much these poisons are affecting so many areas of their lives. They look around and see they are pretty much the same as most other people and that is my point:

You don't want to be the same as over 90 per cent of the population

Most people are missing out on the juice of life. Most people simply survive but don't live. Most people have stress and not challenges. Most people are fat. Most people are ill. Most people end up in hospital or a nursing home. Most people are hooked. Most people are being controlled. Most people are people phobic. Most people reach for a food to try and change the way they feel, and most people don't realize they have a ticket to the big game. You really don't want to be like most people and from now on you don't have to be.

Now that you are breaking free you will always feel more physically and mentally vibrant and much more alive. This gives you the resources to tap into a quality of life you had forgotten existed. So enjoy the journey, don't forget about today, furnish your body with the finest nutrition available and get busy living. I will be supplying you with the full list of simple instructions for lifelong success in a second, before I do I need you to beware. No matter how long it has been since you made the change, the facts about drug foods and drinks **NEVER** change, but their relevance to you will. So in order to make sure your freedom is for life and you don't start to look back with rose-tinted glasses it is essential to heed the final warning …

41

RE-TUNE, RE-TUNE, AND RE-TUNE

Please be aware that the same thing that lured you into consuming these nightmare foods is still out there. The advertising, the brainwashing, the bells, and the peer pressure are all still out there, so be alert and flood your mind with inspiration on a regular basis – in other words, re-tune.

This is a very important ingredient of being slim, healthy, and vibrant for life. In fact this ingredient is the one which makes the difference between slim for life and slim for a month – so understand it and use it. If you miss just one instruction you will get a different end result. Everything I have put in this book is here for a reason and this re-tuning is a very important element of staying slim and free.

There are many people who make changes in life, but so often they are short-lived. They succeed for a while only to find themselves creeping back to their old ways. They claim to have been doing fine for a year but then they just found themselves one day craving other foods. Here's my point – it didn't happen just **ONE DAY.** Each and every day we are bombarded with thousands of images for drug foods and drinks. Each and every day we are surrounded by numerous poor souls who are still rooted in the food and diet trap, each one trying to convince us that we are the ones missing out. Then there are many people who are specifically paid huge sums of money to change the way we think, to get us hooked on their brand of 'food'. The good news is that once you have removed the brainwashing and seen the truth, it takes a lot of images and a long time before your brain gets sucked back in to believing any of it. The point is you don't ever want to get sucked back in again, you want to keep this stuff crystal clear in your mind. As you will by now have realized, as long as you think the right way, it's easy to make the change – it's also very easy for that change to stick. This final ingredient is not in any way a penance or hard work. All you have to do is simply re-tune once in a while.

IF YOUR BRAIN REMAINS CLEAR OF THE RUBBISH THEN YOU STAY SLIM, HEALTHY, AND FREE FOR LIFE

This is why it is essential for you to keep hold of this book – it is a re-tuning tool. If you lend it out, like a CD, you can be almost guaranteed you'll never see it again. You may have read this book and understood it, but when you re-read it you'll understand certain aspects you missed the first time. You also need to re-read it – or at least certain chapters – if you feel any doubt or any of the brainwashing creeping back in. Alternatively, read as much as you can on this subject, go to a few seminars and keep reversing the advertising.

Even if you feel fantastic and don't feel you need a re-tune, it's still good to refresh your memory and keep the lessons clear in your mind. Remember you can't see brainwashing creeping back in, you only know it as a thought or doubt at some point in the future. Should you get it – re-tune and clear your mind. It is good to keep this book's lessons clear in your mind to counter the thousands of false ads and pieces of misinformation we see and hear daily. The more you hear, read, and live this stuff the more it becomes your life. Whatever you focus on becomes real to you, so it's good to refresh your memory and keep focused.

One of the best ways to re-tune is to immerse yourself totally for a day, weekend or even a whole week in the subject. I don't mean sit indoors trying to re-tune and focus, I mean give yourself a real life mental pick-me-up with a seminar, weekend juice detox or a full mind and body detox week (see www.juicemaster.com for full details).

I have quite a few clients who attend one of my retreats a couple of times a year. They not only surround themselves with like-minded people, but they regard it as a form of health insurance. It is a way of not only cleaning the system, but getting back the inspired frame of mind that can so easily slip with the amount of brainwashing and conditioning we are bombarded with on a daily basis. These people see the time and monetary investment as an extremely worthwhile one. It always seems odd to me that if the exhaust goes on your car, you find the time and the money to fix it – yet so many people think twice about investing in the single most important vehicle they will ever have the good fortune to own. Your mind needs investment; if you don't invest, the batteries will wear down and someone else will charge them full of rubbish. And what better place to recharge those batteries than in a sun-drenched country, having freshly extracted juices made for you and attending seminars to keep you inspired and focused?

I realize this sounds a bit like an ad, but I am so passionate about what I do that I want your success to be forever – and I know how important it is to re-tune for that to be a reality. You don't have to come to a seminar or whatever, you can just immerse yourself in one of my books every now and then or just listen to my CD– whatever works for you. But please don't ignore this instruction – it's very, very important. Your health and the way you feel both physically and mentally on a daily basis is the single most important thing in the world and I will do and say everything in my power to make certain you not only get to where you want to go, but that you stay there. And I want to make certain that you do whatever is necessary to ...

Avoid the war

I want you to imagine that there is a war going on where two out of three people die and even those who survive are often very ill or disabled due to the enemy's sustained attack. Now I want you to imagine that you have to go and fight. Every man and woman has been called up and you too are on the list. However, there is a way to get a reprieve, a way to avoid this horrific war: you have to make some fresh beautiful-tasting juice every day, eat some water-rich salad, go out and play, and get a re-tune every now and then.

What do you do?
NOT DiFFiCULT TO ANSWER REALLY iS iT?

The truth is there really is a war going on and the NHS is desperately trying to deal with the casualties every day. The problem is they're so busy treating the wounded that they haven't the time to do anything about actually trying to prevent the war. It really doesn't matter how much money we throw at the NHS, it only goes on treating the casualties. This of course is very necessary. The problem, however, will only ease when we all do our bit to **HELP PREVENT THE WAR**. Every time someone breaks free from the food and diet trap they are doing their bit. You can only be a casualty of war if you are there – by avoiding the war you are, in all likelihood, avoiding the white building with the red cross on it!

There are nearly ten million cases of recognized food poisoning reported each year in the UK alone. There are now over 50,000 deaths directly attributed to obesity, with a cost to the NHS of over £4 billion (conservative estimate). The true death toll and cost will never be known, especially when you think we have recently been given the unenviable title of 'the fattest nation in Europe'! In 2006 1.06 million prescriptions items were dispensed for the treatment of obesity. Over one million tablets to treat a disease simply caused by eating too much of the wrong foods and not moving enough. Over one million pills dished out at a tremendous cost to the tax payer which haven't made even an ounce of difference. We are at a bonkers time in human development and medicine. By law I cannot say a particular fruit or vegetable can treat, prevent or cure a disease, yet **BiG MEDiCiNE** can quite freely dish out over one million pills for the treatment of obesity, even though they create side effects and don't exactly appear to be solving the problem.

I could go on like this forever but the point is: the death toll because of 'food' is more than all drugs on the planet **COMBiNED**, and the true cost to the NHS for treating all drug food and drink related diseases is tens of billions of pounds. The war is raging, but now you can use your ticket to avoid it.

If ever I feel tired and can't be bothered to juice or make a nice soup or salad, I just think about the war and ask myself how much hassle is it really. As far as I'm concerned it's a lot easier to spend ten minutes making a freshly extracted juice or a few minutes putting together a nice salad, than it is to deal with cancer, heart disease, strokes or God knows what kind of other horrific disease. It's amazing how just that thought alone can get you juicing and cooking happily in no time. By keeping your mind free of all the rubbish and flooding it with some mental juice whenever you can, you can achieve optimum health and live your one and only life in a light, slim, sexy, energy-driven body.

Furnish your body with genuine nutrition, keep flooding your mind with the right thoughts, take the time to enjoy the journey and send me a postcard once, not *if*, you get there. I get a real kick every time I hear of the changes people have made because of the information in this book. Since the first version of this book I have received literally thousands of emails, letters, and even genuine postcards. Some of the stories are truly moving and incredibly uplifting. All the tools you need for success you already have, but a reminder of each (the instructions) is to be found over the next few pages, along with some useful information such as what juicer to get, simple rules for juicing and so on. I have also included some frequently asked questions and answers, which are essential reading. The premise of this book is to move away from telling you what you can or cannot eat – what you eat is clearly up to you, I just hope now you have seen the evidence and the trap for what it is, you will now genuinely choose to skip the rubbish and eat well. I am not your keeper and my life will not be affected if you don't change, but yours will. It's all up to you now. However, to give you some idea of how a typical day is shaped, I have written a little 'A Day In The Life Of' as well as the instructions and 'Seven Simple Steps To Be Slim For Life' so you can get an even better feel of how your new day may look. I say 'may look', as it's up to you to shape your day, I can only guide you. Some people work nights, some work on roofs all day, some sit down all day, some like eating their main meal at nights, some at lunchtime and so on. This means the 'day in the life of' I run through, may not work for you, but it will give you an idea of what I am talking about and will give you an opportunity to shape your day and thus your body.

Final Thought

I will leave you with one final thought. When George Burns turned 87 years of age he sent out invitations to all of his friends to come to his 100th birthday party. He hated letting people down and knew by handing out the invites he just had to show up on the day – and of course he did. Enjoy today and always have something to look forward to – it keeps you alive in every way.

Smile, design your own life, and enjoy the journey.

L.i.F.E.
Live In Fearless Excitement

Appendix 1

THE INSTRUCTIONS

The following instructions will mean nothing unless you have read the book. If you have flicked to this page, please go and read the book.

TAKE DECISIVE ACTION

Once you have made the decision to change your diet for life, never doubt your decision. Doubting a decision of this meaning and magnitude is like 'thought cancer' and can spread rapidly. *Knowing*, not *hoping* you are doing the right thing will destroy any doubt instantly. Remember the word 'decision' comes from the Latin meaning 'to terminate' 'to cut off from' – a true decision destroys any doubt and any other possibility has been terminated. It is only indecision that creates doubt and it's only doubt that can cause you to fail in your mission to change your diet for life and be free around all food. When you truly decided to take action you gain power and nothing can shake you. Most people talk a great game; very few take decisive action to achieve their goals.

REMEMBER THERE IS NOTHING TO GIVE UP

The language you use when speaking to yourself or others is more important than people think. If when people offer you some drug-like food you reply by saying, 'No thanks, I've given that up' your brain can easily and falsely start to believe it has made some kind of genuine sacrifice. Just the expression 'given up' implies a sacrifice. This is why, a small instruction it may seem, you should never use the expression 'I've given up'. This is not because you are trying to trick your brain, but because you genuinely haven't *given up* anything worth having. All the emotion and pleasure 'enhancing' abilities of drug-like foods are just one huge illusion. The fact is that for once you are genuinely not 'giving up' anything – you are getting rid of rubbish, rubbish that was making you fat, miserable, and ill. This is the difference between your brain *thinking* it's made a sacrifice and *knowing* it hasn't, and is the difference between 'diet mentality' and one of 'food freedom'. This amounts to the difference between success and failure. The only reason why people struggle when they change what they eat is due to the false belief they have 'given up' – so now you know you haven't, don't start telling yourself you have by using the expression 'I've given up'. Use expressions such as 'I don't have to do that any more', or 'I don't need it any more' or 'I've got rid' – you get the idea. The language you use is vital, so make a habit of using the right terms – if you do you will adjust a lot sooner.

NEVER SAY 'I CAN'T'

This is an essential instruction and once again illustrates the power of language and what an important role it plays. Constant And Never-ending Tantrum is all you can really expect if you start telling yourself you can't have certain things any more. This is diet step mentality and the main reason people struggle when trying to change their diet. Please always remember you *can* have whatever you like, no one is stopping you. But now that you understand the nature of BiG FOOD and BiG DRiNK, and the nature of the food and diet trap, why would you want to? The reason why you have read this book is precisely because you don't want to eat that crap any more, so don't drive yourself nuts by using the term 'I Can't'. Remove the 't' from the word and you have immediately removed the self-imposed tantrum.

DON'T MOAN – REJOICE!

This is another essential instruction and this is where people have got it so wrong for so many years. Remember, you are not making any genuine sacrifice, you're not going to suffer a painful withdrawal and you're doing exactly what *you* want to do. Please realize just how mental and pointless it would be to feel sorry for yourself because you no longer have something you don't want. One of the most insane things seemingly intelligent people do is to spend time moping around for things which they hope they won't have. Enjoy your freedom from the start and rejoice in being one of the few who can see **BiG FOOD** and **BiG DRiNK** for what it is. It is only the moaning that causes anyone a problem when changing their diet; stop the self-imposed moaning and it's ridiculously easy. Remember, if you are having some mental tug-of-war with a particular food or drink in a certain situation you have a choice – either have it and shut up or don't have it and shut up – but shut up! Don't mope and simply rejoice.

DON'T COUNT DAYS

This is again another area where people have it back to front. When people change their diet by using the usual 'Diet Steps' they inevitably count how many days they've been 'on it'. This is because they fully expect to come 'off it' at some stage. When you change your diet as opposed to go on one, there is nothing to come off of. This means counting days is a completely pointless exercise. After all, what are you going to do – count for the rest of your life? And what are you counting for? If you are counting days you miss the point – you have changed your diet and it's for life. The nightmare struggle and diet trap are over and you can now be free.

DON'T AVOID ANY SITUATIONS

Part of the whole diet trap is the belief you have to avoid certain situations when you change your diet in case you are tempted. Avoiding any situation because you have changed your diet will simply give the false impression to your mind that you have made a sacrifice. You have simply changed your diet, you haven't stopped living. I went out more in the first month of change than perhaps I do now. I couldn't wait to be put in situations which, on Diet Mentality, would have normally been my downfall. How can you possibly adjust to a situation if you avoid the situation? This is a mad thing we do and one which compounds the problem and belief that life with rubbish food and drink is great and life without is boring. If you choose to stay in on a diet then you are being boring! The idea here is to get out from the start and go everywhere you would normally go – you are armed with a freedom mentality not a diet one. If you changed your car and were trying to adjust to the new controls, do you think you could ever learn to adjust if you stayed in your house? You need to get in the car and drive the thing – the more you do the quicker your brain adjusts.

DON'T ENVY OTHERS – PITY THEM

One again this instruction is not only vital but also illustrates why diet mentality is so flawed. When people change their diet from crap to delicious and good, they start to envy people who are still eating crap. They envy the very people who they hated being. The mad thing is those people always envy you, even if they don't voice it. This is because the *reality* of consuming junkie foods and drinks never quite matches the *anticipation*. This is due to the anticipation of what you think you'll be getting, based on millions of adverts and taste manipulation moments.

If you are a non-smoker, you wouldn't envy anyone who smokes – so why envy anyone caught in the food and diet trap?

DON'T TRY NOT TO THINK ABOUT JUNK FOOD

I have already covered this, but it needs to be covered in the key instructions. Do not try not to think about drug-like foods and drinks or worry about it if you are a lot of the time. If I had just read an entire book on tennis, then there is no question I would be thinking about tennis a great deal more than I normally would. Fully expect to think about drug-like foods and drinks; it would be strange if you didn't. It's what you think *about it* that makes the difference. If you think, 'thank God I can finally see the rubbish for what it is' – then it doesn't matter if it's in your thoughts 24/7.

NEVER THINK THE GRASS IS GREENER

The grass is not greener on the other side, if it were you would never have wanted to change in the first place. As time goes by you can be easily fooled into thinking that life was rosy when you ate crap and didn't move your body if you happen to be having a bad day. As obvious as this sounds, please remember that there are good and bad days whether you are thin or overweight. We will always experience what I describe as the 'four seasons of emotions' no matter how much money we have or how thin we are. We have all had times when we are having a 'winter' day and get a 'summer' phone call. We have also had 'summer' days and a 'winter' phone call or piece of news that can send us spiralling. The idea is that when you are fit, healthy and have a toned body, you live in summer a great deal more of the time than when you are overweight and lethargic and hating the way you look and feel. The point is there will always be winter moments; the key is to understand that drug-like foods and drinks will not turn winter into summer. It is an illusion: always remember why you wanted to change in the first place.

GET BUSY LIVING

Whoever or whatever created all animals on this planet gave us one fundamental choice on a daily basis – either get busy living or get busy dying. If we were in the wild we would have to be constantly pro-active in order to live; sit around and we get eaten. The same applies to our everyday modern living world. If we simply sit about we don't just stay where we are, we spiral down. It's the same in business, relationships, and your health. You need to be pro-active in order to enhance those areas of your life. I have already gone through this in depth in the book, but one of the key instructions here is to find something that fires you – and to get busy living.

Appendix 2

SEVEN SIMPLE STEPS TO BE SLIM FOR LIFE

1) FOLLOW THE 'NO LABEL DIET'

The whole business of what to eat can be simplified by following not what's on the label, but the label itself. This doesn't include 'mystery food' (food from a cart, stadium, fairground etc.) and your 'no label' foods should be 'organic', 'fair trade', 'grass fed' and so on where appropriate and if possible. Fruits, vegetables and their fresh juices should dominate, with fish being the main source of animal protein and good quality rice being the best form of complex carbohydrates. No label foods also include meat and dairy, but as I illustrated earlier 'grass fed' is best to have a good balance of omega 3 and omega 6, and meat and dairy should only make up a small percentage of your weekly intake. Nuts and seeds are also part of the 'no label diet', but nuts can be quite heavy on the stomach – seeds are excellent. There will of course be times when you eat label foods, that's part of being free, but if the vast majority of your diet consists of 'live', natural 'no label' foods and freshly extracted juices – you are as good as there. Simplicity is the key here and if you think 'no label' what could be easier? This doesn't mean don't look at labels, it just means don't obsess over them and when you do eat label food just choose the best you can. The message is simple, choose food that is as close to its natural state as possible most of the time. There will be times you may fancy a Thai Chi Latte or a quick 'chip butty', the idea again is not to obsess but to be free around all food and use your common sense.

2) CHEW YOUR FOOD THOROUGHLY

Learning to eat in the right way is just as important as changing your diet. Your stomach doesn't have teeth and the enzymes in your saliva are more efficient at breaking down food than those found in your stomach. It seems odd that people say they love food and yet shovel it down without paying any attention to what they are doing. Food is a pleasure and a fuel, which should be savoured where you can. One of the most common traits slim people have is the speed at which they eat. Naturally slim people, on the whole, tend to take their time over food. This not only means you enjoy your food more and actually get to taste it, but it is broken down more efficiently and you feel fuller sooner as your body has had time to acknowledge food has come in.

3) EAT ONLY WHEN YOU ARE GENUINELY HUNGRY

Over the first few days please remember you are starving false hungers in order to leave a genuine one. I hate anyone telling people they should only eat when they are hungry if they don't explain false hungers to them first. Now you know the difference, you will be in a position to genuinely feed a genuine hunger. The key to remember for lifelong success is that you cannot feed an emotion with food. While we consciously know this, the drug-food illusion has fooled many into thinking you can. Remember the only genuine pleasure in eating food is when you end a genuine hunger. If you aren't hungry, what possible emotional benefit do you ever expect to get from the food? Even good food will be stored by most as fat if you put in fuel when the body doesn't require it. Sometimes it can be frustrating that eating something won't actually solve your emotional woes, but it won't. Eat only when you are genuinely hungry, it's the best way to ensure genuine pleasure from the food you eat.

4) STOP EATING WHEN YOU ARE ALMOST FULL

I honestly believe that the unnecessary burdening of the digestive system is the biggest cause of obesity and premature death. I believe it's even more important than what you eat. Having said that, what you eat, as you have seen, often determines the amount you eat. Drug-like foods often create a desperate need for more and so the natural cut off point isn't there. If you can get this step right – and it takes a little training – it could make the biggest difference of them all. If you follow the first three steps, this will be an easy one to adjust to. The power of this principle is perfectly illustrated in the remote Japanese island of Okinawa. People live longer here than any other place on earth and more importantly they actually 'live' to the day they die, as opposed to simply survive. This island has nearly one thousand centenarians (people of 100 years old and over) – that's four times more than the UK and US. It has been shown that Okinawans actually age more slowly than almost anyone else on earth. 'The calendar may say they're 70 but their body says they're 50,' says Bradley Willcox, a scientist researching the extraordinary phenomenon. 'The most impressive part of it is that a good lot of them are healthy until the very end.' Explanations for this mostly centre around the dinner table. Okinawans not only eat more tofu and soya products than any other population in the world, their diet also includes a vast range of different vegetables and fruit all rich in antioxidants. Scientists refer to it as a rainbow diet. However, it's what they *don't* eat that may be at the heart of their exceptionally long, healthy, and slim lives. The Okinawans' most significant cultural tradition is known as hara hachi bu, which translated means 'eat until you're only 80 per cent full'. They consume around 1,200 calories a day, an amount considered dangerous by 'experts' in the UK – despite the fact we die on average at about 80 years old. So if you want to eat a lot it seems the best way to do it is to eat less. By eating less, you live longer so you end up overall eating more! If you can get into this habit you will feel light, be light and if the Okinawans are anything to go by, you will live longer too.

5) MOVE YOUR BODY – DAILY

Walk, run, hop, skip, snowboard, do some weights, rebound– anything – but get your body moving. Movement is like a muscle; if you don't use it – you lose it. Not only for the sake of getting a trim body, but physical movement is essential for many aspects of your mental and physical longevity. Exercise helps to clean the body of dead cells, clears the mind, reduces stress, and speeds up your basal metabolic rate, helping to burn fuel efficiently.

6) GET A JUICER AND A BLENDER

These two machines will do more for your health, energy, and longevity than perhaps any others. I would never get the level of raw live nutrition into my system if I didn't juice on a regular basis. As mentioned you don't need juice every single day of your life, but getting some excellent quality juice inside your system a few times a week will do wonders. Personally I juice a great deal of the time, almost daily. It's not always easy when I am travelling, but I juice as often as I can. When you read 'A Day In The Life Of' coming next, you will see how juicing can make a great start to every day. This isn't a juicing book, but it is one of finding the best way to change your diet and get you fed healthily. With that in mind, get a juicer and blender – they will transform your health and your body in ways you cannot imagine. I have included some wonderful juice recipes to get you started and some juice tips, but if you want to expand your juice knowledge get hold of *The Juice Master: Keeping It Simple*.

7) DO NOT EAT ANY PROCESSED FOOD BEFORE YOU SLEEP

When you sleep your metabolic rate decreases, making efficient digestion harder. If you eat processed food late at night, it can often sit in your stomach and clearly you are doing nothing to burn it off. Clearly there will be times when you do eat before bed, but if you can keep to this step most of the time it will make a difference. Don't get obsessive or refuse a good dinner party – remember this is about freedom!

Appendix 3

A DAY IN THE LIFE OF

There is a saying that if you see someone who has achieved a result you want and you simply follow what they do, you too will achieve the same result. However, I don't know your life and as there are so many variables, please don't simply follow what I do. While this approach may well work for some, it cannot work for everyone. It's about being free to find what works for you and your lifestyle. This typical day doesn't allow for any change of circumstance either, such as dinner parties and holidays.

I also mentioned right at the very start of this book that we all know what to eat, what not to eat and that we should do more exercise. The point of this book is to remove the brainwashing, expose **BiG FOOD** and **BiG DRiNK** and give you the right way of thinking to enable you to find Food Freedom. You already know what to eat and drink to be healthy, but I also understand that if you have been eating the wrong way for so long, it can be daunting to know even where to start.

Here is my typical day, but I have also given some alternatives, which you may well choose instead …

MORNING

- **Hot water with a slice of lemon or herbal tea – usually peppermint.** Hot water tends to 'fire the stomach' first thing in the morning but clearly a little bland. By adding lemon, lime or slice of fennel and at times a little good quality honey, it jazzes up an otherwise bland drink. If I don't feel like hot water, I simply have still mineral water on waking.
- **Some kind of exercise for at least 30 mins – usually a run or rebounding.** I tend to exercise on an empty stomach as I find it easier. Sometimes I will have a small amount of juice before a long run, but usually just some water does me.
- **Freshly extracted juice or smoothie.** The stomach tends to be empty in the morning and this is an ideal time to get maximum benefit from freshly extracted juice. If I don't feel incredibly hungry I have a juice (something like a Veggie Delight, see page 364) or if I am hungry or feel I need more fuel I will have a good smoothie (something like a Turbo Power Smoothie, see page 370). You will notice that I am a keen vegetable juice or smoothie person, but you will also see my recipes have apple, pineapple or both to make sure the veggie juices taste relatively sweet. I would highly recommend vegetable smoothies over fruit. Fruit is great, but we tend to like to eat raw fruit, whereas raw vegetables tend not to be as appealing. You will be amazed at how filling a smoothie made with an avocado can be. (I know avocados are a fruit before you feel the need to call in!) I usually don't have anything else until mid afternoon – that's how filling a good nutritious vegetable based smoothie can be. Clearly you don't have to have a smoothie or juice for breakfast and there are many highly nutritious breakfasts to choose from. If you don't want to juice but want some raw goodness, have fruit. If you fancy egg on toast, just make sure your eggs are the best quality they can be and make sure the toast is bread as close to the grain as possible. If you want oats, have them. Muesli is great, but use soya milk instead of cow's milk. A great breakfast can be sardines on toast. As

long as you keep to the 'seven steps' you can use your imagination and feel free to have what takes your fancy. If you can get into the habit of having a good juice or smoothie, you will find it soon becomes a habit and a great way to start the day. You also know you have done something amazing on the nutrition front first thing in the morning which sets you up nicely for the day.

LUNCH TIME

❦ **Juice/Smoothie/Salad/Soup/Stuffed Pitta/and so the list goes on.** Lunch can be anything. As I am writing this book I happen to be having freshly extracted juices and smoothies all day and then an evening meal, but that's not always the case. This is all about freedom and my lunch often changes depending on where I am and how genuinely hungry I am. One of my favourite lunches when at home is a warm wholemeal pitta bread stuffed with some organic rocket, watercress and spinach salad, along with sun blushed tomatoes, olives, feta cheese, avocado, and lemon juice – delicious and very filling. I use the avocado as the spread, like butter, and add the rest. I also love some toasted rye bread with avocado spread with sardines, pesto, and lemon juice. I also love a bowl of Alpen (no added sugar) with soya milk and sliced bananas. Salads are also great, I have given a couple of examples of good salads in this book (see pages 373–6). I think you get the picture, providing you keep to the seven steps, feel free to enjoy whatever you have. Once again though you will be amazed at how filling a smoothie can be for lunch and if you want to see some good fast results on the weight loss front, having a smoothie for breakfast and lunch and an evening meal will have you in Slim Land in no time.

DINNER TIME

❦ **Exercise.** I often do my second lot of exercise before dinner to shake out the day and give myself an evening boost. I am often near the coast, so I get the opportunity to hit the beach and go surfing. When I am in the city, I either run in the park, hit the gym, do some rebounding or play a game of tennis, squash, football or whatever is on. This not only makes me feel alive, but also keeps my metabolism high for my evening meal. Some people have dinner around 6 p.m. and hit the gym late at night. Personally I like to exercise early and eat slightly later. Clearly this is just a small example and my days are often very different.

❦ **What takes your fancy?** There are so many choices here it's almost impossible to list. I love a good homemade soup with good quality bread in winter. I also adore a nice salad with something hot on top such as salmon, monkfish or organic chicken. Pasta is also good, as long as it's wholemeal pasta. Rice and steamed vegetables, again excellent. The list really goes on and on. I am conscious that I am in danger of repeating myself, but as long as you follow the seven steps, tuck into whatever takes your fancy.

The above is a very quick example of a day in the life of what I do, eat, and drink. My diet isn't set in stone and yours shouldn't be either. This book is about being mentally free and designing your own change of diet and being free around all food. It's about having genuine freedom of choice and about understanding fully that you cannot have freedom of choice without the freedom also to refuse. You are now armed with the right information that will enable you to have genuine freedom to refuse.

For further ideas regarding recipes there are many good books on that subject. I am not a cook and don't pretend to be. I feel that's best left to Gordon Ramsay and Jamie Oliver. Gordon's book *Healthy Appetite* is a good one, but there are many. There are, even if I say so myself, some excellent soup, juice, smoothie, and salad recipes in my other book *Juice Yourself Slim*. Above all, eat natural and keep it simple. I have been to many 'raw food' conventions and to say they make a meal of things is an understatement. Where a simple avocado salad would do, many people overcomplicate the issue.

Appendix 4

FREQUENTLY ASKED QUESTIONS

What do you think of ENERGY BARS?

As with virtually all foods out there, we have the good, the bad, and the ugly when it comes to energy bars. What I hate is the Con-Appetite aspect of this area of 'fast-food'. There are many brands, which have large labels stating how **NATURAL** they are, when they are loaded with sugar. There are very few good quality energy bars on sale in regular stores. Nearly all have cooked ingredients, which in itself isn't bad, but it's best when you can get good raw ingredients. The bars I recommend are those from The Food Doctor, Nakd, and my own range. I am aware that recommending your own range can seem obvious, but I genuinely produced them because what was on the market wasn't good. I have produced two bars: one fruit and one vegetable. They are called Juice In A Bar as I have used dried juice powders. These juices are dried at low temperatures to preserve the enzyme activity and as soon as your saliva comes into contact with them, boom – they come alive. In the Veggie Juice In A Bar there is spinach, broccoli, alfalfa, spirulina, wheatgrass, kale, friendly bacteria, raw almonds, dates, and so the list goes on and on. Uniquely, they have no fillers, such as oats. Oats are good, but they are clearly very cheap. Many 'health' bars are loaded with oats, we have none. Instead: raw almonds, dates, friendly bacteria, and plenty of natural dried juices. They should be available in the supermarkets and service stations by the time you read this book – if not they are on the website. I have looked for the quality of freshly extracted juices in a bar and couldn't find one, so I created it. As awful as the ingredients of the veggie one sounds, it's actually gorgeous. The fruit version contains fruits we can't juice in the UK such as acai and goji berries.

What about supplements?

These can be a minefield. Like energy bars, there are good supplements and really bad ones. I feel if we are eating 'No Label' and 'Organic' and getting plenty of natural juice, supplements shouldn't be necessary. Having said this I do take the odd powdered supplement myself in my smoothies and juices to make sure I get the finest quality nutrition daily, after all I don't want to leave it to chance. I can no longer escape the fact that due to the overuse of pesticides, herbicides, fungicides, and general over farming, our fruit and veg is often a far cry from what it should be. On top of this, some of the most power antioxidant fruits in the world are found many miles from our shores and cannot be shipped fresh. A couple of examples are acai and goji berries. These amazing berries are loaded with disease fighting antioxidants – twice as many as blueberries. However, they go off so quickly after harvesting that unless they are dried and made into a powder, we would never get the benefits of these amazing berries. There are also many herbs and some fruits and vegetables – dandelion and ginseng, for example – which don't juice well or are hard to get hold of. With this in mind some supplements are great. There are many **SUPER GREEN** powders that are superb, such as Udo's Greens, Tony Robbins' Power Greens and I have my own Ultimate Super Food. Once again my development of my own range of supplements came about simply due to the lack of excellent quality supplements on the market. We use no fillers and only the finest ingredients. For more details on all the range see the website. However, I must stress that if you eat organically and get plenty of green juices, you really shouldn't need that many supplements, if any.

Can I have any tea and coffee?

Yes, you can have what you like. I know this concept is hard for some to get their head around, especially if they have been on restrictive diets all their life. However, freedom means being free to do what you choose. If you have read the information but still choose to have the odd cup, then clearly it won't kill you. One cup of coffee or tea a day will not harm. I do strongly suggest that you have a total coffee or tea break as you will see just how easy it can be to do without. You will also see how refreshing alternative teas like peppermint can be. For some, coffee and tea is a massive addiction and they may be on several cups a day, if this is you – skip the lot for a few weeks and see how you feel about it then.

Is yoghurt just as bad as milk?

Yes and no really, it all depends on the particular kind of yoghurt. Most yoghurts are heavily processed and contain quite a bit of sugar. If you want yoghurt then choose the 'live' natural versions. Live yoghurt has what's called 'friendly bacteria' present which can be very beneficial. The friendly bacteria also helps to break down the lactose and I know from personal experience that if you are lactose intolerant, you may well be able to tolerate live yoghurt.

Are there different kinds of milk I can have?

Yes. There are many different kinds of milk on the market that tend to be easier for the body to deal with than cow's milk. There are some good soya milks on sale these days and dairy free milks in most supermarkets. Soya milk with muesli actually taste really good and you can barely notice the difference. In tea and coffee it tends to be a different story, so if you are going to have the odd cup here and there, simply have some semi-skimmed. However, if you are having a Latte in somewhere like Starbucks, get a soy Thai Chi Latte as normal Lattes are loaded with milk, and I doubt the milk is from grass fed cows.

You've talked about how wonderful mother's milk is for babies, but I can't breast feed. What should I feed my baby?

I realize there will be many women reading this book who, for whatever reason, cannot breast feed. If you are wondering what is best to feed your baby, please remember that a baby has the correct enzymes to break down milk – it's only adults who have the problem. In fact it is essential, an absolute must that babies get milk of some kind. If you want the nearest thing possible to mother's milk then goat's milk, organic carrot juice, and water is the best you can get. A goat has one stomach like us so the baby cannot only deal with this type of milk much easier than cow's milk, but it thrives on it. If you are in any doubt please see your GP for some advice.

Is it possible to live on nothing but fruit, veg, and juices?

Yes, without question – as long as you throw in a few nuts and seeds for good measure. Not only is it possible but clearly you would also be extremely healthy. However, although you can, why would you ever want to? Having *nothing* but raw food for the rest of your life – well it's not for me. I once had nothing but freshly extracted fruit and veg juices for three months and trust me, that's a long time to go on nothing but fresh juices. The only reason I did it was to try and clear my skin of psoriasis. I lost far too much weight to the point where I made Posh Spice look fat! You cannot, nor should not, live on juice alone for that long – you need fibre. The maximum time you should have a juice clearout for is 7–10 days. I often have days where I eat nothing but raw foods and drink fresh juices – in fact my intake even when I'm eating cooked foods on a particular day tends to be 70–80 per cent natural fast food. But I am not obsessive and I'm incredibly flexible – it depends on where I am or whom I'm with. If you want to eat nothing but fruit, vegetables, salads, nuts, and seeds and you are perfectly happy doing it then brilliant – it will serve you more than well. But as far as I'm concerned, it is just too restrictive in today's twenty-first century world, especially when we have dinner parties and especially when there is simply no need to. The body was designed to deal with a certain amount of just about anything – so eat, relax, and enjoy!

What about eggs?

I guess if we really thought about what an egg is, we'd probably never go near them. However, eggs aren't a drug-like food and are 'no label' plus quite frankly you can't beat a bit of free-range egg on wholegrain toast after a long run on a Sunday morning. I eat eggs about once every two weeks, if that. The one rule I would have is to keep them out of the frying pan – poach, boil or scamble. Once again 'organic' and 'free-range' applies in this case as, trust me, the things I could tell you about eggs produced from battery hens could fill another book.

What about dried fruit?

Dried fruits are not only delicious, but are very good for you – if used in moderation. My favourite is dried mango – it's simply orgasmic. *Do* check the label though, as many of those on sale contain sulphur dioxide, which is caustic to the stomach. As always, go for the natural, nothing-added variety. The general rule is: if they look too bright and cheery there's probably some chemical involved somewhere.

Note: dried fruits are high in sugar and, although natural, they are very concentrated so please use sparingly. If diabetic or hypoglycaemic – leave well alone.

Fruit is also high in sugar so won't it cause the same problems as white sugar?

NO, NO, NO, NO, NO, NO! Sorry for the outburst, but since the 'eat nothing but fat and protein diet' fads I know several people who are convinced that fruit sugar causes the same problems as the white refined kind and so they eat fried eggs, bacon, and sausages instead of a piece of fruit. For their purposes, as well as yours, I want to make this next point very clear. There is a massive difference between the sugar you find in fresh fruit and the white refined drug variety. The sugar you find in fruit has many different elements to it. It is a whole food, contains plenty of genuine life-giving nutrients and is high in water, which helps to transport the goodness to the cells and flush out the waste. White refined sugars and carbs contain nothing of any value to the body – they are totally empty foods. The only time fruit can be a problem is if you gulp down a pint of juice in a very short amount of time. Once again if you are diabetic – either dilute your juice with half mineral water, or just eat the fruit and juice your vegetables.

This juicing thing sounds a bit of a hassle. Do I have to buy a juicer and juice every day for this to be a success?

No you don't. That may sound a bit strange coming from the **JUiCE MASTER**, but I want to make it clear that juicing is meant to be used as a tool – a catalyst to get you to the land of the slim and healthy. While I wholeheartedly believe in juicing as perhaps the best way possible to get nutrients into an already battered and clogged system, and as an incredible aid to help flush out waste, I'm not so arrogant to say it's the only way. If you prefer to eat all your fruit and are quite happy eating plenty of steamed, lightly cooked or raw vegetables **EVERY DAY** then feel free to do so. Just make certain that at least 70 per cent of what you eat is live natural food, with fish, white lean meat, whole grains, and tiny amounts of dairy making up the remaining 30 per cent. However, I obviously strongly advise using juicing as a tool for your health – especially while you are on the journey to wellness and vibrancy. It's like going first class as opposed to economy! Once you have arrived in the land of the slim and healthy and are 'maintaining' then you may find you are using your juicer slightly less and eating raw more. As with everything – use your common sense.

When looking for 'whole' meal/grain breads and carbs, which ones are okay?

Well the best of the best for health are unleavened breads that contain no flour, yeast, sugars or oils, but still have all the fibre and germ of the whole grain. These breads are made from sprouted grains such as spelt, millet, flax, oats, kamut, and quinoa (you can find these at some super-markets and all good health stores).

Although these are the best, I can almost guarantee, unless you have a real yeast and wheat problem, they will not be the ones you choose all the time. The best choice, I believe, is wholemeal pitta bread. You can warm it slightly in the oven, open it up and stuff it full of water-rich, nutrient-packed salad. Rye bread is also pretty good: toast two slices, spread on loads of creamy avocado and pack out with a water-rich salad. Other acceptable complex carbs are as follows: whole rolled oats, whole-wheat pastas, whole-wheat tortillas, brown rice (not instant), stone ground whole-wheat flour, wholegrain crackers, dark rye crackers, stone ground whole-wheat bagels, stone ground whole-wheat breads, wholemeal breads, whole-wheat croutons.

How much weight can I expect to lose in what time frame?

One of the key instructions is not to be a weight watcher, not to play the 'I'll be happy when' game, but if you want to know how long it's going to take before you personally lose your excess weight, here is a rough idea. The average person I see, who follows the seven steps to the letter, drops about 6–14 lb (2.7–6.3 kg) in weight in the first month and then an average of 2–4 lb (0.9–1.8 kg) a week thereafter. Please understand though that there are no hard and fast rules here, there are many factors to consider. If you are already slim, or only have a few pounds to lose, then clearly you are not going to lose more weight than is healthy following this programme. It's only if you obsess about being a very abnormal Size Zero that you'll end up unnaturally thin. Remember, nature's idea of perfect shape and what the media often portrays can be worlds apart. I once had a young lady phone me and say, 'I'm following everything you said but after the first month I stopped losing weight'. It turned out she was already just 8 stone (50 kg): for her height it sounded about right, maybe even a little too thin – one thing's for sure, she wasn't fat! It would take a completely unnatural diet for her to get to what she believes is an ideal weight. Remember, it may be 'ideal' for fashion editors and models but not for those of us who live in the real world.

Your body may already be its ideal weight and shape, but you are still fighting to achieve what you believe is the 'ideal look'. It's a battle you are bound to lose and why start it in the first place? I will never be a strapping six footer with a body like Brad Pitt – no matter what the hell I eat – and you may never look like whoever, but so what. As long as we are feeling good, looking good, living (as opposed to simply surviving) and are truly free in every sense of the word then we should be grateful for the body we do have, give thanks for our health and rejoice at being alive.

Of course many people reading this book will be overweight and trying to get slimmer. Often people with quite a bit of weight to lose find that they drop a bit of weight and then plateau for a while, to the point where it seems they are 'stuck'. This happens for a good reason. The body does things at its own speed – what's most important to you may well not be what's most important for the wellness of the whole body. There is a good chance that over the years you have damaged tissues or organs and you may also have asthma, arthritis, irritable bowel syndrome (IBS), or other problems. Now as far as your body is concerned, rectifying damage and disease and making you well again might be far more important to it at times than dropping a few pounds. So what usually happens is you drop some weight and then seemingly nothing happens for a short time, then you drop some more and so it goes. As long as you are supplying your body with nutrients and oxygen, and keeping it free from the majority of toxic food products, you can be guaranteed that even if nothing appears to be happening, it is. So trust me, the body will drop excess weight when it feels it's safe to do so, just don't sit around waiting. If you cut your finger you get on with your life and let your body do what it needs to do to repair it – you certainly don't sit there staring at it waiting for it to get better do you? So don't do the same here. Remember – do it right once and you will never have a weight problem again. If you still feel the weight not shifting then get hold of my *7 lbs in 7 days Super Juice Diet* – it's guaranteed.

But I'm not overweight, I read this just to learn more about food. In fact I'm underweight, will this be dangerous for me?

No way. This way of eating, breathing, thinking, and living is healthy for every single human being on the planet and if you are underweight you will not lose more weight on this programme – you will in all likelihood return to a natural, healthy weight. Trying to gain weight for people who are naturally thin is actually often harder than for those trying to lose it. I know people who are overweight don't believe that but it's true. Gaining an appetite is just as hard for a thin person as losing an appetite is for an overweight person. However, eating this way will trigger normal and natural hungers.

What about salad dressings?

I tend to just have a mix of balsamic vinegar, virgin olive oil, and lemon juice. Also try a fresh lemon and lime dressing – it's simple but wonderful. Every now and then I will have a Caesar salad when out and yes I know Caesar dressing is far from the best, but once in a while is fine – remember, feel free.

What about nuts?

Any nut which has been roasted and salted is not only 'lifeless' but very detrimental to the body and because of the white refined salt, also addictive. Natural nuts, on the other hand, are an excellent source of natural fats – Brazils, almonds, pistachios etc., are all superb.

I was on the loo a lot, had a few headaches and felt a bit, well, ill – is that normal on a healthy eating plan?

It can be, but please realize you're not ill – you are getting better. All that's happening is your body is having a good clean out. Don't worry – any discomfort you feel will soon subside and please bear in mind that any physical reactions you suffer are not because you've stopped eating and drinking the rubbish, but because you started in the first place. Your body is full of toxic waste and it needs to go somewhere, so if you do find yourself on the loo a lot during the first couple of weeks – **GOOD**. In no time at all you will be looking and feeling better than you have in years – happy cleaning!

Can I have the odd savoury dip?

Yes, there is nothing wrong with having dips every now and then, but a dip means a dip! Dips are meant to be there for you to dip into every now and then – not to have as your entire meal. Be careful with them; don't get into the habit of having pittas, dips, and nothing else. High water content, 'live' nutrient based meals are the key to lifelong success and if all you have after a hard day at work is dips and bread you will be consuming 0 per cent water-rich, live-nutrient packed food. I am not saying don't have them, but please be aware they fall into the 20–30 per cent category of non-natural food your body can easily deal with. I personally love homemade guacamole – it's creamy, tastes sensational, and is high in water and essential live nutrients. You can use it as a spread, dip, or add water and balsamic vinegar for beautiful salad dressing, or pour straight over jacket potatoes.

When it comes to quick pitta snacks, the key is to warm your pittas in the oven and stuff them full of high-water, nutrient-rich salad or stir-fried veg with perhaps some fresh pesto sauce. You can then use the dips for what they are – dips. Don't make them your whole meal, but it's more than okay to take the odd dip.

Is this stuff safe for my kids?

What, eating well? – yes! It's eating and drinking the 'other stuff' that is not safe for your kids. I have seen many children in my seminars and I'd like to share a letter with you which I received from a young lady of 13 years of age called Patrina:

'Hi Jason … i just wanted to say a big big thank you for what you did for me, i really appreciate it. This new way of eating is great, i have loads more energy. Thank you for sending me that letter it gave me more confidence that i can do it and thank you for recommending the juicer, it's great. i feel like i'm already on my way to the land of the slim. Thanks again.'

Still not convinced?

'Just a quick note to let you know how you changed the life of a 16-year-old girl that attended your seminar. At the time she was around 13 stone [82 kg] and had been having weight problems since she was 10 or younger. You should see her now, she looks fantastic, beyond belief. i told her i was going to send you an email and she said "tell Jason he can send tickets for the land of the slim any time now". i really wanted to say thank you very, very much.' Helen

These are just a couple of the many children I have had the good fortune to coach to health over the years. Children not only thrive on this stuff – they love it. What they hate is being force-fed dead food, especially when it's a sunny afternoon and all they want to do is play. Many times as a child I would literally cry at the Sunday dinner table because I wasn't hungry for food but for oxygen and fun. Being force-fed is not only a nightmare for a child's sanity, but it is extremely unhealthy as you shouldn't eat when you're not hungry. It's made ten times worse when the food is totally lifeless and detrimental to the body.

I'm not picking on parents here, after all they are only doing what they have been taught is best, but if you do have children and also want to set them free – then don't worry on the health front. Most children will quite happily feast on fresh fruit all day given the choice and as for the fresh juices – they love them. Making juice in the morning becomes fun and kids will want to get involved with the process. As for the main meals, they will obviously be eating the same as you, so will be as healthy as pie.

Obviously you will not be able to change everything they eat but if you want a tip on how to make them change, here it is. Children are not stupid and, like us, hate being told what they can or cannot do. Remember **CAN'T** is pure torture, and 'can't' also creates a rebellious mind-set in children. Treat children like adults and explain to them exactly what these foods are doing and why you have chosen to be free from them. You will find that as long as you don't become a member of the 'food police' and keep telling them they can't, they will make the choice themselves – especially when you explain to them just how much better they will look and feel.

Are there any alternatives to salt?

Yes, health – that's a pretty good alternative to this stroke-inducing substance. Lemon juice is the best substitute for salt, as I have already mentioned: it may sound strange, but it really works. If you are going to have salt though, and if we deal with reality there will of course be odd times when you do, then buy the best coarsely grained sea salt you can get. When out in a restaurant use lemon juice where possible, but the little bit of salt you have on a meal out will not make that much difference.

If I do choose to stop eating meat, fish, and all dairy products – where will I get my protein?

A very common question for the very few people who decide to become vegan. In terms of sanity and flexibility I always advise that people don't avoid all animal products, but if you have made that choice, then I want to put your mind at rest when it comes to protein. Our protein is made of something called amino acids – there are twenty-three in all. The good news is that we already have fifteen of them, the bad news is that it is essential to get the other eight from our diet. These eight are known as 'essential amino acids' because without them our health suffers. Despite what many of the 'experts' may say you can easily get all your essential amino acids through eating fruit, veg, grains, and nuts – as long as you eat a variety of these foods. If you have a good varied diet you can be confident that you are getting all the protein you need. If in doubt, use your common sense – the largest and strongest land animal, the elephant, is a vegan!

I hear I can train as a Natural Juice Therapist – where can I find out more?

This training course is the first accredited Natural Juice Therapist program in the world. It took a long time to get it right and I am pleased to say we have many therapists coming through the ranks. All are trained on all aspects in juice therapy as well as the concepts in this book. If you want to know more simply see our website for your nearest therapist or to find out about the course.

Appendix 5

BASIC RULES FOR MAKING JUICES

When it comes to making a tasty juice there is one core rule: vegetable and fruit juices don't mix that well together. Like any rule there are always exceptions. Apples, lemons, limes, avocados, and pineapple all turn an otherwise earthy juice into a sweeter version. Having said that if you were to have an orange and carrot juice it will still be of benefit, but the general rule is not to mix your fruit and veg juice, except apple, pineapple, lemon, and lime.

In order to make sure that your vegetable juices taste wonderful every time here's a tip. Make sure that ½ to ¾ of your vegetable juice is made up of either apple or carrot juice or a combination of these. Virtually every vegetable juice I make has an apple base. You will understand why if you try and do a vegetable juice without it: I once had leek, spinach and celery – it was nearly enough to put me off for life. So other than getting the base right and remembering that as a rule most fruit juices and vegetable juices don't mix very well together, you really are free to concoct your very own juice magic!

Another tip is to make sure you don't peel anything as most of the nutrients are found in the skin. There are some things you will have to peel, such as oranges and grapefruits, but on the whole keep the skin on – especially on vegetables.

I have included a few recipes in this book with instructions, but for advice on how to make a juice in super fast time, tips on cleaning, special bio pulp bags, how to store a juice and so on, go to www.juicemaster.com for a full list of answers to your juice questions.

Appendix 6

RECIPES

Juices

Detox Dream

Freshly extracted apple, cucumber, and celery juice, combined with the zingy zest of ginger and lemon. This beautiful tasting juice will zing your system and help with your body's natural detox.

Juicy Ingredients
2 x apples
2 x slice of cucumber
1 x stick of celery
1 x slice of lemon (with rind on)
1 x inch (2.5 cm) of fresh ginger
Ice

Juicy Instructions
Juice the apples, cucumber, celery, lemon and ginger.
Pour over ice and enjoy.

Dr Juice

The sweetness of freshly extracted apple, carrot, and beetroot juice, blended with the neutral tones of celery and brought to life with the zing of fresh ginger and zesty lemon.

Juicy Ingredients
2 x apples
1 x carrot
½ small raw beetroot
½ stick of celery
1 cm (⅓ in) slice of ginger
1 cm (⅓ in) slice of lemon (with the skin on)
Ice

Juicy Instructions
Place the beetroot, carrot, celery, ginger, lemon and apple into the juicer and juice.
Pour over ice and enjoy.

Carrot 'n' pear twist

This juice is a twist on the famous carrot and apple 'crapple' juice. The pear juice creates a thicker, sweeter juice and the addition of the ginger and lemon gives this juice a wonderful zesty twist.

Juicy Ingredients
2 x medium-sized carrots
1 x pear
1 x cm (⅓ in) slice of lemon with the skin on
1 x inch (2.5 cm) piece of fresh ginger
Ice

Juicy Instructions
Juice the carrot, pear, lemon, and ginger.
Pour over ice and enjoy.

Veggie Delight

A beautiful array of Mother Nature's finest vegetables combined with the natural sweetness of creamy pineapple juice and freshly extracted apple juice.

Juicy Ingredients
1 x apple
¼ x pineapple (leave the skin on)
½ x carrot
½ x celery stick
½ x small raw beetroot
2 cm (¾ in) of cucumber
Handful of spinach (or other green leafy vegetables)
Ice

Juicy Instructions
Juice the apple, pineapple, spinach, carrot, celery, beetroot, and cucumber.

Pour over ice and enjoy.

Creamy nectar

Succulent, sweet pear juice; creamy, tropical pineapple juice; fresh crisp apple juice — all combined together and poured over ice to create a 'creamy nectar' juicy delight!

Juicy Ingredients
1 x apple
1 x pear
¼ x medium-sized pineapple
Ice

Juicy Instructions
Juice the apple, pear. and pineapple.
Pour over ice and enjoy.

Juice Master's Famous Sherbet Lemonade

This juice is as simple as A, B, C to make and contains Vitamins A, B, and C in abundance. This is genuine lemonade at its finest and your taste buds are in for a true taste sensation.

Juicy Ingredients
2 x apples
1 x cm (⅓ in) slice of lemon with the skin on
Ice

Juicy Instructions
Place one apple then the lemon and the other apple into the juicer and juice.
Pour over ice and enjoy.

Smoothies

Magnificent Seven

Seven wonderful fruits and vegetables juiced and blended to create a mighty, magnificent smoothie. Dark red beetroot juice, deep green spinach juice, soft neutral apple, tangy lime, cucumber, and celery juice all blended with the rich and creamy flesh of ripe avocado.

Juicy Ingredients
2 x apples
1 x small bulb of beetroot
1 x handful of spinach
1 x stick of celery
¼ x cucumber
½ x peeled lime
½ x ripe avocado
Ice

Juicy Instructions
Juice the apples, beetroot, spinach, celery, cucumber, and lime.
Pour this juice into the blender, add the avocado and ice and blend
   until smooth.

Creamy honey 'n' berry

Deep, dark mixed berries combined with the freshly extracted juice of crisp sweet apple; a generous helping of bio-live yoghurt; a twist of fresh ginger and then finished with the nectar of delicious soothing honey.

Juicy Ingredients
2 x apples
1 x handful of mixed berries (fresh or frozen)
½ cm of fresh ginger
1 x tablespoon of Bio-Live Natural Yoghurt
1 x teaspoon of honey (manuka honey is best or locally produced honey)
Ice

Juicy Instructions
Juice the apple, berries, and ginger by packing the berries and ginger in between the apples.
Pour the juice into the blender and add the yoghurt, honey, and ice and blend until smooth.

Mango 'Bio-live' Energiser

The soft, tender flesh of ripe mango, perfectly united with creamy banana, thick natural yoghurt, the zesty juice of fresh orange juice, and a gentle squeeze of honey.

Juicy Ingredients

½ x mango (remove the skin and stone or use frozen)
2 x oranges (peeled, but keep as much pith on as possible)
½ x banana
2 x tablespoons of bio-live natural yoghurt
Squeeze of honey (manuka honey is best or locally produced
   honey)
Ice

Juicy Instructions

Juice the oranges and pour the juice into the blender.
Add the mango flesh, banana, yoghurt, honey, ice and blend until
   smooth.

Turbo Power Smoothie

This smoothie is a slight tweak on one of my favourites —
'The Turbo Charge', except this time with no pineapple. This
version is slightly less sweet, yet oh so yummy.

Juicy Ingredients
2 x apples
½ x stick of celery
2 cm (¾ in) of cucumber
Handful of spinach
½ x peeled lime
¼ avocado (peeled with the stone removed)
Ice

Juicy Instructions
Juice the apples, celery, cucumber, spinach, and lime.
Pour the juice into the blender, add the avocado and ice and blend
until smooth.

Blueberry Burst

Sometimes less is more and this recipe certainly supports that statement. Simple freshly extracted apple juice blended with the flesh of ripe banana and dark decadent blueberries.

Juicy Ingredients
2 x tbsp of blueberries
½ x banana
2 x apples
Ice

Juicy Instructions
Juice the apples and pour into the blender.
Place the blueberries, banana, and ice into the blender and blend
until smooth.

Fennel Zest Fuel

A beautiful combination of the juices of sweet pineapple, zesty lime, cooling cucumber, and aniseed-flavoured fennel all blended together with soft, ripe, creamy avocado.

Juicy Ingredients
⅓ x medium-sized pineapple
2 cm (¾ in) of fresh fennel
¼ cucumber
½ peeled lime
¼ ripe avocado
Ice

Juicy Instructions
Juice the pineapple, fennel, cucumber, and lime.
Pour the juice into the blender and add the avocado flesh and ice and blend until smooth.

Super Salads

Green Pesto Power Salad

Avocado, cucumber, and spring onion served on a bed of baby leaf spinach, rocket, and watercress and drizzled with a pesto dressing.

What you need (serves 2 happily)
1 x large ripe avocado
1 x bag (140 g/5 oz) of watercress, spinach, and rocket salad
¼ cucumber
2 x stems of spring onion
100 g (3½ oz) of pesto
2 tbsp of virgin olive oil

What you do ...
Wash the salad leaves and place in a bowl.
Remove the flesh of the avocado, cut into generous slices and add to the salad.
Thinly slice the cucumber and spring onion and add to the salad.
Empty the pesto into a small bowl, add the olive oil and mix well to create a pesto 'dressing'.
Pour the pesto dressing over the salad and serve.

Warm, Organic, Fair-trade Chicken and Avocado Salad

Warm, organic, fair-trade chicken and ripe avocado served on a bed of wild rocket with shavings of parmesan and sprinkled with fresh lemon juice.

What you need (serves 2 happily)
2 x skinless chicken breast (preferably free range, organic)
1 x large ripe avocado
1 x bag (65 g/2⅓ oz) of wild rocket
50 g (1¾ oz) of fresh parmesan
1 x lemon
Virgin olive oil

What you do …
Place the chicken under the grill and grill for 20 minutes until cooked.

Meanwhile simply wash the rocket and place in a salad bowl.

Remove the avocado flesh, chop into generous chunks and add to the rocket.

Remove the chicken from the grill, cut into generous chunks and add to the salad.

Using a peeler or sharp knife, 'shave' thin slices of the parmesan over the salad.

Cut the lemon in half and squeeze the juice over the salad along with the olive oil.

To make this vegan/vegetarian …
Simple leave out the chicken, or replace with an alternative.

Winter Warmer Salad

Oven roasted butternut squash, peppers, red onion, courgette, and baby tomatoes, thrown on a bed of avocado oil dressed salad leaves.

What you need (serves 2 happily)
¼ x butternut squash (peeled)
½ x red pepper
½ x yellow pepper
1 x small red onion (peeled)
½ x courgette
8 x baby tomatoes
1 x bag (100g/3½ oz) of mixed salad leaves
2 tbsp of oil
Avocado olive oil
Black pepper

What you do ...
Pre-heat the oven to 180°C (350°F).
Drizzle the oil onto a baking tray and warm in the oven for 10 minutes.
Roughly chop the butternut squash, peppers, onion, and courgette into small chunks about 1 cm (⅓ in) cubed and place in the baking tray and return to the oven for 25 minutes.
Wash the salad leaves, place in a bowl and drizzle with the avocado oil.
Remove the vegetables from the oven, add the tomatoes, season with black pepper and return to the oven for a further 5 minutes.
When the vegetables are roasted remove from the oven and 'throw' over the prepared salad.

Hot Honey Salmon Salad

Delicate salmon drizzled with manuka honey and served on a bed of watercress, rocket, baby leaf spinach, and cucumber.

What you need (serves 2 happily)
2 x fillets of fresh salmon
1 x bag (140 g/5 oz) of watercress, spinach, and rocket salad
½ x cucumber
2 teaspoons of manuka honey (If you can't get manuka use a good
    quality honey instead)
2 tbsp of balsamic vinegar
1 x lemon
2 tbsp of virgin olive oil
Black pepper
Tin foil

What you do ...
Place the salmon (skin side up) onto the tin foil and cover each
    piece with honey.
Place the salmon under the grill and cook for 10–15 minutes (do
    not turn over).
Meanwhile simply wash the salad leaves and place in a salad
    bowl.
Thinly chop the cucumber and add to the salad.
Make up the dressing by combining the juice from the lemon with
    the balsamic vinegar, olive oil, and pepper.
Drizzle the dressing over the salad and toss well.
Divide the salad onto the two plates, remove the salmon from the
    oven and place directly onto the prepared salad.

To make this vegan/vegetarian ...
Simple leave out the salmon, or replace with an alternative.

Super Soups

Butternut Squash and Carrot Soup

Creamy, smooth butternut squash and carrot infused together to create a genuinely dreamy, sublime, nourishing soup.

What you need (serves 2 happily)
½ x butternut squash
3 x medium carrots
1 x small red onion
1 x vegetable stock cube
1 tbsp of vegetable oil
Crushed black pepper

What you do ...

Peel the butternut squash (remove seeds), carrots, and red onion and chop all the vegetables into small chunks.

Prepare the stock by dissolving the stock cube in 1 pint (0.5 litre) of boiling water.

In a large saucepan heat the oil and add all the vegetables and season with the black pepper.

Gently sweat the vegetables in the pan with the lid on for 15 minutes, stirring occasionally.

Add the stock, bring to the boil and simmer for 10 minutes.

Remove from heat and using a blender (hand or jug), blend the soup until smooth.

Pour into a bowl and enjoy.

'Souper' Green Stuff

The fresh, vibrant, pure tones of Mother Nature's finest chlorophyll rich vegetables, all blended together to create a little taste of Eden.

What you need (serves 2 happily)
6 x broccoli florets (chopped into small pieces)
1 x leek
50 g (1¾ oz) x spinach
1 x courgette
1 x stick of celery
1 x vegetable stock cube
1 tbsp of vegetable oil
Crushed black pepper

What you do ...

Remove the 'top' and 'tail' from the leek, celery, and courgette and chop into thin slices, and prepare the broccoli.

Prepare the stock by dissolving the stock cube in 1 pint (0.5 litre) of boiling water.

In a large saucepan heat the oil and add all the vegetables.

Gently sweat the vegetables in the pan for 15 minutes and then add the stock and seasoning, bring to the boil and simmer for 10 minutes.

Remove from heat and using a blender (hand or jug), blend the soup slightly so it still contains a good chunky texture.

Pour into a bowl and enjoy.

Hunky Chunky Vegetable

A scrumptious vegetable soup containing hunky, chunky vegetables that simply melt in the mouth.

What you need (serves 2 happily)

1 x parsnip

1 x carrot

1 x sweet potato

1 x leek

1 x courgette

1 x vegetable stock cube

1 tbsp of vegetable oil

Crushed black pepper

What you do ...

Remove the 'top' and 'tail' from the parsnip, carrot, sweet potato, leek, and courgette and peel and chop into small chunks.

Prepare the stock by dissolving the stock cube in 1 pint (0.5 litre) of boiling water.

In a large saucepan heat the oil and add all the vegetables.

Gently sweat the vegetables in the pan for 15 minutes and then add the stock and seasoning, bring to the boil and simmer for 10 minutes.

Remove from heat and divide the soup roughly in half.

Blend one half of the soup (hand or jug), then combine the smooth soup with the chunky soup to create something smooth and creamy but that you can really get your teeth into.

Sweet Cherry Tomato and Roasted Peppers

Sweet cherry tomatoes and roasted peppers merge to create a 'souper' scrumptious flavour explosion. This soup is soo delicious, it even made it into our Juice 'n' Smoothie Bars.

What you need (serves 2 happily)
1 x red pepper
1 x yellow pepper
1 x small red onion
2 x cloves of garlic (peeled)
12 x cherry tomatoes (with the stalks removed)
1 x vegetable stock cube
1 tbsp of vegetable oil
Crushed black pepper

What you do …
Pre heat the oven to 180°C (350°F).
Remove the stalk and seeds from the peppers and chop into small chunks.
Peel the onion and chop into chunks.
Place the peppers, onion, garlic, and tomatoes onto a large baking tray and drizzle with the oil.
Place the baking tray into the oven and roast for 15 minutes.
Prepare the stock by dissolving the stock cube in 1 pint (0.5 litre) of boiling water.
Remove the vegetables from the oven and empty into a large saucepan; add the stock and seasoning, bring to the boil and simmer for 10 minutes.
Remove from heat and using a blender (hand or normal type), blend the soup until smooth.
Pour into a bowl and enjoy.

Appendix 7

GET THE RIGHT JUICER ... *FOR YOU!*

Getting the right juicer is crucial to whether juicing makes a regular appearance in your life, or whether the machine gets put in your cupboard and stays there for good! It is extremely important to get the right juicer for *your* needs. Up until now, there have been just two basic types of juicer:

- Masticating (slow juicers)
- Centrifugal (fast juicers)

They both have their pros and cons. The main difference is that 'slow' juicers tend to live by their name: they are slow to use, slow to clean and tend to cost more. However, the *quality* of the juice tends to be superior. Whereas 'fast' juicers are exactly that: fast to use, fast to clean and tend to be cheaper than masticating (slow) juicers. The con with these juicers is the *quality* of the juice. Most have powerful motors that cause the cutting blades to move at incredibly high speeds in order to juice superfast. This creates 'heat friction' and heat affects nutrients. It is well documented that the longer you cook something, the more nutrients you lose. This means the juice oxidises and separates much faster than with a slow juicer and tends to be of inferior quality in comparison. This doesn't mean the juice from fast juicers is void of nutrients; you are just encouraged to drink the juice as soon as possible after making it.

THE GAME CHANGER IN THE JUICING WORLD!

Up until now, these have been the main choices of juicer to get. Both are really good and I have been recommending a *whole fruit* fast juicer for the past ten years and I have also talked about the virtues of slow juicing. The vast majority of people choose a fast juicer because of time restraints, but ideally want the quality of a slow juicer. The good news is that every now and then a game changer comes into the market. The iPod did it and so did companies like Dyson; they completely changed the game in their field and I am pleased to say we have a game changer in the juicing world, too. It's a juicer that almost combines the best of both worlds in juicing: 'slow' and 'fast'.

THE FUSION OF TECHNOLOGIES

From now on when people ask what juicer you have, it will be a case of, 'fast, slow or **FUSION**', The Fusion Juicer is just that: a fusion of both juicing worlds. You can fit a whole apple in it like a fast juicer, but the low-induction motor means it extracts the juice without anywhere near as much heat friction. This means the quality of the juice is comparable to an expensive slow juicer. It's also easy to clean (everything goes in the dishwasher), it's whisper quiet, it looks good and it's **VERY** affordable.

My mission since I started on my own health journey has been to **JUICE THE WORLD** and one of the most important aspects of making sure that mission is achieved is to get a juicer into every household in the world. That can only happen if the juicer is incredible value and affordable by all. But usually the best value juicers aren't the best juicers, and I have, until now, always recommended more expensive juicers. The Fusion

Juicer is not quite as fast as a super-fast juicer and not quite the quality of a £400 slow juicer, but is a beautiful combination of the two. With the Fusion you get a juicer that doesn't heat the juice like a fast juicer but is a million times faster to use than a slow juicer. You get a juicer that produces high-quality juice but for a quarter of the price and from a machine that's easy to clean. You also get a juicer where you can see the juice being made in the juicer itself. This creates theatre in the kitchen and kids love to see the colours going round. If there is any challenge with this juicer it's that you need to learn how to use it, especially if you are used to using a fast juicer. You cannot simply whack hard produce through the juicer and expect it to like it. You can't put pineapple with the skin on, for example, as the low-induction motor wasn't designed for it. It needs to be treated gently in order for the juicer to maximize juice extraction. If you look on my website I have recorded a video of how to use this baby. I also use this juicer for every recipe in my Super Juice Me! app, along with the how to video, as well as a full explanation of the three different types of juicer. Visit: **www.superjuiceme.com**.

Personally, if I were getting into juicing for the first time or looking to change my juicer, the Fusion Juicer would be my choice. I am not the only one who is excited about this juicer: Jon Gabriel, a remarkable man who lost over 200lbs (91kg) with the help of juicing and raw food, said, 'I have been waiting for this juicer for years. Finally a juicer that is fast to use but doesn't create massive heat friction'. I said it was a game changer and it is.

Having said that, juicers are like mobile phones: new ones are coming out all the time, and by the time you read this particular version of this book things might have changed, so before buying any juicer please always visit **www.juicemaster.com** and see what's new in the juicing world! Also, please keep in mind that we are all different, have different-sized families and different needs and desires. For some only a super-fast juicer will do, regardless of quality of juice. For others premium-quality juice is the order of each day, regardless of how long it takes or how much the juicer cost.

GET THE RIGHT BLENDER ... *FOR YOU!*

The other piece of kit you will need for your juicy kitchen is a blender, or 'smoothie maker'. Not all blenders can do the job, so look for one that can also crush ice, blend soft and frozen fruits and demolish an avocado. There are some blenders that claim to be juicers, like the excellent Vitamix blender; but it's still a blender. A juicer *juices* and a blender *blends*. In other words, a juicer extracts the fresh juice from the fibres and a blender blends the fibres with the juice. You need both for a juicy lifestyle. Many people with a powerful large blender feel that by adding all produce whole into the machine and adding water, it means more of the nutrition will be ingested. This is not the case as the body cannot ingest insoluble fibre, it's only the juice contained within that's used. The insoluble fibre is good for 'sweeping' the colon and keeping things moving, but we need very little for that purpose. If anything, there is a danger with adding too much *whole* produce into a blender, adding water and drinking it. One of the main problems is that the body isn't designed to deal with all of that insoluble fibre at once; you would never eat 3 whole carrots, an apple, handful of kale, handful of spinach, and a raw beetroot all at once for example. You may eat one after the other, but you couldn't physically eat all at once (you'd never fit them all in your mouth for one thing!) If you were to drink a blend like the one above *very, very slowly* it would probably be OK, however it's a drink and the natural desire is to down it much, much faster than you would ever eat all of those fruits and vegetables. There is just too much insoluble fibre going into the stomach at once. You may think it's the same with juicing, but juicing removes *all* of the insoluble fibre, so you are only left with easy to absorb nutrition. You will see in the recipes in this book that I often use 'whole' and 'just juice' together, but whenever I use whole fruit or veg in the blender, it's always in an amount I would eat at once. More often than not, you'll see half an avocado or half a banana in the blender, which is then blended with freshly extracted juice. You will never see two bananas, two carrots and a bunch of green leaves, for example. It is important to have some insoluble fibre, which is why I include it in the form of a little avocado or banana, but it is not good to overload your system with too much at once.

There are many good blenders on the market, and again, it's all about the right one for you. If you want super-convenience the Fusion juicer can be bought with the Fusion 'Booster', which is like a blender that doubles up as a drinking bottle, so you can simply blend and go! There are a few blenders like this these days, like the Bullet, but the Fusion Booster is the best value one I have come across so far. Once again, this market is always changing too, so jump on **www.juicemaster.com** to keep up to date with the latest in blending technology.

WANT TO BE A JUICE MASTER NATURAL JUICE THERAPIST?

Due to the genuine health benefits of natural juice therapy and my passion to get this alternative treatment not so 'alternative', I am proud to present the first ever 'Juice Therapist' accreditation. This is a unique opportunity to become an official Juice Master Natural Juice Therapist.

My mission is to 'juice the world', and it's a difficult task to accomplish alone. This is why I am looking for genuine, compassionate and caring individuals to join me on this incredibly rewarding path. If this is something that genuinely juices you, please email us or see juicemaster.com for full details.

The course has been accepted by the CMA (Complementary Medicine Association) and accredited by an English university.

We also run an annual academy at our beautiful health retreat 'Juicy Oasis' in Portugal, where you can spend an interactive, intensive time learning about all aspects of juicing for health. This is a stand-alone event as well as forming part of the Natural Juice Therapy Course. For more information visit **www.juicemaster.com**.

WANT TO CONTINUE YOUR JUICY JOURNEY?

For free recipes, downloads, apps, other books and info on juicing visit:

www.juicemaster.com.

If you are looking for a quick and easy way to get 'juiced' we have two great options:

Get a range of blast frozen, nutrient rich juices and smoothies delivered direct to your door. No shopping, no juicing, no cleaning, no hassle. (3-day, 5-day and 7-day programmes available)

www.juicemasterdelivered.com

Get all the fresh ingredients you need direct to your door, no shopping, no hassle, simply juice! (3-day, 5-day and 7-day programmes available)

www.juicemasterfreshbox.com

JUICE MASTER RETREATS:

For the ultimate juicing and detox experience why not join us at a Juice Master retreat and let our experienced team guide you through our bespoke programme? Our retreats combine juicing, yoga, meditation, mountain walks, mini-rebounding, fitness and inspirational information designed to change the way you think about food.

Jason personally runs just two retreats per year and these weeks focus more on the 'mental' juice giving you the right physiology to change your mindset, deal with your addictions and truly educate you to live a healthier life.

For more information visit **www.juicyoasis.com**

Follow us on Twitter **@juicemaster**

Or find us on Facebook: **Facebook.com/juicemasterltd**

Or on Google +: **plus.google.com/ljuicemaster**

Jason Vale has been described as one of the leading
authorities on health, addiction and juicing. His books have
now sold over 3 million copies and been translated into
many languages. Other titles include:

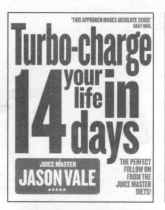

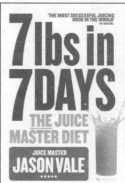

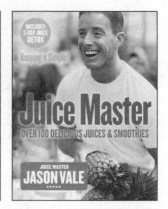

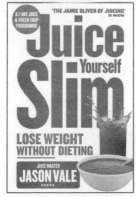

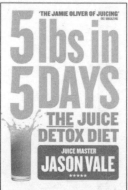

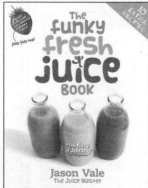